Economic Aspects of Health Care

Milbank Resource Books

David P. Willis, *Series Editor*

Economic

Aspects of Health Care

A SELECTION OF ARTICLES FROM THE
MILBANK MEMORIAL FUND QUARTERLY

Edited by John B. McKinlay

Published for the Milbank Memorial Fund
by   PRODIST   New York   1973

PRODIST
a division of
Neale Watson Academic Publications, Inc.
156 Fifth Avenue
New York, N. Y. 10010
© 1973 Milbank Memorial Fund
Manufactured in U.S.A.

Library of Congress Cataloging in Publication Data

McKinlay, John B.   comp.
  Economic aspects of health care.

  (Milbank resource books)
  1. Medical economics—Addresses, essays,
lectures. I. Milbank Memorial Fund quarterly.
II. Title. [DNLM: 1. Costs and cost analysis—
Collected works. 2. Delivery of health care—
Collected works. 3. Economics, Medical—Collected
works. WB50 M158e 1973]
RA410.M32   338.4'7'362108   73-19789
ISBN 0-88202-054-4
ISBN 0-88202-052-8 (pbk.)

Foreword to the Milbank Resource Books

Since 1923, the Milbank Memorial Fund has published a *Quarterly* journal in response to the premise that "the lack of application of knowledge which is in the possession of experts . . . is about the most difficult thing with which the world has to contend." This early statement of purpose, somewhat disarming in its simplicity and hopefulness, is even now characterized by an essential wisdom. Eminent scholars in a range of fields dealing with the health of the public have responded generously over the past 50 years, making the *Quarterly* a notable forum and repository of knowledge. More recently, teachers, researchers, policymakers, public administrators, and especially students, have had to contend with an even more elemental difficulty, i.e. gaining convenient access to the rich resources contained in these 50 volumes.

Many of these articles are widely recognized as classic statements. Their seminal significance makes them as viable as they are venerable. In response to continuing requests for accessibility and economy, the Milbank Memorial Fund is undertaking to republish selected papers as Resource Books.

A venture of this nature has limitations which must be faced with cautious confidence. In order to expedite publication, articles in this series are drawn exclusively from the universe of the *Quarterly*. Nevertheless, the broad range of topics addressed over the years presents an extraordinary diversity from which to select. A number of selections were originally contributed several years ago, and no pretense is made for their being either the last word or even the latest word in their substantive content. T. S. Eliot, when asked why one should read earlier writers since we now know so much more than they did, replied, "Precisely, and they are that which we know." The reader is reminded that all of the authors represented here have progressed in their thinking and have advanced their subsequent work in other journals and books.

Milbank Resource Books are envisaged as introductory readers for students with varied interests in the organization and delivery of health services. In selecting articles for individual volumes, the respective editors attempt to balance general theoretical concerns or overall principles with illustrative practical examples. The division of each volume into different sections advances this perspective.

It is planned to keep this series active and responsive to changing needs. Suggestions for future volumes will be welcome.

Contents

MANPOWER:
SOME ILLUSTRATIVE ECONOMIC ISSUES

Introduction

When considering the economic aspects of the health care "industry" in the United States, two features stand out above all others — its enormity and its phenomenal rate of growth. This industry is clearly one of the largest in the country, involving around 90 billion dollars a year and accounting for about 8 percent of a gross national product of over 1,000 billion dollars. It is "labor intensive" and consumes a high proportion of the most qualified labor. National data reveal that, while the population doubled over the last forty years in the United States (from 100 to 200 million persons), public and private expenditures for all health care, including personal health services, increased about twentyfold. The health care system stimulates and utilizes the most advanced technology and purportedly supplies services for important and unavoidable social needs. There are no indications that overall demands for it are declining in any detectable ways.

Of course, these massive totals tend to disguise their meaning for individuals with needs. One way around this difficulty is to consider per capita expenditure for health. In 1949–50, annual per capita expenditures were estimated to be about $79; in 1964–65, this estimate was $198; it reached $327 in 1969–70 and has increased to over $400 during 1972-73. To place these figures in context it may be useful to consider two recent government-sponsored studies. The first is a study from the Census Bureau which shows that, while the income of the median American family rose for the first time above $10,000 in 1972, the gain over the previous year was wiped out by inflation. In other words, when the 1972 median income is converted into "constant dollars" of equal purchasing power, it works out at almost precisely the 1971 figure. The study also shows that the estimate of 25 million people below the poverty level is the highest total since 1967. Until 1970, this number had for a decade dropped annually from a total of about 40 million in 1960, despite a natural population increase. The latest figures represent a 5 percent increase in the number of people below the poverty threshold although population growth has slowed markedly.

The second study from the Labor Department, consistent with the findings of more modest investigations, reveals that a changing population and a changing industrial structure are producing a clear and persistent trend toward inequality in the distribution of income among wage earners and salaried workers in the United States. This trend is toward concentration of an increasingly large share of average wage and salary income among people in occupations that already bring higher pay. Using national census data, this study explodes the myth that the gap between the rich and the poor is actually narrowing. To the contrary, this study indicates that, from 1958 to 1970, the share of aggregate wage and salary income earned by the lowest fifth of male workers declined to 4.60 percent from 5.10 percent. During this same period, the share for the highest fifth of male wage earners and salaried workers rose from 38.15 to 40.55 percent. It would seem therefore that, while annual per capita medical expenditures have increased dramatically, there certainly has been no compensatory increase in income. In fact, for lower socioeconomic groups, there appears to have been a concomitant decrease in the spending power of earned income.

There are no clear signs that the demand for health care will either level off or decline. In fact, the predominant market price economic system which prevails in the United States is likely to ensure that a decline in demand does not occur. For example, the entrepreneurial pharmaceutical industry appears to be devoted to the task of making people overly conscious of health concerns and to engendering a regular reliance on "over-the-counter" medications. This relatively unregulated multi-billion dollar industry, with considerable ingenuity, has managed to produce more than 100,000 nonprescription items. Over 4 billion dollars each year is extracted from the public for varieties of vitamin pills, mineral supplements, laxatives, sleeping pills, and painkillers which have been repeatedly found to be largely ineffective. Despite Food and Drug Administration studies which show that nearly all of these items are worthless, they continue to be promoted to a gullible public. Through beguilingly ingenious advertising the pharmaceutical industrial complex has been able to engineer a state in which, for example, a recent FDA interview survey report ("A Study of Health Practices and Opinions") could uncover the following:

— Three-quarters of the public believe that extra vitamins provide more pep and energy.
— Thirty-five million adults use vitamin and mineral supplements without skilled medical advice.
— One-fifth of the public is convinced, unjustifiably, that cancer, arthritis, and other diseases are caused, at least in part, by vitamin and mineral deficiencies.
— One-third of the public holds "fallacious concepts" about weight control, most commonly that there are special medicines which cause people to reduce.
— Fifty million adults would not be convinced by almost unanimous expert medical opinion that a hypothetical "cancer cure" was worthless.
— Three Americans in every eight subscribe to the view that advertisements for health products must be factually correct or such agencies as the FDA and the FTC would not permit their presentation.

An additionally disquieting feature of the U.S. health care economic system relates to gross maldistributions of trained health personnel. Such maldistributions are various in form and differ according to the type of health occupation being considered. *First,* with regard to physicians, there are clearly disproportionate numbers in certain specialties — specialties, incidentally, which tend to inflate the costs of medical care. *Second,* there are disproportionate numbers of health care personnel in certain geographic areas, with the result that the nature of equity and access varies from area to area (for example, one could contrast urban with rural settings). *Third,* there are considerable changes over time in the shape of the health care occupational structure which are not necessarily dictated by need or demand. At one time, a particular specialty may be well represented, while at another it may appear almost nonexistent. For example, it has been estimated that the ratio of primary care physicians to patients in the United States has approximately halved between 1940 and 1970, while the demand for them has increased.

Why do these maldistributions exist and what can be done to rectify them? The answers to these questions lie, in large part, in the types of incentives and rewards that presently exist in the U.S. health care system. It is, for example, probably true that urban health care personnel earn more than their rural counterparts. In some instances these is a clear incentive to move to urban areas through the granting of an urban living allowance. There are clearly many other noneconomic incentives operating, such as the prestige derived from an affiliation with a notable urban hospital or university, the availability of support facilities, and, most likely, the social-emotional satisfactions which accrue from regular association with professional colleagues. While disparities in earnings between different areas and selected specialties could be resolved through the application of economic expertise, they are probably not the most important contingencies in decision making with regard to either location or career choice. The additional factors already mentioned are obviously not as amenable to economic intervention. As a first step, however, and to the extent that they are fostered and reinforced by professional training and activities, they can probably be significantly modified. Unfortunately, we have hardly begun to consider such possibilities.

In introducing this volume on *Economic Aspects of Health Care* I have touched on four important issues. To recapitulate, they are:

a) The enormity and rate of growth of the health care sector of the U.S. economic system.
b) The phenomenal and unrestrained rise in annual per capita expenditure in the face of inflation (which wipes out the positive effects of any increase in earnings).
c) The existence of a largely unregulated pharmaceutical industry which is successfully engineering a potentially harmful demand for worthless items which seemingly bear little relation to undisputed medical need.
d) The maldistribution of health care manpower, resulting in gross and unjust disparities in equity and access.

I am clearly not suggesting that these are the only economic issues of importance, nor is any allocation of priority intended. Rather, they provide a perspective on the types of issues discussed in the rest of this volume. Many other equally important concerns could have been addressed. For example, one could highlight the wasteful duplication of services (especially hospital facilities) or the financial absurdities in much modern hospital architectural design (most hospitals are outmoded before their construction is complete). One could explore the funding of health-related research and the ways in which the granting system contributes to the inflation of personal medical expenditures. Alternatively, attention could focus on the prevalence and economics of unnecessary medical treatment and ritualistic surgery. One could highlight the costs of medical education and investigate the extent to which students are informed of the necessity and expense of various treatments and procedures. Finally, from a more macro-economic perspective, one could examine the linkages between the health sector and other related sectors of the economic system (especially education, industry, defense, insurance, and welfare). And even if all these additional issues were satisfactorily addressed, we still would be nowhere near exhausting the reservoir of important concerns which await investigation.

Readings in this volume are divided into two main sections. The first section consists of a set of papers dealing with general economic considerations in health care. The article by Boulding on the concept of "need" for health services provides a useful starting point by discussing, among other things, how needs are created and who has a mandate to determine which needs and/or demands are important and how they should be serviced. Fein considers questions regarding equity and access in health care and some implications of a system of universal financing. In particular, he makes insightful comparisons between the systems of health care financing in the United States and Great Britain. The two selections by Fuchs analyze, in a general manner, both the contribution of health services to the overall American economy and the relationship between the health sector and other interdependent economic sectors. Feldstein's discussion is at a more specific level: research on the important question of "demand" for health services. Falk focuses on the current crises in medical care, on the causes of the crises, and on financing which is geared toward explicit solutions. Piore argues for rationalizing the mix of public and private expenditures on health, while Thompson examines the perennial question of the "reasonable costs" of hospital services.

The papers comprising the second section focus on issues regarding health manpower. Hiestand considers aspects of research into health manpower, while Kissick investigates trends in and requirements for manpower in a rapidly changing health care system, and some of the factors which impede the full realization of manpower potentials. Butter and her associates examine the effects of manpower utilization on the cost and productivity of a neighborhood health center and describe a methodology for evaluating the use of manpower in ambulatory health facilities. A number of potential applications of this methodology are also proposed. Finally, with Tancredi and Woods we turn our attention to the ways in which mandatory licensure systems affect health manpower utilization.

JOHN B. McKINLAY, PH.D.
Department of Sociology
Boston University

General Considerations

THE CONCEPT OF NEED FOR HEALTH SERVICES

KENNETH E. BOULDING

The concept of need is often looked upon rather unfavorably by economists, in contrast with the concept of demand. Both, however, have their own strengths and weaknesses. The need concept is criticized as being too mechanical, as denying the autonomy and individuality of the human person, and as implying that the human being is a machine which "needs" fuel in the shape of food, engine dope in the shape of medicine, and spare parts provided by the surgeon. Even if the need concept is expanded to include psychological and emotional needs, the end result would seem to be a wire run into the pleasure center of the brain which could provide a life of unlimited and meaningless ecstasy. Demand, by contrast, implies autonomy of the individual, choice, and a tailoring of inputs of all kinds to individual preferences. Only the slave has needs; the free man has demands.

In spite of the economist's uneasiness about it, a considerable demand exists for the concept of need. As even the most liberal of economists cannot deny the right of a demand to call forth a supply, the development and elaboration of concepts of need can hardly be denied. The demand, however, may be for a number of different concepts, and a single concept will not serve the purpose. The demands for this concept are quite varied, and the supply must be correspondingly differentiated. No single concept of need exists, and especially no single concept of need for health services.

One demand for a concept of need arises because the concept of demand itself has serious weaknesses and limitations. It assumes away,

3

for instance, a serious epistemological problem. The very idea of autonomous choice implies first that the chooser knows the real alternatives which are open to him, and second that he makes the choice according to value criteria or a utility function which he will not later regret. Both the image of the field of choice and the utility function have a learning problem which, by and large, economists have neglected. This problem is particularly acute in the case of medical care, where the demander is usually a layman faced with professional suppliers who know very much more than he does. The demand for medical care, indeed, is primarily a demand for knowledge or at least the results of knowledge. In the case of ordinary commodities the knowledge that is required is fairly easily available and the market itself is a learning process. If one buys something he does not like he will not buy it again. In the case of medical care, however, as in the case of certain other commodities such as automobiles, the learning process can easily be fatal, in which case it is not a learning process at all. In any case the experience of the market cannot teach people what they have to know in regard to the choices they have to make, or even what preference functions they should use in evaluating these choices.

The concept of need which emerges from the criticism of demand is that of professional choice. It is implied to some extent in the very idea of the patient or the client, and it is expressed in the aphorism that doctor (or father, or lawyer, or preacher, or president) knows best. One's demand for medical care is what he wants; his need for medical care is what the doctor thinks he ought to have. The demand for medical care leads to the proliferation of drug stores, patent medicines, osteopaths, chiropractors and faith healers.

That is the market for medical care and it is a large one. It spills over into the medical profession itself, in private practice and the reputation of particular doctors and surgeons, in the prestige of Harley Street and its equivalents in many cities, and it includes both the medicine cabinet in the bathroom and the psychiatrist's couch. It can be thought of as an "industry" or segment of the economy; it is subject to the general principles of the price system, in the sense that wherever a demand is sufficient to make a supply profitable it will arise, even though this principle has to be limited also by the power of the ingenious supplier to create his own demand.

In contrast with the market in medical care, an increasingly professionalized, socialized, organized structure satisfies what the professional conceives of as needs. The periodic medical examinations in corporations and universities, the veterans' hospitals, the school doctor, public health, the professional public provision of clean water and sewage disposal—all this represents a professionalized sector of the economy, characterized by professions which set their own standards of what they ought to do and which are financed by taxation or near-taxation. Among these are Blue Cross and other health insurance plans, Medicare, or even private clinics supported by monthly assessments. Here the activity originates from the profession rather than from the client, from the supplier rather than from the demander. In its extreme form it takes on the flavor of, "What you need is what I as your professional advisor have to give you; what you want is quite irrelevant."

The idea of professional need always rests on some definition of homeostasis or state maintenance of the client, his property or his environment. The professional defines a certain state of his client and his related systems as a state of "health" which he has a professional interest in maintaining. The course of operations of any system, however, involves consumption. That is, the state of the client and his environment changes in some way and become "worse," or diverge in a downward direction from the ideal. The ideal in this case is the professional's ideal, that is, his impression of what state should be maintained. The maintenance of a state, however, requires certain inputs to replace what has been lost by consumption. It may also require the professional handling of certain outputs, such as excreta, which must be removed and disposed of if the organism or organization is to continue to maintain its state of activity. A very fundamental principle in nature implies that any state of activity can only be maintained by a throughput involving both inputs and outputs. In part that may be because inputs come in packages in practice, only part of which can be utilized, and what is not utilized must therefore be excreted as output. Even more fundamental reasons, however, dictate the presence of output in the form of excreta, whether gases from automobile exhaust, carbon dioxide given off in breathing or waste products of the digestive process. The transformation of chemical into mechanical energy, on which all organization seems to depend almost universally, seems to require an input of oxygen and an output of an oxide.

This suggests that certain minimum mechanical, chemical, biological, physiological, even economic and sociological requirements exist for the functioning of any organism or organization. That in turn suggests that the concept of professional need can be broken down into two further problems; one the problem of what might be called homeostatic need. That is, what is actually required to maintain a given system in operation. The other is the problem of perception or knowledge of homeostatic need. That is, can the system itself be trusted to maintain the inputs and outputs necessary to satisfy homeostatic need, or is a professional required with a wider body of knowledge who can perceive and prescribe the homeostatic needs? Homeostatic needs can be divided into two categories, those which can be taken care of by the organism itself and those which require a professional decision.

These categories can be illustrated by pointing to certain undignified analogies between the human being as an organization and an item of material capital such as an automobile. Both require inputs of air if they are to function, and the air must be reasonably pure, though usually only automobiles are provided with air filters. Each of them pollute the air they breathe with the byproducts of combustion, and unless fresh air can be constantly supplied continued operation will become impossible. Both the man and the automobile require food; carbohydrates, proteins and fats in the case of the human, gasoline and oil in the case of the automobile. A certain parallel can even be drawn between the vitamins of the human and the various additives of gasoline. The parallel is particularly striking in Scandinavian countries where automobiles are "buttered," not greased. Food input is usually administered on a fairly nonprofessional basis. The automobile owner buys gas for his car in very much the same way as he buys food for himself, with a certain amount of professional advice but not much professional interference. In the course of operation of the system, internal stocks of food are used up fairly continuously and they have to be replaced at intervals. The automobile takes its dinner at the gas station, which is a kind of automobile restaurant.

The input of food and of fuel and the output of its waste products are not, however, sufficient. In the course of operation, both of the automobile and of the human, wear and tear occur. Consequently, not only are gas stations, restaurants and food stores needed, but also garages and hospitals. At this level need becomes professionalized. The greasing every thousand miles or the annual physical examination may be fairly routine, though at this point one begins to think of medical care for either automobile or man rather than simple fueling and feeding. The professional need is most apparent in breakdown, that is, when the subject simply refuses to function even when fueled and fed. Then the car goes to the garage, where mechanics perform operations on it, and the human goes to the hospital where surgeons perform operations on him. The atmosphere of the garage, indeed, is curiously like that of the hospital. The garage is permeated by the same air of professional importance, the same feeling that the customer is rather in the way, the same rather offhand bedside manner, the same assumption that the customer or the patient is, professionally speaking, an ignoramus, if not a fool. In fact, the principal difference between the garage and the hospital seems to be that the hospital is cleaner and more expensive. The concept of professional need appears in the helplessness of the customer. All he knows is that he hears a funny noise in the gear box or has a pain in his stomach. Once he puts himself into the hands of the professional, demand disappears and no substitute exists for trust in the professional's concept of need.

The difficulty with homeostasis as the basis for a concept of need is that homeostasis is never really successful. No matter what occurs in the way of inputs, virtually all known organisms and organizations exhibit the phenomenon of aging, which is closely related to the phenomenon of growth. Aging is common both to machines and to biological organisms, and it might almost be defined as that adverse change in state of the organism which no known input can remedy. In biological organisms, growth is actually rather similar. It can be thought of, indeed, as a kind of negative aging. The inputs of the growing child have to be sufficient not only to provide for replacement, but also to provide for growth. Growth, however, is almost as unpreventable as aging. Mechanical organizations such as the automobile are not generally subject to growth. They are more like the moth or the butterfly in that they emerge fully grown from the chrysalis of the factory, and henceforth are subject only to aging. Up to now very little is known about aging, at least in the case of the biological organism. It can perhaps be hastened by certain inputs or outputs or by certain deficiencies in input, which is also true of the automobile. In both cases, a life of hard work and poor nutrition results in premature aging. Up to now, at any rate, any inputs which would postpone the aging process beyond the allotted span have not been discovered. If they are, as seems not impossible, at least in the next 100 years, the human race will probably be faced with the greatest crisis of its history, for no existing human institution would survive in its present form the extension of active human life even to 200 years.[1]

Aging introduces a very tricky problem into the concept of need for maintenance, which is difficult enough even in the case of the machine, more difficult in the case of the horse, and a problem of excruciating delicacy in the case of the human being. The problem with the machine is at what point in its history it should be scrapped. The formal answer to this is fairly easy: a machine should be scrapped when its present value as a functioning apparatus, derived by discounting the future costs and benefits to be allocated to it, has fallen just below the net value of a possible replacement. The net value is defined as the present discounted value of future benefits less that of all future and installment costs of the replacement plus the scrap value of the machine which is replaced. With no technical progress and if the machine is replaced by one exactly like it when new, the main factor determining the age at which it will be replaced is the increase in the maintenance cost and perhaps a decrease in its output as it gets older. Where technical change occurs a machine may be scrapped because of obsolescence, that is, because of a rise in the net value of what might replace it.

A machine is generally regarded as having no value in itself, that is, its value is purely instrumental; hence the owner feels no qualms about scrapping it if he feels such action is necessary. Even horses, however, when they can no longer fulfill their economic function, are sometimes put out to pasture in honorable retirement at some cost to their owners. In the case of the human being, the problem of the person himself becomes very acute, because persons cannot be regarded as purely instrumental. That is, they are not merely good for something else, they are good in themselves. They are, in other words, something *for which* other things are good. Whereas the death of a machine is determined mainly by economic forces, this principle as quite inapplicable to persons, where, in theory at any rate, the person supposedly possesses a positive value even up to the moment of death, and death, therefore, is always regarded as a loss. When death occurred mainly in childhood or middle life, this principle could evoke no criticism. As medical science, however, has successively eliminated the causes of early death, the fiction that death is always an "act of God" is increasingly difficult to maintain.

At this point the concept of professional need for medical care becomes most difficult. Should the medical profession devote a relatively large proportion of its resources, as it does now, in keeping miserable and senile elderly people alive, when their capital value even to themselves has become negative? Men, even physicians, have a reasonable aversion to playing God and to introducing a nonrandom element in what has hitherto been sanctified as random. The only solution may be to substitute an artificially random process for the natural randomness by which death came in the past. If death could be arranged by drawing a random number, perhaps by hiding one euthanasia pill in the nursing home diet each week, the Godlike power of the medical man might be laid on the shoulders of Chance, and death might be restored to its former dignity.

A proposal such as the above will seem deeply shocking to many people, and indeed, is put forward only in the form of a most tentative question, intended merely to illustrate a problem which is likely to be more and more prevalent. One principle in the spirit of the Hippocratic Oath to be argued for very strongly is that the person himself must decide at what point death or the chance of death is preferred to life, and no one else should have the right to make this decision for him. At this point, surely, demand must take precedence of need, and the autonomy of the patient be reasserted. Even at the moment of making this assertion, however, and nailing it to the masthead, realistic doubts arise. At what point, for instance, do people become incapable of making decisions for themselves? That is a question of immediate practical importance for the medical profession, for even if they do not have the power at the moment of consigning people to eternity, they do have the power of consigning them to what is often the living death of the mental hospital, and the moral problems of the latter are surely of the same order of magnitude as those of the former. Nevertheless, people do become incompetent and incapable of managing their own affairs. Society has decided that mental hospitals must exist, and along with them the machinery for committing people to them. Who is better able to estimate that professional need than the medical profession, especially when its decisions are mediated through the apparatus of the law? One sobering thought, however, is that a person virtually ceases to be a legal person when he ceases to have demands and has only needs.

Some of the above problems may well reflect a lag in society in the development of a professional sense of what the needs of the incompetent and the aged in fact ought to be. A marked shift has taken place in the care of the aged, from the family into hospitals and

9

nursing homes. Even two generations ago most people died in their own beds in the bosom of their families, amid the consolations of religion and the ministrations of a beloved family physician. Such, at least, is the idyllic picture; the reality was probably more disagreeable. Nevertheless, of the people who die of old age today, most die in nursing homes, old people's homes, and hospitals, away from the comforts of the familiar and the ministrations of kin. No great deal of thought has been devoted to the needs of the departing, and none at all to the need for death. Death, however, is a medical matter. It is certainly part of the need for medical care, if such exists, and it deserves to receive a great deal more care and attention than it has in the past. That is not to suggest that the medical profession should abandon its concern for the needs of the incompetent, the aged and the dying; rather that more attention be given to this problem, both in medical research, so that vigor and physical well-being can be prolonged until the end, and in social and moral research that can devise economic, financial, architectural and social institutions which will give dignity and serenity to the last years of life and will not deprive its end of the majesty which is due it.

At the other end of human life, the increasing control, which the biological sciences seem to be opening up in genetics, presents even more difficult problems in regard to the need for medical activity. If the rights of the living and the dying are hard to determine, the rights of the unborn are an even more difficult problem. The whole problem of population control, in fact, in regard to both quantity and quality, is moving more and more onto the shoulders of the health sciences, and it is a problem for which they cannot escape responsibility. In the last 15 years, the spectacular decline in infant mortality which followed the introduction of malaria control in the tropics has created social problems which seem to be virtually insoluble in the next 15 to 20 years.

One must think here in terms of the homeostasis, not merely of the individual, but of a whole society. When, as a result of the introduction of certain public health measures, a society which previously was in approximate demographic equilibrium, with high birth rates and high death rates, suddenly finds the death rates drastically reduced while the birth rates continue high, an enormous long-run social disequilibrium is created which may have quite unforeseen consequences, both for good and for ill. Many societies in the tropics are now increasing in population at unprecedented rates—between

10

three and four per cent per annum—and this in itself places an enormous burden on the poor society which is anxious for development. When the population doubles every 20 years a whole new country must be built, and the whole physical apparatus of a society doubled in a relatively short space of time, even if per capita capital is not to decline. If the country is already fairly thickly populated, with no unused land areas of any magnitude, the sheer problem of doubling the food supply in 20 years is almost insoluble, and a slow and deadly reduction in nutritive levels can easily follow.

Add to this gloomy picture the fact that in these countries most of the working force was born before the great decline in infant mortality and hence is small. That small working force has to support an enormous number of children and young people—in many of these countries more than half the population is now under the age of 18. Furthermore, very large teenage generations now exist which cannot be absorbed in the traditional structure, especially of the village society, and are forced to migrate to the towns. The towns, because of the phenomenon of what has been called the "rural push," are growing much faster than the population itself, some of them as much as 15 per cent annually which means doubling every five years. Under these circumstances providing housing and municipal services is impossible, and enormous slums and shack towns spread over the landscape like a blight. These circumstances dictate an extremely pessimistic forecast for the next 25 years for many of these countries. On the other hand, if a massive campaign for birth reduction takes place now, so that birth rates could be halved in five or ten years, then the next generation will be a large labor force able to cope with the smaller numbers of children and that will be the moment when these countries may be able to make the leap into the modern world. In the absence of substantial reduction in birth rates, however, the outlook is bleak indeed. Enormous famines, disastrous internal strife and even total civil breakdown may be expected. All this may well be the result of the World Health Organization's malaria eradiction campaign in the years around 1950.

On the other side of the picture, without a substantial increase in the expectation of life, and particularly without the elimination of mortality in the productive years, economic development is also very difficult. An essential step toward the modern world is the introduction of modern medicine and the elimination of the appalling waste of human knowledge and human capital which occurs in

11

countries where human life expectancy is little more than 30 years. The ideal situation would be a sharp reduction in the death rate and an equally sharp reduction in the birth rate, so that the demographic equilibrium was not unduly disturbed. Even if this happy result were unobtainable, a certain disturbance of the demographic equilibrium is entirely desirable in the interest of development, and a public health campaign is at least a start in disturbing the low-level equilibrium of a traditional society.

These problems present great difficulties, even for social scientists, and up to now at any rate the medical sciences have been extraordinarily lax in attending to them. Medicine has considered health mainly in terms of inputs to an individual, not to a society. The possibility of an acute conflict between the health of the individual and that of his society is a problem that has received scandalously little attention. Now the tables have been turning, and birth control has become fashionable and respectable, almost to the point of being advocated as a panacea for all developmental difficulties. Quantitative population control, however, is only a part of the general problem of what might be called societal health, which is not the same thing, incidentally, as public health. Public health concerns itself primarily with the environmental factors affecting the health of the individual. Societal health deals with the factors that determine the health of the whole society, and societies can be sick even when the individuals in them are medically well.

The problem of qualitative population control is beginning to rise seriously onto the human agenda. The eugenics movements of the nineteenth century were premature, and based on wholly inadequate genetic concepts. With the enormous advance in genetics in this century, however, the problems of the genetic composition of future populations are no longer as random as they used to be. Indeed, a recurrent nightmare is that all the medical advances will eventually prove ineffective simply because the improved techniques of individual survival will enable more and more adverse genetic strains to penetrate the population. In his argument against that position, Medawar says that if a genetic adaptation to medical knowledge produces more people who have to be kept alive by "artificial" means, nothing is particularly wrong with that, because genetics always adapts itself to the environment and medical knowledge is part of the environment of man.[2] The argument, however, is not wholly satisfactory, simply because of the cost of medical care for those whose genetic constitution

12

requires it. If the existence of medical care produces a population of the genetic composition which requires it, the whole system seems to be self-defeating. Whatever level of medical care is established, no matter how high and how elaborate, one can argue that in the long run the genetic composition of the population will deteriorate to the point where the established level of medical care becomes necessary. In this case the level of medical care creates its own need. No objective need exists which determines the level of medical care.

Looking to the rather long run, therefore, one would expect to find large payoffs in research devoted to altering the genetic composition of the population in directions which would minimize the cost of medical care. Conceivably, genetic control might eliminate medical care almost entirely, except for accidents; for some genetic constitutions are extraordinarily resistant to disease, and if these could be propagated in the population, the need for medical care would correspondingly decline.

In the next few decades, the possibility of changing genetic constitutions even after birth is not wholly off the agenda, although it certainly seems to be difficult. Even without that, however, the possibility of genetic control at the moment of conception opens up an enormous and rather frightening horizon to the human race, even though this would also open up enormous possibilities for good. Certainly the elimination of the more obvious genetic-related diseases or conditions would be a great gain. The ethical problems involved at this end of the scale, however, are just as severe as those at the other end relating to death. At what point, for instance, in the life history of a person does he have any rights? Opinion seems to have shifted in this regard toward the moment of birth as the point at which human rights are acquired. The increasingly favorable public opinion in regard to abortion would seem to imply that the embryo has no rights, whereas the infant does, as infanticide is still severely censored. If, however, the process of conception can be controlled and, for instance, selective gene structures implanted in the egg, the question of the human rights even of the fertilized egg becomes acute. That again is a problem because the ethical standards and ideas of the human race have been adapted to processes of birth and death which in the past have been essentially random, and substituting nonrandom for random processes always produces an acute moral crisis. Perhaps some consensus might be salvaged with elimination of certain obviously maladaptive genetic traits, for instance mongoloidism and obvious feeblemindedness. Even considering the elimination of haemophilia, enough distinguished people have had this disability to suggest that something might be lost by eliminating it. The ethical problems become even more acute with the proposal to alter genetic structures positively. The production of a race of supermen who would supersede the present generation might not be regarded favorably by ordinary mortals.

Underlying all this discussion is a seldom-discussed specter regarding the idea of health itself. Even assuming the very simple position that need involves merely the maintenance of homeostasis, the question as to what state of the organism is to be maintained still has to be answered. That is like the problem of at what temperature the thermostat should be set. Every homeostatic mechanism implies an ideal, and the question of the critique of the ideal itself, therefore, cannot be brushed aside. In particular, the conclusion cannot be avoided that within limits which may be quite broad, health is a matter of social definition. Societies and cultures do exist in which what is now defined here as ill health is somewhat admired. One recalls W. S. Gilbert's pale young curate, whose tubercular charms in the eyes of the village maidens even outweighed those of gilded dukes and belted earls. In some societies, epilepsy is regarded as a sign of divine favor. The limits of what is socially defined as physical health are so narrow that not much of a problem arises.

With mental health and human behavior in society, however, the limits seem to be broader, and the matter of social definition more important. For instance, should the problem of homosexuality be considered a problem in mental health, to be "cured," even if no cure seems to be currently available, or should it be regarded as a legitimate variation of human behavior, to be accepted and regulated by custom and law? A rather similar problem involving the acceptance of deviant subcultures has descended upon society with the development of the psychedelic drugs such as mescaline and LSD. Some claim that these are legitimate avenues to the expansion of human consciousness and others claim that these are dangerous drugs the use of which should be prohibited by law, except under medical supervision, and that unauthorized users should be punished as criminals. A similar conflict of voices is raised on behalf of marijuana, some people claiming that it affords a legitimate expansion of human consciousness and is no more dangerous than alcohol. The prevailing sentiment, however, is to lash out at the use of these drugs with all the ferocity of criminal law.

The failure to deal with alcohol, which has been with the human race for a long time and is certainly the earliest of the psychedelic drugs, is not an optimistic indication that society will be able to deal with a succession of new chemical and perhaps electrical devices, such as the "pleasure wire," which produce various types of euphoria. One remembers with a slight shudder the use of soma as a social tranquilizer in BRAVE NEW WORLD. Even in the medical field, not very much is known about the impact on society of the enormous use of the tranquilizing drugs both in medical practice and in private life in the past few years. The frightening possibility of a society steeped in agreeable chemical illusions to the point where it becomes quite incapable either of recognizing or solving its real problems is by no means a matter only for science fiction.

Different societies have given very different answers to these questions, and they constitute merely one aspect of a much larger question as to the boundary between health, morality and law. In many fields the problem is defining the point at which behavior which is in some sense disapproved or regarded as below normal is defined as sickness or is defined as turpitude. In this society a long-term movement has attempted to push this boundary to define fewer things as turpitude and more things as sickness. Nevertheless, no golden rule dictates where this line should be drawn. In Samuel Butler's EREWHON, crime was treated by doctors and illness by policemen, and one has an uneasy suspicion that this might work too. The problem of the overall effects upon society of its system of punishment is very little understood, and the line between the need for medical care and the need for criminal prosecution is really quite hard to draw.

A question which is even more fundamental and still more difficult to answer, but which should not remain unasked, is whether the concept of ill health can be applied to moral and political ideas themselves. For instance, do diseases of the moral judgment exist, and if so, are they subject to epidemics? How are these epidemics spread? The rise of National Socialism in Germany and McCarthyism in the United States, of witch-hunting, war moods and irrational hatreds in innumerable societies, indicates that the concept of disease in the moral and political judgment is worth taking seriously, even though it is very hard to define. One may be able to define something like mass infections of unrealistic images of the world, if only one could be sure what is realistic. Whether these phenomena fall under the purview of the medical profession is, of course, a debatable point. The medical profession has long been required in forensic medicine to

15

advise on the medical status of a possible criminal act. Perhaps, one day it may be called in to determine the medical status of a political act or even of a moral exhortation. The difficulty here, and it is a real one, is that, up to now at any rate, a clear physical correlate of mental, moral and political ill health does not exist. The idea is not wholly far-fetched, however, to suppose such physical correlates do exist and that the discovery will be made one day of a drug against malevolence or another that increases good will. Even if the physical correlates are hard to find, the status of psychoanalysis as a medical speciality suggests possible extensions into therapeutic communication in moral, political and social systems.

Society is so accustomed to thinking of the problem of the inter-relations of government, science and medicine in terms of the impact of government on science and medicine that people are at a loss when asked to consider the impact of science and medicine on government. Nevertheless, that may well become one of the major questions in advanced societies in the next generation or two. Political decisions are still made largely in the light of what might be called folk knowledge or at best literary knowledge. The scientist is supposedly to serve the values and interests of the folk but he is not to insert any values and interests of his own. He is supposedly an instrument of the state or at least of the people and not an autonomous creator of values and needs. That is the point of view of the famous aphorism that the scientist in government should be on tap but not on top, and that he should be a humble servant of folk and national values. That, however, is a most unrealistic estimate of the present situation. Science is not a passive servant of existing values. It has its own culture, it creates its own values, and because of its enormous impact on the world, it compels a re-examination of values everywhere.

The role of the social sciences in this respect is even more striking than that of the physical and biological sciences. The physical or biological scientist operates in a different field from that of the politician. The special skills of the scientist in, say, physics or physiology give him very little comparative advantage in attempting to answer a question in social systems. In respect to the economic system or the international system, the physicist or biologist has as much right to be heard as any intelligent citizen, but no more. The social scientist, however, occupies the same field as the politician and is in direct competition with him. The possibility of severe conflict between the folk culture and the scientific culture is thus present at this level. Up to now the conflict has been muted only because it has hardly begun; because the social sciences are only barely at the point where they can begin to challenge the folk wisdom of the politician. Economics already has a kind of establishment of "Lords Spiritual" in the Council of Economic Advisors and in the Joint Economic Committee in Congress. The impact of this establishment is already noticeable in economic policy, and the United States is by no means the most advanced country in this regard. The other social sciences, and least of all what might be called the sociomedical sciences of clinical psychology and psychiatry, still seem to be a long way from any such status. The possibility, however, that one of the needs for medical care may be defined in the future as political mental health, though it may sound absurd at the moment, should not be taken lightly. Society is already beginning to see that the automobile is a problem in public health; to regard the Department of Defense as a similar problem is a simple logical extension of this position, for the present international system is almost certainly more dangerous to health than the automobile and far more dangerous than most communicable diseases.

Even at this point, the ambiguity can be maintained between demand as defined by the consumer and need as defined by the professional. All fields of life seem to feel the necessity for working out an uneasy compromise between these two concepts. Undiluted consumer sovereignty, whether in economics or politics, where it takes the form of the absolute sovereignty of the voter and the sovereignty of the nation, is ultimately intolerable and leads to corruption and disaster. On the other hand, total professionalization, in the case of the doctor, the economist, the sociologist or the political scientist, is likewise intolerable, if only for the reason that having that much father-image is intolerable; and the revolt against paternalism, no matter how benign, is an essential aspect of the human identity. Somewhere between the proposition that the customer is always right and the proposition that the public be damned must be an uneasy Aristotelian mean, and toward this the concept of professional need for medical care or for anything else uneasily steers itself.

The word need has a number of meanings, and the idea of homeostatic need or professional need which we have been discussing does not exhaust it. Another very important connotation of the word is that implied in the word "needy." One's need in this sense is not merely what some wise professional person thinks one ought to have, but what one

17

cannot afford because he is poor. In this sense also, need is thought of as something which stands in contrast with demand, and the need for a concept of need arises because of certain deficiencies in demand as a principle of allocation. The concept of need as a criticism of demand here refers to the fact that effective demand is closely related to income and to the distribution of income. Need is an equalitarian concept. It recalls the famous communist slogan, "From each according to his ability, to each according to his need."

Demand, perhaps because of its very stress on autonomy and freedom, is libertarian rather than equalitarian, and liberty is seldom equally divided. If medical care is distributed according to demand, the rich will get most of it and the poor very little. One of the main concerns of society for the need for medical care, therefore, is the fact that a sizeable proportion of the population is "medically indigent" in the sense that its income is not large enough to provide a demand for the minimum medical care which a society, or a profession, identifies as need. That may be a part of the general problem of the social minimum. At present nearly all societies have a deliberate policy to establish a minimum standard life below which citizens are not supposed to fall. Whether the policy is in fact successful is another matter, for in almost all cases some people do fall below the minimum, and all the machinery of society is not powerful enough to elevate them. Nevertheless, the principle of a social minimum has been established for a long time and today is almost universally accepted.

Even the acceptance of a social minimum, however, does not necessarily resolve the conflict between need and demand. Some argue that insofar as the problem is one of poverty, the only solution to this is to make the poor richer, either by giving them money, by improving their skills or by integrating them more fully into the culture around them. Once the poor have been made richer, the problem of the need for medical care resolves itself essentially into the problem discussed earlier of a consumer's demand versus professional need, between which poles some uneasy compromise must be reached.

In the case of medical indigency, however, the temptation is to deny consumers sovereignty as the price of the relief of indigency, and to say that the poor must have what the professionals think is good for them whether they want it or not. This is part of a very old and still unresolved question as to whether the grants economy should content itself with grants of money, leaving the recipient to spend it as he will, or should consist essentially of grants in kind supplying needs as defined

18

by the professionals. Those who are somewhat liberal are inclined to emphasize demand even in the case of the indigent, and to give them at least some freedom to reject medical care if they prefer a short life and a merry one, though the liberty to preach against such behavior should also be preserved.

One of the great problems of the grants economy—which appears in the relief of medical indigency just as it does elsewhere—is that it can easily result in quite unintended administrative distortions of the price structure which in turn can cause social loss and quite unnecessary individual misery. If, for instance, a grant system bases a grant on a cost of service which is wrongly estimated, it can severely discourage the services which are undervalued and unnecessary and encourage the services which are overvalued. For example, certain casual administrative regulations in the social security system have stimulated a profitable practice of keeping indigent patients in nursing homes in bed, simply because the nursing homes are paid an extra amount for keeping people in bed. Hence nursing homes make more money on bed patients than on ambulatory ones. As a result of the strong financial pressure patients are kept in bed, in spite of the fact that this may be quite unwarranted medically and may contribute to the already bad enough miseries of old age and incompetence.

Generally any system which sets out to administer a price structure will get it wrong so that some things will be underpriced and some overpriced. The same problem may be seen in the universities, where teaching is underpriced relative to research, or where good administration is underpriced and bad administration overpriced. Under these circumstances a kind of universal Gresham's Law operates: the overpriced bad always drives out the underpriced good. No proposition as far as is known says that this problem is insoluble. Unless it is solved, however, socialized and administrative medicine will operate under some handicaps. The uneasy compromise between need and demand takes the form that if needs are to be well satisfied, demand, if it is not to be free, must at least be simulated. If administrative terms of trade are established in the system, it must also have an apparatus that can get feedback from their consequences and review them and adjust them rapidly in the way that the market does.

The last question of this discussion relates to the problem of the effectiveness of medical activity and research. Probably only in the last 100 years has the medical profession done more good than harm in promoting health. Now, although the direction of the effect is not in

19

doubt, a certain amount of doubt remains about its magnitude. Certainly the most spectacular productivity of human activity in the production of health is only indirectly related to the medical profession as such. That is the kind of activity involved, for instance, in antimalaria campaigns, in cleaning up water supplies, in improving nutrition and even in teaching more desirable habits of child-rearing. This fact should not be surprising, nor does it redound to any discredit to the medical profession. Nothing is wrong with the assumption that the business of the doctor is sickness rather than health, just as the business of the garage mechanic is the repair of automobiles, not their production, or the provision of roads on which they may safely be driven. The medical profession is only a single input in the enormous network of social inputs which together determine the general level of health of the population. No one wishes the medical profession to lose its interest in sickness, for that is when a doctor is most needed. On the other hand, one also likes to see a strong interest in preventive medicine and in public health and in what might be called the larger environment of the health sciences. The need is also strong for the development of a social science of health, not only in economics but also in sociology and psychology. Considerable strides have been made toward this, but not in many centers in the world—to bring even one to mind is difficult—is the social science of health studied and taught as a whole.

One would like to see a research operation of at least the magnitude of the Rand Corporation, the object of which would be to study health in all its aspects, social, biological and physical, in a manner permitting a good deal of interchange among specialists. Such a study would clearly reveal that the need for medical services will depend on a very large number of other variables, economic, sociological, biological, and on the whole system of this planet. That answer may not satisfy those who are seeking quick results to solve administrative dilemmas, and the importance of administrative shortcuts cannot be denied. Nevertheless, in the long run, a very substantial intellectual endeavor still awaits mankind in the study of this problem, and at the moment its solution is not near.[3]

The Rand Corporation is used merely as a symbol of the magnitude of the research effort in the social science of health which would probably be profitable. Whether the effort should be concentrated in a single institution or scattered around the academic community is a matter of research strategy on which may rest very valid differences of opinion. Something is to be said for the theory of the "critical mass," especially in interdisciplinary research; and the extraordinary fruitfulness of the Center for Advanced Study in the Behavioral Sciences at Stanford, indicates that a critical mass of this kind may actually be quite small under some circumstances. On the other hand, a research strategy should certainly not be confined to any particular institution, and should envisage the whole intellectual community as its field. Research strategies which are too specific can easily do more harm than good, and even the concept of the need for research needs to be looked at with a slightly quizzical eye. The growth of knowledge is much more like an evolutionary than it is like a mechanical process, and this means that it is fundamentally unpredictable. This can be seen very clearly by asking the question, can anyone predict what will be known 25 years from now? The answer is obviously no, or it would be known now. If the results of a research program are known in advance, the point in doing it has been lost. Hence the growth of knowledge must always contain what is called fundamental surprise, and any research strategy must be built around the capacity to expect and react creatively to surprise.

If any research strategy emerges out of these considerations, it is that one should be extremely suspicious of research devoted specifically to finding out the need for medical care. Too much of such research has already been done, all of which has outlined "needs" which are absurdly inflated, and which, if allowed to be fulfilled, would justify themselves with the greatest of ease. A research program which concentrated solely on quantitative estimates of need would inevitably neglect the problem of demand and the problem of the price structure. A great deal in research depends on how questions are framed. If the question is asked, how does one use a combination of the grants economy and the price structure in producing a system of medical care that compromises between needs and demands, a much richer and more satisfactory answer will likely result than if one simply asks, what is the need for medical care? Almost everyone who has raised children has heard the anguished cry, "But I need—" and soon learns to interpret this as meaning, "I want something badly but I am not prepared to pay the price for it." This cautionary note seems a suitable place to end what is mainly an appeal to move gingerly into an inevitably uncertain future, without forgetting that the movement must be made.

REFERENCES

[1] Boulding, K. E., The Menace of Methuselah, *Journal of the Washington Academy of Sciences,* 55, 171–179, October, 1965.

[2] Medawar, P. B., THE FUTURE OF MAN, New York, Basic Books, Inc., Publishers, 1960.

[3] *See* Ginzberg, Eli, The Political Economy of Health, *Bulletin of the New York Academy of Medicine,* 41, 1015–1036, October, 1965.

ON ACHIEVING ACCESS
AND EQUITY IN HEALTH CARE

RASHI FEIN

This paper addresses some of the issues related to health care in the United States. In so doing, I give primary emphasis to questions involving access to health care. Even so, I limit the discussion of any particular topic to its most important facets. The principle of selection involves various criteria: insofar as possible, I discuss those issues that are important at a system level (particularly as they impinge on the allocation of resources), that involve economic arrangements influencing behavior and performance, and that can be illuminated by the economist's perspective. I attempt to give primary emphasis to those variables whose influence is far ranging.

In so doing, of course, we cannot examine every network of interrelations. Although this simplifies the discussion, we pay a price for incompleteness. There is little choice, however. One of the difficulties with the health field stems from the fact that everything is interrelated: that intervention on one front has "side effects" on other fronts; that intervention designed to accomplish one purpose sometimes fails to do so because other factors that appear unrelated are not changed. To discuss everything is impossible. On the other hand, to say *nothing* because we cannot discuss *everything* is irresponsible.

Finally, we will have to reach judgments even in spite of the relative weakness of the data available for analysis. We know far less, for example, about the availability of services (particularly if corrected for quality differentials) than we would like to. So, too, with the impact of differences in utilization on levels of health. The current refrain often seems to be, "But we have no output measures." That, regrettably,

23

is frequently the case. Nevertheless, just as we cannot be silent because of the complexity of intertwined relations, neither can we be silent because of insufficiency of data. We can use experience and judgment to arrive at (tentative) conclusions. Not knowing everything does not mean we know nothing.

ACCESS AND EQUITY: FINANCIAL CONSIDERATIONS

Why Be Concerned About Equity?

The first question we address is, "Why is so much attention devoted to the health sector; why all the fuss about equity?" This issue is often raised by those who regard health as important, but who believe the relation is very weak between medical care expenditures and services (inputs) and health (outputs). They argue that monies that might go to the health sector to achieve equity might be better spent in other areas—e.g., housing, nutrition, education— even if the goal that is being sought is better health. All of us have heard the analysts who question the value of increasing the availability of health resources or services. We have heard distinguished leaders of medicine note that most disease is self limiting and that in a high proportion of cases physicians cannot intervene effectively.[1]

Some remarks are in order on the question of the importance of medical services. I do not intend to review the evidence on whether medical services make a difference (and to what degree) to the health of a population. Rather, I propose to consider the significance of the fact that the public believes the services to be important and, therefore, desires a greater equity in their distribution.

In the case of health and medical care, we are dealing with a sector in which, because of customs and folkways, image may be even more important than reality. Because some (even if relatively little) medical care deals with matters of life and death, because of fear, because of infatuation with science and technology—as well as because medicine oftentimes does help some individuals and, therefore, each individual can hope that it will help him—persons have come to believe that medical care services and intervention by the physician make significant contributions to health. This view is not likely to change.

It is quite likely that public policies will reflect what the public believes to be the case even if analysts find little evidence to support the public view. Part of the reason that policy will respond to public belief relates to the attitudes that surround questions of health and of

24

life and death. Part of the reason relates to the different perspectives of the public and the analyst. This difference in perspective, and in criteria used in decision making, lies at the heart of some of the major difficulties in allocating resources to the health sector.

The analyst is likely to examine issues—e.g., the impact of medical care on health—in terms of group phenomena. He is interested in a *rate* of return, in what happens on the average. The citizen—importantly, the provider as well as the consumer—is far more interested in the individual case. His behavior is responsive to the fact that intervention can make a difference in one case rather than to the fact that it makes a difference in only one per cent of the cases. If each individual believes or hopes that he may be the one who will benefit and if we do not know who the one will be and, therefore, require that the service be available to all who might benefit, we have a situation made for conflict. The analyst may say that *only* one per cent of the cases will benefit. The physician (trained to think in terms of the individual patient) and the patient (for obvious reasons) will focus on the fact that in one per cent of the cases there will be a benefit. Neither will want to be denied the resources needed for the particular case at hand. That case, after all, may be the one in a hundred.

This, I believe, is one of the basic difficulties in formulating and administering public policy in the field of health care. We reject market mechanisms that might allocate resources to and within the health sector, in part, because market results are at variance with our values. We say "medical care is a right" because we do not believe medical care should be rationed in terms of income. As a consequence, we need to develop other allocative and rationing mechanisms. Often these alternative processes will involve government regulation and program development. Government, however, will find it difficult to limit the resources allocated to the health sector and thus, in effect, to ration services.[2] In making public policy, provider and consumer attitudes (concern about the individual) weigh against the analyst's benefit-cost ratios (reflecting concern about populations).[3]

Furthermore, when the consumer hears the analyst say that, in the light of the rate of return, we need not devote additional resources to the health sector (or to particular parts of it) he recognizes that the constraint on resources implies rationing. Existing American health care financing mechanisms provide little assurance that the rationing mechanism will not be income related. Medical care, of course, is rationed in other economies and under other health care financing mechanisms: when central government allocates a given amount of resources to the health sector and when this amount is less than either consumer or provider could or would like to utilize, some "rationing" will take place. The issue, therefore, is not rationing itself, but the nature of the rationing process. Are the rationing decisions related to income or to medical needs or priorities?[4] Thus, groups who today receive less than what they consider their fair share of services are hardly likely to be impressed by an argument that they translate: "Some people do get more of certain services, but after all the services don't—on the average—yield high benefits (relative to their costs). Therefore, though the rich may 'waste' their money in purchasing the services, we shall not invest government funds to increase the availability of the services. The poor should not be distressed—they are not being denied things of considerable value."

In recent years, much of what has been said about medical services could have been so translated. This, however, means maintaining the status quo. It is not surprising that the translation is not likely to find favor among those whom the status quo has not served relatively well.

For these (and other) reasons, arguments that equity is not that important will not find favor among the general public. Most consumers will remain more concerned about distributional equity in the provision of health services than about equity considerations in the provision of most other goods and services. They will behave as if medical services do count for more and public policy will respond to their concerns.[5]

The issues raised in the above discussion are important in considering public policy. Should government allocate resources as the public might prefer, even if those resources will not accomplish that which the public desires? What, for example, is the proper mix for an antipoverty program, that which the analyst feels will eliminate poverty or that which the poor value highly? The two are not always the same. We avoid these important issues by suggesting that if government cannot "educate" the consumer or beneficiary it will have to respond to his images, tastes, values and beliefs.

What is the present situation in regard to equity in access to care? There are two parts to this question: the financial constraints and the delivery system performance. We shall need to examine both for we cannot assume that solving the problem associated with financing care would make services available, nor can we assume that increasing the supply of services would enable persons to purchase them. Let us begin with the easier part: the financial barrier. I use the term "easier" because restructuring the financing of health care is, in many ways, easier to achieve than is a restructuring of the delivery system. The fact that we are debating national health insurance (NHI) rather than a national health service (NHS) is not a coincidence.

Why Provide Specific Financing for Health Services

Surely we need not belabor the point that financial barriers to health care exist in the United States. Little would be gained by once again citing the data that all of us already know. Prepayment and voluntary health insurance, largely the result of labor-management agreements, have reduced the financial barrier for many, but not for all Americans. Medicare, Medicaid and a variety of categorical programs addressed to particular population groups or to particular diseases have also helped. Yet, even so, financial problems remain. These are of two kinds: (1) the ability to pay for care, (2) the impact of payment on family income and assets.

In this connection, it is useful to remind ourselves of some of the history of the Medicare debate. That legislation was justified on the basis of two arguments. The first derived from the fact that many persons, ages 65 and over, were unable to obtain an appropriate amount of health care because they lacked the financial resources to purchase the care. The second justification was that, even though individuals might be able to pay for care, their financial resources were so limited that the care would cut heavily into their discretionary income.[6] Thus, the debate related both to the financial ability to pay for the care that was needed and to the impact of large and unpredictable medical expenses on the financial status of the aged.

In a situation that has the characteristics of a lottery in which some will be heavy losers, there will be great concern about developing insurance safeguards. That concern is undoubtedly increased by the fact that the lower the individual's income, the greater the losses as a percentage of that income.

In some cases, the lack of money to pay for medical care (given required expenditures on housing, clothing and food) will prevent people from seeking care. In other cases, the monetary conditions result in a psychological barrier: individuals will postpone seeking care in the hope of avoiding an expenditure that would be large in relation to disposable income. In still other cases, persons may seek and pay for care but with a significant impact on their discretionary income.

27

It is necessary to distinguish between these different situations if we are to develop a public policy designed to meet the various financial problems. If I am correct, the public is concerned not only about the impact of the income distribution on the utilization of medical care, but also about the impact of the utilization of and expenditures on care on the income distribution itself. It is the second problem that calls for specific financing programs for health services rather than the provision of money to achieve a more equal distribution of pre-illness income.

Were we dealing with a category other than health care, it would not be as clear that the financing or provision of the specific good or service would be necessary. Outside of the health care sector, for example, it is often argued that an income distribution problem can (and should) be met by the provision of money.[7] This would permit the consumer to determine whether he chooses to spend those funds on the product that others had in mind or on some other product that he prefers. It is sometimes suggested that these considerations should also guide us in relation to health care, and that government should not provide assistance for specified services or support specifically for health expenditures. Instead government should provide individuals with money that they could use to purchase care (or insurance), but that they could also use for other goods and services if they so preferred.

If, however, our concern is the *ex post* income distribution, it is not sufficient to provide *ex ante* income (valuable as that may be) inasmuch as the sick would "lose" the money and the well would retain it. A solution to the various problems requires that health services, like education, be provided free.[8] Even if we cannot eliminate the "lottery" that causes some to be ill and others well, we can eliminate some of the monetary losses associated with the lottery.

There are additional reasons for the view that targeted dollars are required: (1) There is evidence that taxpayers prefer to support programs not people. The categorical, targeted legislation fares better than does the broad and all inclusive. Cancer support would fare better than national health insurance; the latter better than general income maintenance. Taxpayers want to retain a measure of control over the uses to which their dollars are put. (2) Unless funds are channeled through a single payment mechanism, it is difficult to achieve important changes in the health delivery system. (3) In the absence of government intervention, private expenditures on health care may be suboptimal because of "externalities;" i.e., my well-being is affected by the next person's state of health (and the next person does not consider that when he determines his health expenditures).

Some Equity-Equality Issues

What is meant by equity in the provision of health services? Were we speaking of tax matters and of dollars rather than services, the criteria would be simpler. In the health field a consensus on definitions is sorely lacking, in part because we have failed to specify objectives and the criteria by which to measure their attainment. Is our concern solely with the health producing aspects of the service or do we care— and if so, how much—about the amenities and the conditions under which the money or service is provided? What is the relation between equity and equality? Is equity realized when equal numbers of dollars (or services) are available for the health care of different persons, or when equal numbers of dollars (or services) are utilized, or when equal health outcomes are achieved?

As can be seen, the issues we discuss are not unique to the health sector. In different forms they are found in other sectors. The fact that they have not been solved adequately in other sectors can give us little comfort. Yet, we can gain some useful perspective from the experience elsewhere. In the field of education, for example, we find similar problems—and this in spite of the fact that in many important respects the educational sector is easier to understand than is the health sector. In the early 1960s, the definition of equality in education related to per pupil expenditures. Though we have not achieved even that limited goal, our definitions have changed and become broader. From a criterion of equality in dollar *inputs,* we moved to a definition of equality in terms of *outcomes.* At present, it is argued that there should be inequality in dollar inputs per student; inequalities that compensate for the dispersion of advantages and disadvantages that, in turn, make for variation in output per dollar of input and in outcomes. As they have in education, the newer definitions of equality will overtake the health field.

In education, we are still groping for answers to problems associated with equity and equality, with "basics" and "extras," in the public sector. Recent court decisions will help in the search for answers, but the achievement of equality at a basic minimum level is only one part of the problem. How do we deal with the fact that some persons will be able to purchase even more services than the basic minimum, that some communities will be willing and able to do more? If a community has no public kindergarten should we (can we) deny some individuals the opportunity to organize and finance their own kindergarten, i.e., to have a private kindergarten? If the school system does not provide librarians for all schools (and chooses, therefore, not to supply them to any) should we deny some (generally, upper income) mothers the right to volunteer their services as librarians in *their* school? The difficulty in saying "no" is clear. The implications of saying "yes" should be equally clear.

The battle of equity and equality has not yet been fought in the field of health in the United States. One can predict that, at some point in the future, it will be fought. If society, looking at the benefits to society, should decide not to provide various health services to the population, will it permit individuals who want those services and can afford to purchase them in the private market to do so? What if those services involve matters of life and death? If society were to conclude that it would not finance kidney dialysis for all who need it, will it finance it for some (and, if so, how will it select the "some")? Will it permit individuals who have the resources to finance the service privately? If society should decide that it will not invest significant resources in keeping individuals alive in the latter stages of a terminal illness, will it allow the individual who has the resources to do so?

Nor is this a problem that exists only in the case of exotic and expensive procedures. It should not surprise us that in today's market, a blend of the public and the private, similar issues arise in Medicare. If a physician, more highly qualified and providing a higher quality of medical care, charges more than the prevailing and customary charge in the community, the patient must pay the difference. This can be interpreted to mean that the Medicare program is prepared to pay for an average level of physician competence for all individuals while permitting individuals interested in a higher quality of care, *and who can pay* for that higher quality, to seek it out. Even though Medicare does, therefore, bring an adequate or average quality of service to all, it does not bring equality. It is clear that it does not provide what public officials often set as a goal: the highest quality for all. With limited resources one cannot have the highest quality for all. If the quest is for equality, the slogan might well be: the highest quality for none. That, however, is hardly a slogan that will find its way into a Presidential message (in part because it is not of such slogans that Presidents are made).

It is not clear, of course, that the objective is full equality. It may be that a more limited objective—say the elimination of income as a rationing device—is sought. With scarce resources, society may decide not to withhold services from everyone because it cannot provide services to all, but instead to provide them to some who are selected on a basis other than their ability to pay for the services. Tables of random numbers or other criteria could be used to determine the allocation of the scarce resources.

Though I have raised these issues because it seems to me that, at some point, the body politic will wrestle in some continuing fashion with many of them, we should not be misled. The fact that there is no consensus on these matters and that they cannot all be solved does not imply that we cannot move forward. We are not required to have a solution to every possible dilemma before we develop a public policy to resolve those that we can do something about.

In considering equity, we can adapt some of the approaches used in discussions of tax equity. We can distinguish between horizontal and vertical equity. By horizontal equity we mean that the health care system shall provide essentially the same set of health services (or a distribution of services that equalize outcomes) for persons in approximately the same economic circumstances. Most often horizontal equity considerations are assumed to relate to questions of access affected by the availability of services (e.g., rural-urban differences). These, of course, are important. Horizontal equity, however, is also affected by the nature of government support for the purchase of health services. If such support, as in the Medicaid program, leaves the states free to determine eligibility and the level of benefits (i.e., if the system is based on matching grants rather than on 100 per cent federal funding) horizontal equity will not be achieved. Indeed, the existing inequities are likely to be compounded. The achievement of vertical equity requires government involvement in the financing of care. The achievement of horizontal equity requires that it be the federal level of government. This is not surprising for horizontal equity requires that the residents of different states be treated in like fashion (i.e., as Americans). Only the federal dollar can insure that that occurs.[9]

Vertical equity, "fairness," in the provision of services for persons in different economic circumstances, is more difficult to define. Because health benefits must be financed, an examination of the progressivity of the distributional impact must consider the distribution of the tax, premium or other device that finances the benefits as well as the distribution of the benefits themselves (the availability and distribution of the services). It must also consider the proportion of health care costs that is covered by the program. We achieve relatively little even if we devise a highly progressive tax structure, but one that finances services that play only a small part in the consumer's budget. If our goal is equity in the distribution of health expenditures, we must consider the distribution of total health care costs in relation to income.

Paying for Medical Care: Present Patterns

At the present time, the individual's medical care costs are often met both by out-of-pocket expenditures and by voluntary health insurance benefits. Out-of-pocket expenditures occur because voluntary health insurance coverage usually involves deductibles and co-insurance, is not comprehensive in its scope and sets upper limits on benefits. This approach has a long tradition and has found its way into public programs, e.g., Medicare.

Deductibles and co-insurance are supported on two rationales. The first is that the larger the amount the individual must pay on an out-of-pocket basis, the smaller the premium charge (or tax) can be. The second rationale is based, if not on empirical analysis of the demand for health care, on well-established economic principles. It is assumed that if the individual is required to share in the cost of care at the time that the care is sought his utilization of care will be reduced. In the absence of deductibles and co-insurance, care is "free." At that zero price the individual would seek more care than if he were required to pay a small sum, sufficient to deter him from seeking unncessary care, but insufficient to deter him from seeking care when it is required. This second rationale is closely associated with yet another that is put forward: if the consumer is required to pay a share of the cost, he will be more cost conscious than would otherwise be the case. This cost consciousness, in turn, will induce providers of care, including hospitals, to exercise price restraint and to compete on a price basis.

Although these arguments carry some weight, it is possible to advance arguments on the other side of the co-insurance and deductible issue. It is clear, for example, that a fixed deductible and a fixed percentage co-insurance cannot hit with equal impact on families in different income brackets. The amount that is appropriate for one family (i.e., it deters only unnecessary medical care) may be trivial for another (serving not to deter at all) and too large for yet another (serving to deter even important care). It is true that, in theory, this particular objection can be met by letting the size of the deductible

32

or the per cent of co-insurance vary with the income of the family. Yet, deductibles and co-insurance may entail significant administrative costs and the more refined the approach, the greater the costs of administration. Nor do we have the requisite information to construct a sliding scale that would have the particular impacts we desire. One must, therefore, ask whether the claimed benefits of deductibles and co-insurance are sufficient to justify the costs.

We have little information concerning the degree to which utilization would be affected by different co-insurance and deductibles.[10] We also lack information that would enable us to assess whether an increase in utilization is unwarranted. Costs of travel and waiting time, possible loss of income from work, fear, concern and so forth, all associated with visiting the physician, may lead persons to underutilize medical care services. If utilization should be higher—even then it would be at a zero price—one would not want to erect a financial deterrent.

We can also indicate some doubt concerning the effectiveness of deductibles and co-insurance as cost-control devices. Even in spite of existing financial barriers, the health sector has not had an enviable cost-control record. Furthermore, though we know relatively little about how prices and expenditures are determined in the marketplace, what we do know suggests that the physician is the critical actor in the determination both of unit costs (the price of the product) and total cost (unit cost times quantity, the degree to which the product is utilized). The largest savings on the expenditure side are likely to come as ways are found to affect utilization (rather than price). Since utilization is largely physician (not patient) determined, efforts to contain the total costs of a program require that the programs be structured to provide incentives to change *physician* behavior.[11] Deductibles and co-insurance (at levels that do not deter necessary care) are not likely to do that.

Costs associated with treatment for conditions not covered through the insurance mechanism are also part of out-of-pocket expenditures. The failure of insurance to be comprehensive in scope has taught us that the medical care system can be distorted by virtue of what is and what is not covered through insurance. Economics does make a difference. In theory, such distortions could be for good or for bad. One could, presumably, structure a health insurance program so as to reduce unnecessary and expensive procedures. It would, however, be difficult to leave the most expensive procedures without coverage. Even though, for example, some may overutilize expensive hospital pro-

33

cedures, others utilize the services because they need them. Shall they be uninsured?

As contrasted with other types of insurance, our problem is compounded by the fact that the provider and consumer help determine whether the insured service is utilized. If some services are insured and others are not we are likely to find distortions in utilization. Because we are called on to insure expensive procedures, we are providing incentives for their use. One is, therefore, almost inevitably led to comprehensiveness of coverage, in part for medical reasons, in part to prevent unfavorable impacts on the allocation of resources within the medical system and in part to achieve the equity we spoke of earlier.

There is a third element of medical care that is paid for by the patient on an out-of-pocket basis: those costs that occur after the insurance has reached the upper limits on the number of days of hospital care or on the total cost that will be covered. In many ways this is the anomaly in the insurance field. Had health insurance not originally been developed by the hospital sector as a way of protecting itself from bad debts, we would likely have had larger deductibles and greater protection at the upper end. Since most patients spend a limited amount of time in the hospital, the emphasis, however, was on shallow-end coverage. The consequence—incorporated into federal legislation in the Medicare program and duplicated in a variety of proposals that have been offered to the Congress—is that those who stay in the hospital the longest time (and who often are most sick) run out of benefits. Insurance, in general, tries to protect against high expenses that occur relatively infrequently and the occurrence of which is not under the control of the person having the insurance, but that upper-end coverage that is lacking. The costs associated with exceeding the upper limits may not significantly affect the distribution of medical care costs by income class (because the upper limits are seldom reached). Nonetheless, the costs are a severe problem for those who must bear them and require relief.

Paying for Medical Care: Future Possibilities

In my view, a comprehensive insurance program is called for with coverage at both the upper end of the cost spectrum (if high-cost services are to be available) and at the low end (there is little evidence that deductibles and co-insurance yield important benefits). I refer to coverage both at the upper end and at the lower end, so I could, of course, be asked about my trade-offs: would I rather have the one or

34

the other? If the question assumes that, for political reasons, we cannot have both upper- and lower-end coverage, it is meaningful to pose the issue. This is not the case, however, if the question assumes that we can afford one or the other, but not both. Costs are incurred whether or not they are covered by a national program. We are not talking about new dollars (except to the extent that utilization is increased, and that increase may be one of the desirable consequences of the program). In largest measure we are talking about old dollars in new clothes. The question is how shall the cost be borne; i.e., shall the expenditures for medical care be private or public?

For the legislator, the trade-off question is meaningful. Legislative bodies are concerned about increasing taxes even if these taxes pay for services that would otherwise be paid for by private expenditures. Part of the dilemma of the legislator is the result of the fact that he has failed to educate the public as to what the issues are. Education is never easy, and the task is made even more difficult by the cynicism and mistrust that is the legacy of our recent past. Yet, it is a task that cannot be avoided except at the risk of creating more mistrust.

Quite often, the difficulty in explaining what the public might receive for its taxes lies in the fact that expenditure programs are not tied to specific tax revenues. This is one of the strengths of our fiscal system. It permits the Legislative Branch to choose between programs (presumably) to maximize welfare. Nonetheless, the absence of a link, at least in the consumer's mind, does make it more difficult to associate particular benefits with the general taxes that we pay. These considerations are relevant in examining the method by which funds might be raised for a program that would distribute the costs of medical care more equitably.

The most progressive part of our tax system is the federal personal income tax. Given a progressivity goal, one could, therefore, argue in favor of financing a national health insurance program out of general revenues, in large part, derived from the federal personal income tax. Furthermore, appropriations from general revenues increase the competition between dollars for health and for other programs. This can have a significant and desirable effect on the Congressional desire to control costs. Arguing against the use of general revenues to support the program is the lack of a visible link, as seen by the taxpayer, between the tax and the program. Such a link might increase the public's understanding that public dollars for health compete with private expenditures and, thus, would be useful in generating consumer concern about

35

cost control. It is possible, therefore, to argue that general taxation increases Congressional concern about prices and costs, whereas the levying of a special payroll tax increases the consumer's concern. If it is necessary that all parties understand that there is no such thing as a free lunch, it may be desirable to use both types of taxation in funding a national health insurance program.

The payroll tax, in its present form, however, is hardly a tax that can be considered progressive. Its deficiencies are well known: e.g., it does not take account of family size, often discriminates against multiple-earner families, considers only certain kinds of income. It is proportional up to the wage base and then regressive. Raising the wage base would help, but other adjustments are also desirable: e.g., low-income families could be given a refund for the payroll tax deducted. Over the last decade we have had a number of personal income tax cuts even in spite of the social needs pressing upon the nation. The nonprogressive payroll tax has, therefore, come to have an even larger impact on the tax burden by family income. Today a family of four earning $4,000 pays $32 in federal income tax. Yet it pays over $400 in payroll taxes (if we include the employer's contribution). If income tax rates reflect our judgments about the tax levels that are fair or appropriate at the various income levels or about the relative tax burden by family income, we can hardly add a very substantial payroll tax and assume that we are not distorting the very standards that we have set.

The payroll tax does have important political strengths. It is to be hoped, however, that we would not embark on payroll taxation as the method of financing national health insurance with the belief that a few years later we could amend the payroll tax to improve it. Such amendments will not come easily. The time to press for a more equitable payroll tax is before the program is enacted.

Earlier we have discussed the importance of cost control. Although indicating that it would be useful for the consumer to recognize the link between costs of the program and tax levels, one can hardly expect that the individual will be influenced in his utilization of medical care services by such considerations. This is the case for two reasons: first, because no individual believes that his utilization will affect the general price level, the total utilization and the tax rate. Little personal gain is to be derived from acting in a socially responsible fashion. Second, decisions regarding utilization are more often made by the physician rather than by the patient. Consumer awareness about costs should be increased. Ultimately, however, costs will depend on how the system is structured and on physician behavior. We must, therefore, now turn to those things within the system that can affect the physician in his determination of appropriate utilization.

We are also compelled to turn to the question of system because the financing of services is only one part of the equity consideration. We cannot assume that if financial barriers are removed, the distribution problem would be solved through market adjustments—as might, for example, be the case with food. To assure a more equitable distribution of food is relatively simple (conceptually, if not politically). In general we need only provide families with sufficient money (or with food stamps, if we want to reduce the possibility that the "currency" provided would be used for nonfood purchases). We are not required to open grocery stores. We can assume that a food distribution network exists or will expand to meet consumer demand. The level of skill demanded of grocery store managers does not necessitate a long lead time to train supply (surely not as long as that required to educate and train physicians). Nor, in contrast with physicians, would we have to attract managers to the Ozarks from New York. In the case of health services the situation is quite different—and particularly so in a system as highly fragmented as ours. Access to health services requires that health resources be available (not simply that the "health stamp" be distributed to families). Physicians are people, not commodities. They prefer certain locations, certain kinds of situations, certain types of associations. Under those conditions, providing equal access (however we choose to define it) requires that we address the delivery system's characteristics. We thus turn our attention to some of the issues related to the allocation of resources to and within the health care system.

ACCESS AND EQUITY: SYSTEM CHANGE

The health system is a complex network many parts of which we do not fully understand. In the search for equity we must consider that system and the allocation of resources within it for access is, in part, determined by the allocation of resources. That the system suffers from a variety of ailments in its resource allocation is clear. What is unclear is which of the problems are interrelated and to what degree. We are, therefore, often at a loss to understand the nature of the required therapy. Too often we tend to approach each ailment or misallocation as if it requires direct action and intervention. Seldom do we explore the possibilities that actions on another part of the system may, in an indirect manner, affect the variable that is our concern.

The bias in favor of direct intervention is clear. It seems simpler to attack a problem in a frontal fashion. The disadvantages should also be clear. Too often the problem we see is really a manifestation of more basic difficulties and is the logical consequence of a more basic structural deficiency. It may, therefore, resist intervention, recur again or require periodic intervention as it manifests itself in some new manner.

To suggest that one knows the single root cause of our difficulties and that that cause can be described in specific terms would be foolish. Nor is it even clear that there is one single cause to all our problems. Actions on a number of fronts are required, though little in the American tradition suggests that, even if we had the understanding, a rational and organized approach would be followed. We are far more likely to move in fits and starts, first in one area then in another. Nonetheless, it is useful to recognize the interrelations within the system. At the margin this knowledge can affect our public policies. It can prevent us from dissipating energy on policies that would have little impact, could enable us to devote our effort to actions that have basic effects, could keep us from taking an action in one area that negates what we are doing elsewhere in the system. It should be clear that as we examine basic problems and discuss them in more specific terms than "what we need is a reorganization of the delivery system," we cannot help but be controversial. The existing system has its rewards for many providers and consumers. It is hardly to be expected in a field as important to the consumer and as rewarding to the producer as is medicine, that important changes will be welcomed by everyone. At the minimum there is the fear of the unknown. At the maximum there is the recognition that the particular individual may not gain through change.

The fact that controversy is present means that the health sector is politicized, a phenomenon not to be deplored but welcomed. No longer can the sector be viewed as belonging solely to the "experts." What is to be deplored is that many first-class analysts have played the role of second-class politicians. Desirous of change and improvement, they have presented analyses and recommendations that are far reaching but that stay within the limits of what they conceive of as political reality, within their definition of what is possible. This is regrettable, on at least two grounds. The quest for political acceptability has tended to focus the discussion on technical matters, as if there were no ideology. As a result, the most important areas of controversy, the ones that require debate and on which people disagree, have been neglected. The effort to "sell" a program steers one to the technical nonideological issues and replaces passion with blandness. This lowers the quality of the discussion and does less than is required for the education of the public. In addition, there is little to suggest that the political analysis is necessarily correct. Too often the analyst, in playing politician, rejects proposals that have greater political viability than he imagines. Although it is true that one can offer proposals so politically unrealistic that the advocate as well as the proposal is rejected, that danger, it seems to me, should be considered important only in the center of the political arena; i.e., on the Washington scene. The problem, perhaps, is that too high a proportion of those concerned with American medicine are (imagine themselves to be or hope to be) directly or indirectly part of the Washintgon scene.

We need only remind ourselves of Phases I and II, to recognize that one can underestimate what is possible. Similar examples exist in other areas. Before the health analyst rejects a proposal as politically unrealistic he might ask whether it is more "daring" than a trip to China, a proposal to impose a moratorium on a category of court decisions, a budget deficit of over $25 billion. Surely, asking that question will suggest that one need not be inhibited about being "far out" in his suggestions.

Regulation and the Market

What are some of the more basic elements of the health care system that would benefit from change? What organizational and financing structures have influences so pervasive that changing them might result in fundamental changes in the allocation of resources and, therefore, in access?

Many of our difficulties in the health sector relate to the fact that we operate in a never-never land, somewhere between the free market and the results it might bring and government regulation and its consequences. Rejecting the market because the characteristics of health care suggest that market results would not meet our preferences, rejecting tight government regulation because of American traditions and the difficulties inherent in the regulatory process, we have found ourselves in an untenable situation. Our difficulties will not disappear;

indeed, they could grow even more severe with the enactment of measures limited to the financing of the purchase of health services. Many persons would be aided by such legislation, but unless these programs (or accompanying legislation) address some of the issues that affect the delivery of services, we will provide a good deal less health or equity than we should with the resources available. This, after all, has been the record of Medicare and Medicaid. To suggest, as some do, that these programs have only caused inflation is fallacious. They have offered financial protection to many and have provided additional services to some. Nevertheless, it is also true that while helping to solve some problems, they have contributed to the worsening of others. In my view their pluses far outweigh their minuses. Nonetheless, it is clear there have been minuses. Furthermore, they have, unfortunately, led to a certain disillusionment.

During the decade of the 1960s—in the days of the optimism of the New Frontier and the Great Society—we enacted a wide variety of social programs in a number of areas. The characteristic of many of these programs was that the federal government appropriated funds with which to buy goods and services from the private sector. It did not produce the goods or services itself, nor did it take over the control of the particular sector. Medicare and Medicaid are examples of this approach, but the examples extend beyond the field of health. The programs were underfunded and, in some cases, poorly managed, but those were not the only difficulties they faced. Watching dollars flow out of Washington and observing that the dollars would not change delivery systems (on observation that should not have come as a surprise) many who believed in the aims of the legislation gave up hope too quickly and began to consider the virtues of the market as a regulatory device. This process was accompanied by a disillusionment with government itself. Considered impersonal and unresponsive, bureaucratic and inefficient, the call was for withdrawal: "Give it back to the market, call in the for-profit institution, sell the city hospital (or post office), turn to a voucher system in education, and so forth."

It is perhaps the case that we had chosen the most difficult of all worlds. I do not suggest that to operate a nationalized sector effectively is easy. Indeed, that is not the case. Neither do I suggest that the solutions arrived at through normal market forces (and it is not clear what these are in the health sector but surely they are not those of pure competition) are desirable. That, too, is not the case. But operating a mixed economy (perhaps in the health field the phrase "mixed-up" economy would be more appropriate) may lead to higher costs with relatively little increase in output or redistribution for the increased dollars. It leads to a high level of frustration.

It is difficult to administer effective regulations—regulations designed to allocate resources and to make a real difference. In part, this is because regulation runs counter to a number of our traditions. In part, the difficulty stems from the fact that we know less than we should like to, especially about the production function for health. Regulating the construction of health facilities, for example, requires more than just a "feel" for the "right" number of hospital beds. No regulator can easily withstand the political pressure if his chief weapon is his intuition. The recognition that he lacks technical knowledge that might buttress his case against political pressures tends, therefore, to cause the administrator to shy away from regulation. Instead of saying "no," he says "yes." Instead of redistributing resources he calls for more dollars and more resources in the hope that some of these will trickle down and solve the particular problem with which he was initially concerned.

To say that today's health economy is substantially unregulated (where it counts) is, however, not to imply that government regulation that says "this you must and that you can't do" is the only solution. Much that is wrong today in the health sector derives from the fact that the structure of the health industry provides the wrong incentives. It is possible, therefore, to effect change, not by regulation but rather by substituting a different set of incentives and permitting the system to adjust to these incentives. If such a mechanism could be developed, it would have a number of advantages: it would appear (and often be) less arbitrary; it would provide us with "signals" as a feedback to tell us how the system is operating.

Let us examine some of the issues. In so doing, we shall focus on the physician because he is the critical actor in the health care system, because access to his services is a key equity issue and because, in large measure, he determines the utilization of other parts of the system.

Fee-for-Service: Physician Control of Market Forces

Much of our difficulty relates to the set of incentives that impinge on the physician and the setting in which they operate. Physicians are self-employed, small businessmen and, in many critical ways, are viewed in that light. They are among the relatively few Americans who are self-employed: of the 75 million persons employed in nonagricultural industries in 1970, only 5 million were self-employed. Though there is a trend toward grouping of physicians, many of them still practice in solo, independent practice. They are subject to relatively little control or oversight. The quality of their performance may be good or bad—there is no real way to know because a data system does not exist that will record relevant information or a mechanism for performance review by impartial observers. Once licensed, they remain licensed without reassessment of their performance. With licensing and entry restrictions (generally justified as protecting the consumer and maintaining quality) but without continuing or periodic quality assessment, we have a system that, to a significant extent, protects the producer by sheltering him from the forces of competition while not requiring performance standards.

Though many small business markets bear some resemblance to the physician market (though with different supply constraints), those sectors, most often, must meet a market test. That, perhaps, is the critical difference in health services. Consumer ignorance of medicine and health, combined with fear and customs, prevent the consumer from performing his own quality assessment, from evaluating physician performance, from examining prices. More than that is involved, however. The consumer's utilization of services is largely dependent on *physician* decisions. The physician (businessman) is one of the relatively few American entrepreneurs who can expand the demand for his services (and without advertising or at the expense of a competing firm). The power to influence, if not determine, the level of demand is a strong power, indeed. That there are inducements to expand demand is also clear. The system of payment, fee-for-service, is at issue. Given a payment system that has characteristics of a piece-rate wage, the power to determine the number of pieces (with "piece" defined as a procedure rather than the attainment of a desired outcome, say "cure"), and little control of quality (including excess visits or surgery and unnecessary procedures as poor quality), it is easy to see that normal market forces are not likely to involve the kind of adjustment processes that operate to equilibrate other markets. The essential factor is that the physician can control his market to a substantial degree, administering price, quantity and quality.[12]

Today's system preserves the freedom of physicians to practice where they want, the kind of medicine they want (by specialty), as well as with population groups they prefer. The physician is free to allocate his resources as he sees fit. This is a freedom given to few others in the society. Even though it is the case that government regulation does not often direct labor (allocate it by skill, occupation or location) or business, other regulatory devices (called economic incentives) do operate. They provide for allocations that are acceptable or that we believe tend to distribute the supply of services in relation to consumer demand. The quest for profits, the desire to take advantage of economic opportunity, to win the test of the marketplace, is the lubricant that, presumably, makes the story end happily. It is not clear, of course, that there are as many happy endings as our illusions suggest. Unfortunately, there is increasing evidence that rigidity in various economic sectors interferes with the adjustment process. Bigness, for example, plays its interference role; discrimination plays its interference role; licensing restrictions play their role; differential tax rates play their role; government regulation, often times converted to the protection of the regulated, plays its role. Nonetheless, the small business retail service sector does exhibit a number of competitive characteristics. Some establishments succeed and others fail. The fact that some fail means there is a test. The health sector, however, is different. It does not even offer the illusion that the forces of competition are at work to respond to consumer demand. Furthermore, meeting consumer demand for health care, as expressed in the marketplace, would not be sufficient. Today our concern is with consumer need. We cannot as readily accept the nonadjustment process that prevails in the health market.

Suppose, however, we do not consider the physician as a businessman. Surely then his freedom, say, to settle where he would like, to specialize as he might like, is the same freedom others have—or so it might appear. Is that the case, however? As already noted, the vast majority of Americans are not self-employed. Most Americans take jobs, and this is true at all levels of the occupational ladder, including professionals. They enter fields in relation to income potentials and a projection of job opportunities. Their choice of a place to live is, in part, determined by job opportunities. In many cases, of course, these job opportunities exist all over the nation; e.g., school teachers, clothing salesmen and so forth. In other cases, the range of choice is limited. If one wants to be an aeronautical engineer, chances are one cannot live in South Hill, Virginia. If one wants to be a Supreme Court Justice, one must reside in the Washington, D.C. area. The allocation of labor and of its productive services is determined by market conditions. Many of us may be unaware of the economic controls over our behavior because they are so much a part of the system that we do not recognize them explicitly, and because they appear impersonal and not arbitrary. The young man in a small community in New England who would like to live in that small community but who would also like to be a petroleum engineer most probably does not consider that his "freedom" is restricted because he must choose between the two. Physicians in academic medicine hardly consider their freedom restricted because they cannot be both in academic medicine and in Springfield, Massachusetts (there is no medical school there). The crux of the issue is that most physicians are not employees and, therefore, meeting a test of demand by employers; but at the same time as self-employed individuals, they are not required to meet the rigorous market demand tests that other self-employed individuals face. They are insulated from the forces of competition.

The largely unrestricted freedoms physicians have are not the freedoms most Americans have. Yet we have somehow come to believe that to restrict the physician's freedoms is to single him out and engage in discriminatory action. Physicians, in criticizing the organization of medical care in other nations, often complain about the loss of freedom (say, to be a neurosurgeon and to practice in a particular city whose hospitals have no unfilled posts in neurosurgery). They would do well to consider that if the market in medical care were truly competitive (the results of "free enterprise," which the very same physicians praise) significant (albeit impersonal) economic controls would influence their decisions. It is not surprising that physicians prefer the United States pattern under which they can control the market forces. What is surprising is that the layman has come to accept that situation as an essential freedom.

The market for some other professionals may exhibit characteristics similar to that which the physician faces, but his advantages are somewhat greater. These derive from two considerations: the first relates to the fact that the physician, though he does not have total control over the market, can exercise greater control than most and, thus, reduce the economic differentials that might otherwise obtain. The second relates to the fact that, in general, we consider medical services to be more important than various other services; indeed, it is because we so consider them that the physician faces a relatively inelastic demand curve for his services and that he can push that demand curve to the right.

The picture we draw is an extreme one. There are limits, of course. The physician does not have complete control (or freedom), but he does have sufficient control to affect the market so that the signals that

44

it would normally send regarding shortage and oversupply are missing. Within the limits of the existing supply of physicians, the pressures to reach an equilibrium position that reflects needs are far too weak. One can hardly imagine that, it we had ten times as many physicians, they would be distributed as they are today. Market adjustments would take place. We do not, however, have ten times as many physicians, nor could one responsibly advocate a policy to solve market disequilibrium by increasing supply until, on some trickle-down or overflow basis, our poorer areas would be served. The costs of producing that manpower, as well as the cost of "overdoctoring" in areas that would be even richer in physician supply than they now are, can hardly lead us to advocate that solution.

Finally, of course, we must recognize the unhappy set of coincidences that exists. If, after all, we argue that part of the problem is that the pressures to fill medical needs can be resisted because of the nature of the medical marketplace, that in no way suggests that they must be resisted. After all, there is no inexorable law of nature that says that physicians' desires must be at variance with society's needs. One could imagine a world in which both society and physicians placed a high value on primary care and in which physicians wanted to practice in inner cities and in rural areas. In that case, physician control would be less troublesome because, even in its presence, physicians would be moving to the very areas where they were needed. But the world does not end that happily because of two factors in physician preferences.

Specialization and Location

The first factor is that for a variety of reasons an increasing proportion of physicians moves away from primary care and in many cases into specialties not closely related to the primary care function (e.g., pediatrics, obstetrics and gynecology or general internal medicine). Despite the fact that leaders of American medicine and observers of the American medical scene may deplore the movement into specialties and the emphasis on surgery and on subspecialties, the energy devoted to discussing the problem has failed to change the pattern of movement. The pressures seem to be too great. One such pressure comes from the larger society from which medicine does not stand independent. The forces at work to increase specialization in other areas of activity also affect medicine. As knowledge explodes and is transmitted in innumerable journals, the pressure to specialize grows greater. As the number of specialists increases, the generalist comes to be considered as

45

the nonexpert, and this in a society that places a high value on expertise.

These pressures are further reinforced by the process of medical education. The National Institutes of Health have helped enlarge the subspecialties and create a research endeavor and a reward system that many students have seen as denigrating the physician who delivers general care and is not doing research. The culture of the medical school, the nature of its faculty, the heavy emphasis on clinical teaching in the hospital (the world of the specialist), all tend to reinforce the pressures that already exist. Trained in the hospital where one sees the sickest patients, where things are happening, where time is compressed (which is one of the reasons the hospital is used as a training institution), it is no small wonder that specialists become the role model. These pressures in themselves might be sufficient, yet the nature of modern medical practice adds to them. There are significant disadvantages to being a primary care physician, particularly in individual solo practice, a type of practice that places heavy demands upon the physician.

The fact that the physician can validate his decision to be a specialist, in part by control of the market, leaves little hope that, in the existing system, the primary care needs will be met (except, perhaps, in the hospital outpatient department, which has special characteristics that would enable it to "succeed" or by new nonphysician kinds of personnel).

The second factor that inhibits the development of a more equitable geographic distribution of physicians is that physicians, like most Americans, prefer locations other than the rural area or the inner city. Furthermore, this is reinforced by the bias in medical school admissions in favor of applicants from families in the upper part of the income distribution, whose background is not likely to be the rural area or the inner city. In addition, the decision to specialize affects the geographic distribution because the specialist needs a different population base and may require different facilities, a network of relations with other physicians and so forth. Finally, the nature of practice—particularly the way medical services are disorganized at the present time—makes solo practice in the inner city and rural areas less desirable: the risks are greater, practice is hard and frustrations are many. With greater mobility than most persons physicians are able to satisfy their geographic and location preferences.

46

The critical issue, however, is not that physicians decide to be specialists and offer less primary care than needed. Nor is it that the geographic supply is maldistributed. These are results not causes. They are the outcomes of a process that permits the physician to determine the allocation of resources (his as well as much of the health sector) without the constraints set by the normal requirements of meeting consumer demand (which he can influence) or government regulation (which is weak at best and often absent). Because the allocation of resources determines access, the other side of the equity coin, we face the prospect of continued inequity even in the face of more comprehensive financing mechanisms.

It can, of course, be argued that under a system of universal financing, the distribution of physicians by specialty and by location would show some improvement. Surely there are physicians who, today, do not practice in locations with a high proportion of low-income families because of the difficulty that they envision in achieving a desired income level. Given an alternative financing pattern, we could expect some improvement in the maldistribution. Medicaid, after all, has made services available to some who otherwise would have gone without services. Yet the Medicaid story suggests the difficulties involved in using this approach to solve a distribution problem: the re-allocation of resources is not likely to take place in an efficient manner, quality differentials remain and so forth. We cannot assume that we will achieve the desired distribution and equal access by giving the poor money so that they will be better able to compete with the nonpoor. Even though the dollars of the poor are as green as the dollars of the rich, the poor are not likely to compete on equal terms. This is especially the case if the nonpoor can outbid the poor because they have more dollars with which to purchase the limited supply of services; i.e., if a private market continues to function.

Maldistribution: the Difficulty of the Direct Approach

If equity and access are to be achieved, the distribution of physicians and of their services must change. Such changes will not come through exhortation. Intervention is required. The question is, "What kind of intervention, direct or indirect?"

Three approaches, not involving a restructuring of the basic organization of the medical system, can be examined. The first attempts to select medical students with characteristics that, it is hoped, will alter the probabilities of various specialty and location choices. The second attempts to use the regulatory process (and coercion). The third attempts to use incentives (most probably economic in nature).

American medical education uses the first approach to a limited extent and in a rather haphazard fashion. On occasion, applicants from rural areas are given preference. A number of schools give preference to minority applicants, hoping that this will increase the services available to inner core city residents.[13] There is little hard data, however, that would provide confidence in selecting applicants with specific characteristics in an effort to change the geographic and specialty distribution of physicians. Furthermore, even were such data available, it is likely that the individual medical school admissions committee would prefer to maintain traditional standards "relying" on other medical schools to make the adjustments. Finally, the stock of physicians is so large, relative to the annual inflow of new United States graduates, that change in the distribution of the total number of physicians would occur very slowly even if new admissions' policies were established and these were successful in attaining their objective.

The regulatory process, applied to specialization, would also require collective action. One could hardly expect individual hospitals or medical schools—except in rare instances—voluntarily to limit the number of residencies available in the various fields. However much physicians in Medical School X may feel there are too many residencies in the nation in Specialty Y, they may also feel that their residency provides better training than the next school's and that that school should make the needed changes. Responsible action on the part of one medical school is insufficient, and competitive forces are not likely to bring responsible action by all medical schools. Furthermore, we cannot help but recognize that in the heavily hospital-oriented present system of medical care house staff members provide a significant number of services. Voluntary action on the part of the hospitals in the absence of new financing mechanisms, and a greater emphasis on nonhospital care is, therefore, unlikely. The system is too intertwined to permit of action on one front alone.

Government, because it is involved with all parts of the system, could apply the regulatory process. The difficulties in this regard are clear: applied to specialization on a yes-no basis, government would receive few "signals" back to inform it that adjustments are called for. This common problem in regulation may be even more severe in the health sector. To apply regulation to locational decisions—extremely difficult

48

to imagine, given American traditions—is also difficult. One can picture a system of coercion; e.g., two years' service in various locations. Such an approach may have merit, if we are unprepared to attempt more basic institutional reform, but it is an incomplete solution because, like other regulatory or coercive devices, it does not attack the cause of the problem.[14]

A third alternative approach to changing the manpower distribution involves the use of economic incentives. Here, too, one can generate little optimism. We have little information on the level at which incentives would have to be set to materially affect the distribution. We do, however, know this: incentives are expensive. Extra payments to physicians to enter certain fields and to practice in certain areas cannot be offered as rewards only to those whose behavior we are trying to change. They must be offered to all. In the first place, we cannot tell whose behavior is changing and who would have "done the right thing" anyway. In the second place, it is difficult to justify an administered payment mechanism that rewards the individual who is induced into a field, and discriminates against the one who would have entered it voluntarily. Incentive payments, therefore, must be given to all. They must reward those who would have accepted smaller payments with the same amount required to induce the marginal individual to change his behavior. Finally, given the high income of physicians and present tax rates, economic incentives in the form of higher income (as contrasted with, say, vacations) are not likely to have much influence.

Alternatives to Fee-for-Service: The Advantage of Prepaid Group Practice

These direct approaches to the distribution question, however, are not the only ones we need consider. Our earlier discussion suggested that many of our difficulties (and not only ones involving the distribution of physicians) stem from the fact that physicians are not subject to various market constraints (that they can influence demand and price). Is not the better approach to change these conditions? We need to intervene on the organization side rather than try to correct the consequences of the unfavorable organization.

The elimination of the fee-for-service payment mechanism would go a long way toward eliminating the incentive to overdoctor and the incentive to create one's own ma: et demand. Today, fee-for-service may lead the consumer to restrict his demand, but it provides the physician with the incentive to expand it. Because the physician is more powerful in the physician-patient relationship, the consequences are apparent. Given a different method of payment, the incentives would be altered.[15]

We can consider various alternatives to fee-for-service. Two such alternatives are capitation and salary. In either case the physician's income no longer depends on the volume of services rendered to the patient. Furthermore, if the supply of dollars available is related to the number of patients (including adjustments based on the relation between their demographic characteristics and needs; e.g., age) the available dollars will serve to cause labor market adjustments. Such a payment mechanism could be adjusted at periodic intervals in response to the way physicians distribute themselves. It cannot, however, respond to validate those decisions by making unlimited dollars available.

To say that the incentive has been changed is one thing. To say that the new incentive is neutral is fallacious. The situation that leaves the physician dominant *vis-à-vis* the patient remains, but now the patient faces a physician whose incentives are to underdoctor. This, however, seems a better situation for a number of reasons. In the present system medical ethics do not seem to be at variance with the danger of extra procedures: is it unethical to ask for one more test, one more visit, one more procedure? One should certainly like to believe that the medical ethic would inhibit the physician from underdoctoring; i.e., not doing things he should do.

Yet, this is not necessarily the case nor can we be assured that it is. Furthermore, we have already alluded to the fact that today's system exerts little control over and provides little knowledge about quality. A different payment system in itself does not insure a change in this situation. Other changes are required, though even then we cannot be fully optimistic as long as our knowledge about quality (the input and output relationship) is meager. Nonetheless, if the physician is in a situation in which data review is possible, peer review is present, consumer involvement likely and standards are set, the outcome is likely to be improved. Such a situation prevails when physicians are grouped together.

To suggest that grouping physicians and using salary payment mechanisms assures quality performance would be fallacious. We have, after all, had sufficient experience in recent years to be sensitive to these matters. Our schools and prisons, for example, place institutional constraints on salaried workers (who, in many cases, are professionals). Yet performance is not always responsive to the needs of the persons

50

to be served. Our universities are staffed with salaried professionals, yet we know little about the output of the faculty. One cannot assume the prepaid group will do significantly better unless attempts are made to structure the environment, to gather data and monitor performance, to build in consumer review and involvement. Even so, we may fall short of the desired goal. We can note, however, that if we fall short it is, in large measure, because of the behavior of physicians. Is there any reason to prefer today's approach, which relies on fee-for-service to insure better performance? Does a fee-for-service mechanism in solo practice provide assurance that patient interests come first? The answers are hardly in the affirmative. That problems will remain, even in a prepaid group practice setting, is clear. That such a setting offers greater potential for solution of problems should also be clear.

The prepaid group practice model in which there is a fixed sum of dollars and a defined population would affect physician distribution markedly. Physician distribution would take place in accordance with supply and demand conditions (but the demand conditions would be heavily influenced by needs and by the dollars made available through the national health insurance program). If group practices had little need for the services of additional neurosurgeons, medical students would (of course, with lags and slippages) adjust their plans accordingly. Income of neurosurgeons would tend to fall if an excess supply were competing for available opportunities, thus providing yet additional "signals" to prospective entrants into the field. A similar situation would prevail as regards geographic location decisions.

The prepaid group practice model yields an additional benefit: the creation of a unit of responsibility (larger than the single practitioner, smaller than a regional authority) to which the consumer can relate. We need such institutions, for the physician-patient relationship is not a relationship of equals. The patient may, and sometimes does, have complaints and dissatisfactions. Yet, he finds it most difficult to voice them to his physician. Nor does one change physicians easily. In the absence of an institutional responsibility, the patient must deal with the physician in a one-to-one relationship. This may be appropriate for medical affairs, but it is inappropriate for other matters. The prepaid group practice—with consumer involvement—provides a mechanism that permits someone to speak for the patient (and permits the patient to speak to someone other than the physician). The individual patient is not dealing with the individual physician.

The discussion of prepaid group practice could examine a number

51

of additional issues: hospital utilization, use of nonphysician personnel and so forth. Rather than extend the detail we have focused on what we consider the critical variables: the advantages of institutional responsibility with the potential that provides for institutional decision-making on allocation of resources within the institution and for consumer involvement in the delivery system; the constraints of a predetermined budget, and the potential advantages of such constraints on rational decision making; elimination of fee-for-service with the potential advantage of salary and capitation is changing the behavior of the physician and the allocation of physician manpower. Various of the advantages can be obtained under other arrangements, but it is not clear that other arrangements can permit all of the advantages to be obtained.[16]

SOME CONCLUDING THOUGHTS

We turn to the implications of a system of universal financing in conjunction with a delivery system in which physicians are paid on a salary or capitation basis.[17] In such systems the potential for an equitable distribution of health resources and services would be present. Departures from equity would depend in part on the degree to which a privately financed sector were permitted (or, if not permitted, to the degree that a black market might exist) and in part to the degree that the quality of services provided might vary with the attitudes of physicians to particular patients. These departures would be significantly less than is the case today, than would be the case with universal financing and a continuation of fee-for-service or with prepaid group practice and a continuation of private financing of medical care.

What would such a system cost? There is no specific answer. We recognize that the aggregate to be devoted to health can be determined in two ways. The two approaches are perhaps illustrated by the contrast between the United States and Britain. In the United States we are able to estimate *ex post* what we have spent (and then only with a considerable time lag). These estimates are derived, essentially, by adding up the expenditures as determined by the millions of decisions made by consumers, providers and other participants in the health care system. There is no decision making at the macro level; the macro is the sum of the micro. Even Phase II will not change this picture, for Phase II controls prices, and the total expenditures are determined by price and quantity.[18]

52

The British approach contrasts with that of the United States: aggregate expenditures are determined by government, and a host of microdecisions are made within the constraint that has been established. One could say that in the United States the real decisions are made by the actors in the health system drama and the Treasury must adjust to those decisions. In Britain the decisions are made by the Treasury, and it is the people in the health service drama who must adjust.

Under a national health insurance program, it would be possible to decide the level of resources that would be made available to the health sector in any particular year. This would be an important advantage. I do not suggest that discipline be exerted in quite the way that it is in Britain. Traditions in our health care sector are different. Furthermore, a national health insurance program rather than a national health service would permit of many more leakages and slippages and, very likely, a much larger role for private expenditures. Nonetheless, it would be possible to exert greater control than is the case at present in the determination of the allocation of resources to health in a given year. The determination of expenditures at central level for the given year is, however, not the only issue. We must also ask how the microdecisions adjust to the macro during the year and what pressures, therefore, build up to change the allocation to the health sector in subsequent years. Over the long run, government cannot make macrodecisions that must be translated into microdecisions that are unacceptable to providers or consumers. Similarly, providers and consumers cannot make microdecisions requiring an unacceptable macroresponse.

In a national program we will have to face these questions. Their solution will require changes in attitude and behavior and a restructuring of the total reward system (not simply economic rewards) in medicine. We will also have to develop ways to provide signals regarding consumer preferences within constraints that equity not be violated. How, for example, will consumers indicate their preferences for more resources in the health sector in the absence of supplementary private or local government expenditures? At present we have few answers to these kinds of questions for they are relatively new to us.

Perhaps the answers for America will ultimately lie in a more equal distribution of income between the various states and regions. Were that achieved (and it is achievable), less reliance would have to be placed on the transfer powers of the federal government *vis-à-vis* the health sector. Greater consumer participation and control of a variety

53

of institutions at local level would then permit diverse tastes and desires to send their signals to local and regional decision makers. We are far from that equality today and federal intervention is, therefore, called for.

These issues are not uniquely health issues. They are among the most important issues facing our society. Cast in different clothes, they are the old issues—as yet unresolved—of how much we are one nation and one people. They are yet another formulation of the question to what extent are we Americans, to what extent North Carolinians or Californians.

The health system can address some of these questions but the limits on its answers will be given by the total society. The sector can only change as part of a process of organic development. It is a part of our social order not apart from it. It is difficult to be optimistic about solutions to our health problems—but, perhaps, because it is difficult to be optimistic about America. Yet, because of the link between the two have we any real choice in our behavior? Optimistic or pessimistic, we have to continue to try to find the answers to our problems. To give up is to say we are certain we would not succeed in our search. Can any of us be that certain?

REFERENCES

[1] It is depressing to report, however, that analysts in various other applied fields seem to reach the same conclusions about their field; e.g., in the recent past the education economist has questioned the benefits of general increases in the resources devoted to education. Oftentimes this seems to be the case because of strong skepticism about the structure and effectiveness of particular government programs. Sometimes the absence of output measures seems to be at issue. An important research question is whether the disenchantment with increased resources in various fields tells us more about the field itself or more about those who are disenchanted. Perhaps analysts suffer from an overdose of skepticism ("if we can't document it, it isn't so"). Perhaps in their commendable zeal to be hardheaded, they have become hardhearted.

[2] It has proven impossible, for example, for government to withhold expensive procedures offering little (but some) likelihood of success under the Medicare program.

[3] In addition, it is unfortunately the case that benefit-cost ratios tend to emphasize the maximization of output rather than its distribution. Equity is sometimes neglected because it is difficult to quantify.

[4] In the absence of radically new financing mechanisms, income and price rationing is likely to become more, rather than less, important. Medical science and technology make possible diagnostic, curative and life-prolonging interventions that often turn out to be costly and that create an ever-increasing problem for significant parts of the population.

[5] This may strike some as a "straw-man" argument. I do not believe that to be the case. Quite often colleagues and students, not especially involved in the health area, place relatively little emphasis on a more equitable distribution of health services, not because they are less "decent" or "humane," but because they do not consider those services that important. They then wonder why there is all the pressure, say, for national health insurance.

[6] This line of reasoning was used in appealing to the children of the aged for support for the legislation. It was suggested that, in many cases, the financial impact of illness of their parents would fall upon them.

[7] But the income distribution problem is a simpler one because, once determined, the distribution is not affected by the "involuntary" consumption of the good or service itself, by untoward events; i.e., by the "lottery" effect.

[8] Some would argue that this is true only for "essential" services. Defining "essential" is difficult. We cannot ignore our earlier discussion on the importance of public attitudes.

[9] Stuart, B., Equity and Medicaid, *The Journal of Human Resources*, 7, 162–179, Spring, 1972.

[10] See two recent studies: Scitovsky, A. A. and Snyder N. M., Effect of Coinsurance on Use of Physician Services, and Phelps, C. E. and Newhouse, J. P., Effect of Coinsurance: A Multivariate Analysis, both in *Social Security Bulletin*, 35, June, 1972. The coinsurance provision was 25 per cent. This high rate did lead to a substantial decline in the demand for physician services.

[11] Some important insights into these matters are provided by Victor Fuchs in Eilers, R. D. and Moyerman, S. S., NATIONAL HEALTH INSURANCE CONFERENCE PROCEEDINGS, The Leonard Davis Institute of Health Economics, 1971, pp. 184–207.

[12] It is important to realize that a number of different factors help create the situation that makes the consumer relatively powerless: medical ethics, the white coat of the physician and so forth. The economic relations reflect other relations.

[13] This, of course, is not the only rationale for increasing the proportion of minority students in medical schools. At least two other rationales can be offered. One involves the educational impact on nonminority students; the other involves the attempt to overcome the legacy of discrimination.

[14] Such an approach may have benefits other than on the distribution side of the question. One should be clear what those benefits might be if one supports this mechanism.

[15] Although it is possible, within limits, to alter the specialty and geographic distribution of physicians even with retention of fee-for-service, by fixing the total number of dollars available to the health system (or to physicians) for the care of a given population, the preservation of fee-for-service means the preservation of fee-for-service incentives. Given that the consumer is not in a position to determine which particular service he needs, and in the presence of competition between physicians for scarce dollars, we could have continuing problems with, say, excess surgery. Furthermore, if fee-for-service is preserved,

we have little assurance that all members of the community would have equal access. If the community includes poor and nonpoor, the former are likely to suffer in the competition (because the physician can still maintain his income by increasing the quantity of services made available to the nonpoor). If we agree that any system of medical care will entail rationing, our aim ought to be to structure the system in such a way to increase the probabilities that the rationing of scarce resources will be in terms of medical need. The retention of a fee-for-service arrangement will not induce the needed changes in the medical ethos. It hardly impels the physician to consider the group as well as the individual patient.

16 A separate discussion is required for the special problems of rural areas. It should be clear, however, that there would be a potential for organization and linkages of rural practitioners to group practices and other institutions in the urban setting in the mechanisms we describe.

17 Prepaid group practice is the element that offers various protections to the consumer. In theory, solo practice with capitation or salary—with adequate monitoring and if the number of dollars available in an area were controlled to prevent misallocations—could yield results similar to group practice along a number of axes. We believe prepaid group practice has a number of additional advantages not discussed in this paper.

18 Indeed, even if Phase II is successful in combating inflation in prices it may work in a perverse fashion in controlling the increase in health expenditures. Price control can lead to higher utilization. Reductions in the unit cost of a day in hospital can be realized by an increase in occupancy rates, but this will increase total expenditures in the health care system. Part of the difficulty arises because of the confusion about prices and expenditures, which is reenforced by the fact that, in measuring price, we are often measuring the wrong variable. We measure the price (unit cost) of a service, not the price (total cost) of taking care of a particular condition.

THE CONTRIBUTION OF HEALTH SERVICES
TO THE AMERICAN ECONOMY

VICTOR R. FUCHS

INTRODUCTION

Good health is one of man's most precious assets. The desire to live, to be well, to maintain full command over one's faculties and to see one's loved ones free from disease, disability or premature death are among the most strongly rooted of all human desires. That is particularly true of Americans who, on the whole, eschew the fatalism or preoccupation with the hereafter that is characteristic of some other cultures.

These sentiments are widely held. Therefore, is not the question— what is "the contribution of health services to the United States economy?"—presumptuous? Who can place a value on a life saved, on a body spared from pain or on a mind restored to sanity? If not presumptuous, is not the question a foolish one, and likely to evoke an equally foolish answer?

When an economist enters an area such as health—so tinged with emotion, so enveloped in an esoteric technology and vocabulary—he runs a high risk of being either irrelevant or wrong. What, then, is the justification for such an inquiry? The principal one is the fact that the question of the contribution of health services is being asked and answered every day. It is being asked and answered implicitly every time consumers, hospitals, universities, business firms, foundations, government agencies and legislative bodies make decisions concerning the volume and composition of health services, present and future. If economists can help to rationalize and make more explicit

57

the decision-making process, can provide useful definitions, concepts and analytical tools, and can develop appropriate bodies of data and summary measures, they will be making their own contribution to health and to the economy.

Plan of the Paper

This paper has limited objectives. It does not pretend to offer a measure of the contribution of health services. Even partial completion of such a task would require a major effort by a research team over a period of several years. Statistics are presented, but for illustrative purposes only.

The primary purpose is to set out in nontechnical terms how the problem looks to an economist, to discuss definitions, concepts and methods of measurement, to indicate sources of information and to suggest promising research approaches. The paper offers a highly personal view of the problem rather than a synthesis of all points of view. Some discussion of relevant literature is included, but no attempt has been made to be exhaustive. Moreover, the paper is limited to the assigned topic and does not provide a general review of the health economics literature. An overall survey of the field, through 1964, is available in Klarman.[1] In addition, useful bibliographies may be found in Mushkin,[2] Wolf[3] and the proceedings of a 1962 conference on the economics of health and medical care.[4]

First this paper will consider the meaning of "contribution." Then it will go on to discuss the inputs to health services, the outputs of health services (with special emphasis on health) and the contribution of health to the economy. The paper concludes with a brief summary and suggestions for research.

THE CONCEPT OF CONTRIBUTION

One frequently reads discussions of the contribution of an industry couched in terms of the number of jobs the industry provides, the volume of capital investment of the industry, and the value of its purchases from suppliers. Such use of the term is ill-advised.

In economic terms the contribution of an industry to the economy should be measured in terms of its output (what does it provide for the economy?), not in terms of its input (what drains does it make on the available supply of resources?). The fundamental fact of economic life is that resources are scarce relative to human wants. Despite a great deal of loose talk about automation and cybernetics, the desires for goods and services in this country and the world exceed the available supplies. Indeed, if this were not the case, no reason could be found to study the economics of health or the economics of anything else. Additional resources would be devoted to health up to the point where no health want would be unmet. That this cannot be done at present is obvious. The reason should be equally obvious. To devote more resources to health services, the people must be willing to forego some other good or service. To the extent of the unused capacity in the economy, some increase could be obtained without diversion from other ends. The extent of this unused capacity, however, relative to the total economy, is very small at the present time.

What is the output of the health industry? No completely satisfactory answer is available. One possible way to think about the problem is to distinguish three different kinds of output that flow from health services. They are health, validation services and other consumer services.

Probably the most important of these, and certainly the one that has received the most attention, is the contribution of health services to health. However, to define the output of the health industry in terms of some ultimate utility, such as health rather than health services, runs counter to the general practice followed by economists in the study of other industries. For the most part, economists follow the dictum, "whatever Lola gets, Lola wants." They assume that consumers know what they want and know how to satisfy these wants. They further assume that goods and services produced under competitive conditions will be sold at a price which properly reflects (at the margin) the cost of production and the value to the consumer. The health industry, however, has certain characteristics, discussed by Arrow,[5] Klarman[6] and Mushkin,[7] which suggest that special treatment is required. In the present context, three important differences could be emphasized between the health industry and the "typical" or "average" industry.

Consumer ignorance. Although expenditures for health services account for more than six per cent of all personal consumption expenditures, consumers are, for the most part, terribly ignorant about what they are buying. Very few industries could be named where the consumer is so dependent upon the producer for information concerning the quality of the product. In the typical case he is even subject to the producer's recommendation concerning the quantity to be purchased. A recent report by the American Medical Association says flatly, "The 'quantity' of the hospital services consumed in 1962 was determined by physicians."[8]

The question is even more complicated, as indicated in the following statement by J. Douglas Colman, president of the New York Blue Cross:[9]

> We must remember that most elements of hospital and medical care costs are generated by or based on professional medical judgment. These judgments include the decision to admit and discharge patients, the decision to order the various diagnostic or therapeutic procedures for patients, and the larger decision as to the types of facilities and services needed by an institution for proper patient care. For the most part, these professional judgments are rendered outside of any organizational structure that fixes accountability for the economic consequences of these judgments.

One reason for consumer ignorance is the inherent uncertainty of the effect of the service on any individual. How can the lay person be expected to know the value of a particular procedure or treatment, when in many cases the medical profession itself is far from agreed? Also, many medical services are infrequently purchased. The average consumer will buy many more automobiles during a lifetime than he will major operations. Therefore, he cannot develop the necessary expertise. Furthermore, the consumer is often not in a good position to make a cool, rational judgment at the time of purchase because he is ill, or because a close member of his family is ill. Finally, the profession does little to inform the consumer; in fact, it frequently takes positive action to keep him uninformed. This leads to the second important difference.

Restrictions on competition. In some other industries where the possibilities for consumer ignorance are considerable, the consumer obtains protection through the competitive behavior of producers. If the producers are engaged in vigorous competition with one another, some of them, at least, will go out of their way to inform the consumer about the merits of their product and those of the competition. Also, middlemen, such as retailers, are usually involved, one of whose main functions is to provide information and dispel consumer ignorance. In the case of physicians' services (and this is the keystone to health services because of the dominant role of the physician in the industry) the reverse is true. In the first place, severe restrictions on entry are assured through the medical profession's control of medical schools, licensing requirements and hospital appointments. Advertising is forbidden and price competition is severely frowned upon. Critical comment concerning the output of other physicians is also regarded as unethical.

A good example of the conflict and confusion on this point can be found in the report previously cited. An extensive discussion of medical care in America is presented, and an attempt is made to identify it with the competitive free enterprise system. The report then goes on to say, "The Medical Care Industry has as its prime social goal the development and maintenance of optimum health levels."[10] The authors apparently fail to realize the inconsistency of this statement with their attempt to place the industry in the context of a market system. In such a system, industries do not have "social goals." The goal of the individual firm is maximum profit (or minimum loss); the achievement of social goals is a by-product of the profit-seeking activities of individual firms and industries.

Numerous arguments can be advanced in support of each of the restrictive practices followed by the medical profession. (Arrow's discussion of the role of uncertainty in health is particularly relevant.[5]) In the present context, these restrictive practices mean that an appraisal of the industry's ouput and performance by economists cannot be pursued using the same assumptions that would be appropriate in appraising the output of a more competitive industry.

The role of "need." Health services are one of a small group of services which many people believe should be distributed according to need rather than demand (i.e., willingness and ability to pay.) Other services in this category, such as education, police and fire protection, and sanitation are typically provided by government. For a time philanthropy and the generosity of physicians were relied upon to achieve this distribution for health services, but now increasing reliance is being placed on taxation or coverage in compulsory insurance schemes. If "need" is to be criterion, however, a closer examination of the role of health services in filling that need seems in order.

If a person "demands" an article of clothing or a haircut or some other good or service, in the sense of being willing and able to pay for it, usually no special cause for concern or inquiry arises on the part of anyone else regarding either the need underlying the demand or whether the purchase will satisfy the need. However, if a service, such as health, is to be provided to others on the basis of "need," then those paying for it would seem to have some right to inquire into the actual presence of "need," and an obligation to determine whether or how much the service actually satisfies the need. Because need is often the criterion for obtaining health services, much of the payment for these services is by a "third party." This means that the consumer

61

has less incentive to make certain that the output (what he is getting) is truly worth the cost.

These characteristics of the health industry indicate why output cannot simply be equated with expenditures. However, that does not mean that economic analysis cannot be applied to this industry. On the contrary, precisely these special characteristics make the industry an interesting subject for economic analysis, both from the scientific and public policy points of view.

Total versus Marginal Contribution

In studying the contribution of health services to health the *total* contribution must be distinguished from the *marginal* contribution. The total contribution can be appraised by asking what would happen if no health services at all were available. The results would almost surely be disastrous in terms of health and life expectancy. A reasonably safe conclusion seems to be that the total contribution is enormous. A modern economy could not continue to function without some health services.

The marginal contribution, on the other hand, refers to the effects on health of a small increase or decrease in the amount of health services provided. To expect a small change in services to have a large effect on the level of health is, of course, out of the question. But that is not what is being measured. Rather, the question is, what is the relative effect on health of a small relative change in health services?

The reason this question is crucial is that changes are usually being made at the margin. Most decisions are not of the "all or nothing" variety, but involve "a little more or a little less." The goal of an economic system, in terms of maximum satisfaction, is to allocate resources in such a way that the last (marginal) inputs of resources used for each purpose make contributions that are proportionate to their costs.

HEALTH SERVICES

"Health services" can be defined as services rendered by:

1. Labor: personnel engaged in medical occupations, such as doctors, dentists and nurses, plus other personnel working directly under their supervision, such as practical nurses, orderlies and receptionists.

2. Physical capital: the plant and equipment used by this personnel, e.g., hospitals, x-ray machines.

3. Intermediate goods and services: i.e., drugs, bandages, purchased laundry services.

This definition corresponds roughly to what economists have in mind when they refer to the "health industry." Payment for this labor, capital and intermediate input is the basis for estimating "health expenditures."

This definition seems satisfactory for the purposes of this paper, but some classification problems are worth mentioning. First, some health-related resources might or might not be included in health services, such as the provision of a supply of sanitary water. A second problem arises because a portion of the personnel and facilities in hospitals is used to produce "hotel services" rather than health. This paper will not exclude such inputs from health services, but will try to allow for them by showing that part of the output consists of other consumer services (see Figure 1).

One of the greatest problems concerns the unpaid health services that people perform for themselves and for members of their families. According to present practice in national income accounting, this labor input is not included in health services. Therefore, this "home" production must be treated as part of the environmental factors that affect health.

Approximately two-thirds of the value of health services in the United States represents labor input. Somewhat less than one-sixth represents input of physical capital and the remainder represents goods and services purchased from other industries. These are all rough estimates. Information about the volume and composition of health services must be derived from a variety of official and unofficial sources. No census of the health industry compares to the census of manufacturing, trade or selected services. As the importance of the health industry grows, the government may wish to reconsider whether a periodic census of health should be undertaken.

Present sources of information are of two main types: those that give information about expenditures for health services, and those that report on one or more aspects of inputs of resources. A good example of the former is the material supplied by Reed and Rice.[11] A few problems arise when these data are used to measure inputs of health services. First, some of the items represent investment expenditures by the health industry rather than payment for current services. Expenditures for construction and medical research are the most important ones in this category. No particular economic justification may be found for treating these as inputs in the year that the investment takes place. On the other hand, current input of capital may be understated to the extent that hospital charges do not include an allowance for depreciation and interest.

The expenditures shown for drugs, eyeglasses, etc., do not all represent payment for intermediate goods purchased from other industries. A substantial portion (probably about one-half) represents the labor services of pharmacists, opticians and the like and the services of the plant and equipment used by this personnel.

The net cost of health insurance represents output of the insurance industry. It may be thought of as an intermediate service purchased and resold by the health industry.

A final point concerns the failure of expenditures data to reflect contributed labor. This results in an underestimate of labor input, especially in hospitals.

Other sources of information on expenditures for health services include: the Office of Business Economics,[12-14] detailed annual data on personal consumption expenditures for health service; the Social Security Administration,[15] special emphasis on government spending for health services; the Public Health Service,[16,17] expenditures cross-classified with characteristics of the individual incurring the expense; the Health Information Foundation,[18] and Bureau of Labor Statistics.[19,20]

The decennial population census[21] is an excellent source of information about labor inputs to health services. In addition to providing a complete enumeration of the number employed and their geographical location, numerous economic and demographic characteristics are described in considerable detail. With the aid of the 1/1000 sample of the 1960 census,[22] comparisons may be made within the health industry and between health and other industries on such matters as education, earnings, age, sex, race and hours of work. The labor input to health services may be defined as all persons employed in the health and hospital industry, plus those persons in medical occupations employed in other industries. Health employment, so defined, amounted to almost three million in 1960. This represented almost five per cent of total employment.

Another good source of data on labor input is provided by the Public Health Service.[23] This source is particularly useful for those interested

64

in such characteristics as physicians' type of practice, specialization, medical school and location of practice.

Information on capital inputs to health services is more difficult to obtain. The annual guide book issue of *Hospitals* reports the book value of hospital plant and equipment.[24] This was given as 21.3 billion dollars in 1963. This figure is biased downward as a measure of present value, because of the rise in prices of construction in recent decades. It is biased upward to the extent that hospitals have failed to make deductions for depreciation. This same source also provides useful data on labor input by type and size of hospital.

Some information on the capital inputs associated with the labor input of physicians can be gleaned from the reports of the United States Internal Revenue Service.[25] According to these reports, 163,000 returns were filed for unincorporated businesses under the heading of "physicians, surgeons, and oculists" in 1962. These returns showed business receipts of six billion dollars. They showed net rent paid of 250 million dollars (most of this represents payment for capital services) as well as depreciation charges of 190 million dollars. Some information for other types of health services, such as those provided by dentists and dental surgeons, is also available from the same source.

One important source of information about inputs of equipment and intermediate goods that has not received much attention is the quinquennial CENSUS OF MANUFACTURER.[26] The latest one (1963) provides considerable data on shipments by manufacturers of drugs, ophthalmic goods, dental equipment and supplies, ambulances, hospital beds and many other health items.

Real versus Money Costs

One problem in measuring inputs that has already been alluded to in connection with volunteer labor is the need to distinguish between "real" and "money" costs. The person who is not an economist usually thinks of the cost of health services in money terms; when more money has to be spent, costs are said to be rising. This approach is readily understandable and for some purposes useful and proper. The analysis of many problems, however, requires a stripping away of the money veil and an examination of "real" costs. The real cost to society of providing health services, or any other good or service, consists of the labor and capital used in the industry, plus the cost of producing the intermediate goods and services. For instance, if the workers employed in a given hospital are unionized, and they negotiate a large increase in wages, the money costs of that hospital clearly rise, other factors remaining unchanged. But the real cost of that hospital service has not changed at all.

In a perfectly competitive market economy, money costs usually provide a good measure of real costs. But in the health industry, with its curious mixture of philanthropy, government subsidies, imperfect labor markets and contributed labor time, concentration on money costs alone may frequently be misleading. Good decisions about the allocation of resources require information about the real costs involved.

One important element of real cost is often overlooked, namely, the time of the patient. When the patient is ill, the value of this time (measured by alternative opportunities) may be very low. But, in calculating the costs of periodic medical examinations and routine visits, omitting this cost would be a mistake.[27]

HEALTH

Any attempt to analyze the relationship between health services and health runs headlong into two very difficult problems. The first concerns the definition and measurement of levels of health, or at least changes in levels. The second involves an attempt to estimate what portion of changes in health can be attributed to health services, as distinct from the genetic and environmental factors that also affect health. This section discusses the question of definition and measurement of levels of health.

What is Health?

Definitions of health abound. Agreement is hard to find. The oft-quoted statement of the World Health Organization[28] is framed in positive (some would say Utopian) terms—"A state of complete physical and mental and social well-being." Others, e.g., Ffrangcon Roberts,[29] simply stress the absence of, or the ability to resist, disease and death.

A few points seem clear. First, health has many dimensions—anatomical, physiological, mental, and so on. Second, the relative importance of different disabilities varies considerably, depending upon the particular culture and the role of the particular individual in that culture. Third, most attempts at measurement take the negative approach. That is, they make inferences about health by measuring

66

the degree of ill health, as indicated by mortality, morbidity, disability, etc. Finally, with respect to health, as in so many other cases, detecting changes in health is easier than defining or measuring absolute levels.

Indexes of Health

The most widely used indicators of health levels are those based on mortality rates, either age-specific or age-adjusted. The great virtues of death rates are that they are determined objectively, are readily available in considerable detail for most countries, and are reasonably comparable for intertemporal and interspatial comparisons.

Health experts rely heavily on mortality comparisons for making judgments about the relative health levels of whites and nonwhites in the United States, or of smokers versus nonsmokers, and for other problems. A recent survey of health in Israel, for example, concluded:[30]

> The success of the whole system of medicine in Israel is best judged, not by an individual inspection of buildings or asking the opinions of doctors and patients, but by an examination of the health statistics of the country. Infant mortality is about the same as in many European countries, and life expectancy is equal to, or better than, most.

The tendency in recent years has been to dismiss mortality as a useful indicator of health levels in developed countries because very little intranational or international variation occurs. These reports of the demise of mortality indexes are premature.

Differences within the United States are still considerable. The most important differential is race, but even considering rates for whites only, the age-adjusted death rate (average 1959–61) in the highest state is 33 per cent greater than in the lowest; the highest infant mortality rate is 55 per cent above the lowest; and the death rate for males 45–54 in the worst state is 60 per cent higher than in the state with the lowest rate.

Comparing the United States with other developed countries, the differences are even more striking, as shown in Table 1. For males 45–54, (a critical age group from the point of view of production), the United States has the highest rate of any country in the Organization for Economic Cooperation and Development (OECD), and has a rate which is almost double that of some of the other countries. Such gross differences surely present a sufficient challenge for scientific analysis and for public policy.

Another argument that seems to underly the objections to mortality

67

TABLE I. DEATH RATES IN OECD COUNTRIES RELATIVE TO THE UNITED STATES, AVERAGE 1959–61

Country	Age-Adjusted Death Rate*	Infant Mortality	Mortality Males 45–54	Mortality Females 45–54
United States	100	100	100	100
White	96	88	94	87
Nonwhite	138	164	155	220
Iceland	78	62**	62	81
Netherlands	82	63	57	65
Norway	82	74**	54	58
Sweden	86	63	52	69
Greece	86	155	56	64
Denmark	90	85**	59	78
Canada	92	107	76	79
Switzerland	94	83	67	75
France	96	105	89	83
Italy	98	166	74	77
Belgium	102	113	82	79
United Kingdom	103	87	76	85
Spain	104†	178	75†	84†
West Germany (excluding Berlin)	107	129	77	84
Luxembourg	107	122	96	89
Ireland	109	118	74	105
Austria	110	142	87	87
Japan	115	127**	83	102
Portugal	131	328	84	84

* Age-adjustment is by the "indirect" method. For each country, United States age-specific death rates were applied to the actual population distribution and the result was divided into the actual number of deaths to obtain the mortality ratio, i.e., the age-adjusted death rate in index number form.

† 1957–59 average.

** 1958–60 average.

Sources: Age-Adjusted Death Rate, Mortality Males 45–54 and Mortality Females 45–54: United States Deaths: United States Public Health Service, VITAL STATISTICS OF THE UNITED STATES, 1959, 1960, 1961. United States Population: United States Bureau of the Census, 1960 CENSUS OF POPULATION, Volume I, Characteristics of the Population, Part 1, United States Summary. OECD Countries: Population and Deaths: World Health Organization, ANNUAL EPIDEMIOLOGICAL AND VITAL STATISTICS, 1959, 1960, 1961. Data for Luxembourg from United Nations, DEMOGRAPHIC YEARBOOK, 1960, 1961.
Infant Mortality Rate: United Nations, DEMOGRAPHIC YEARBOOK, 1961, Table 17.

indexes is that age-adjusted death rates (and average life expectancy) have been relatively stable in the United States for the past decade. The real costs of health services have increased over this period, and medical science has certainly made some progress; therefore, one may assume that some improvement in health levels occurred that was not captured by the mortality indexes.

This type of reasoning begs the question. Possibly the increase in health services has not resulted in improved health levels and the scientific advances of recent years have not had much effect on health. An alternative explanation is that changes in environmental factors in these years have had, on balance, a negative effect on health, thus offsetting the favorable effects of increases in services and medical knowledge. The latter explanation seems to be a very real possibility. Health services do not operate in a vacuum, nor can they be regarded as being matched against a "health destroying nature" that remains constant over time. An apt aphorism attributed to Sigerist states that "Each civilization makes its own diseases."[31]

Most of the suggestions for new and better indexes of health involve combining morbidity and mortality information. An excellent discussion of some of the problems to be encountered, and possible solutions, may be found in Sullivan.[32] One particularly intriguing approach, suggested by Sanders,[33] consists of calculating years of "effective" life expectancy, based on mortality and morbidity rates. Such an index would measure the number of years that a person could expect to live and be well enough to fulfill the role appropriate to his sex and age. This approach could be modified to take account of the fact that illness or disability is a matter of degree. The years deducted from life expectancy because of disability should be adjusted by some percentage factor that represents the degree of disability. The determination of these percentage weights is one of the most challenging research problems to be faced in calculating a health index.

HEALTH SERVICES AND HEALTH

Writing this section would be more appropriate for a physician than for an economist since the relation between health services and health is a technical question best answered by those whose training is in that technology. All that is intended here is to record some impressions of an outsider who has reviewed a minute portion of the literature from a particular point of view.

The impact of health services on health depends upon two factors: 1. How effective are the best known techniques of diagnosis, therapy, etc.? 2. How wide is the gap between the best known techniques ("treatment of choice") and those actually used across the country? The latter question has been reviewed extensively in medical literature under the heading "quality of care";[34] it will not be discussed here. A useful introduction to the first question is provided in Terris.[35]

The belief that an important relationship exists between health services and health is of long standing. Reliable evidence to support this belief is of much more recent origin. For thousands of years sick people sought advice and treatment of physicians and surgeons, but many of the most popular remedies and courses of treatment of earlier centuries are now known to have been either harmful or irrelevant.

If this be true, how can one explain the demand for health services that existed in the past? Two possible explanations seem worth noting; they may even continue to have some relevance today. First, doctors probably received a great deal of credit that properly belonged to nature. The body itself has great healing powers, and most people who successfully consulted physicians would have recovered from or adjusted to their illness without medical intervention. Second, and probably more important, is the intensive need "to do something" that most people have when faced with pain and the possibility of death.

In more recent times, the value of health services for certain illnesses has been established with considerable certainty; but broad areas of doubt and controversy still remain. The following discussion considers a few examples of each type.

Infectious disease is an area where medical services are demonstrably effective. Although the decline of some infectious diseases (e.g., tuberculosis) should be credited in part to environmental changes such as improved sanitation, the important role played by improvements in medical science cannot be downgraded. For many infectious diseases the health service is preventive rather than curative and "one-shot" rather than continuous. Such preventive services do not occupy a large portion of total physician time, but the results should nevertheless be included in the output of the health industry.

Examples of the control of infectious disease through immunization are: diphtheria,[36] tetanus[37, 38] and poliomyelitis;[39] chemotherapy is effective in tuberculosis[40] and pneumonia.[41] The decline in mortality from these causes has been dramatic and some correlation can be observed between changes in the rate of decline and the adoption of specific medical advances. For example, during the 15-year period, 1935 to 1950, which spanned the introduction and wide use of sulfonamides and penicillin, the United States death rate from influenza and pneumonia fell at a rate of more than eight per cent per annum; the rate of decline was two per cent per annum from 1900 to 1935. In the case of tuberculosis, considerable progress was made throughout this century, but the relative rate of decline in the death rate accelerated appreciably after the adoption of penicillin, streptomycin and PAS (para-aminosalicylic acid) in the late 1940's, and of isoniazid in the early 1950's.

70

Even more dramatic examples are the death rate patterns of syphilis and poliomyelitis, where the introduction of new forms of treatment for the former and immunization for the latter were reflected very quickly in precipitous drops in mortality. To be sure, the diseases mentioned have not been eliminated. Partly for sociocultural reasons, the incidence of syphilis has actually increased in recent years. In other cases, modern treatments of choice are losing their effectiveness because of the development of resistant strains of microorganisms.

The situation with respect to the noninfectious diseases is more mixed. Some examples of demonstrable effectiveness are the following: replacement therapy has lessened the impact of diabetes,[42] dental caries in children are reduced by fluoridation[43] and medical care has become increasingly successful in treating trauma.[45] The diagnostic value of the Papanicolaou test for cervical cancer is established[46, 47] and the incidence of invasive cancer of this site has been reduced in the 1960's, presumably due to medical treatment during the pre-invasive stage disclosed by the test. Also effective is the treatment of skin cancer.[48]

Less heartening are the reports on other cancer sites. The five-year survival rate for breast cancer (the most common single organ site of malignancy in either sex) is typically about 50 per cent. Moreover, a review of the breast cancer literature found such striking uniformity of results, despite widely differing therapeutic techniques, that the author was prompted to speculate whether such end results record therapeutic triumphs or merely the natural history of the disease.[49] Some writers stress the importance of prompt treatment for cancer; others question whether elimination of delay would dramatically alter survival rates. The problem of delay itself is complex, and not simply attributable to ignorance or lack of access to health services: "Physicians with cancer are just as likely to delay as are laymen."[50]

Heart disease is another major cause of death where the contribution of health services to health leaves much to be desired. Despite the contributions of surgery in correcting congenital and rheumatic cardiac defects[51] and the decline in recurrence rates of rheumatic fever,[52] apparently no curative treatment has been found for rhematic fever.[53, 54] The treatment of coronary heart disease is only partially effective.[55] The value of antihypertensive drugs in preventing early death in case of malignant hypertension seems assured, but these drugs may be harmful in nonmalignant hypertension.[56] The value of

71

anticoagulants in reducing complications and mortality with acute myocardial infarction has been questioned by recent reports.[57, 58]

Definitive therapy is still not available for widespread afflictions such as cerebral vascular disease[59] and rehabilitation results indicate that only the more severely ill may benefit from formal therapy (the others seem to recover spontaneously).[60] No cure is known for schizophrenia. The tranquilizing drugs and shock therapy have had a significant impact in shortening hospital stay, yet they do not seem to lower rehospitalization rates below those achieved with other methods.[61]

Health services have always been assumed to be very valuable in connection with pregnancy, but a recent study of prenatal care reveals little relation to prevention of pregnancy complications or prevention of early pregnancy termination, except in uncomplicated pregnancies of 30 weeks' gestation and over.[62] The latter cases do not clarify whether the medical care component of prenatal care, as distinct from nutritional and other components, is due the credit.

Innovations in health services are not limited to improvements in drugs, surgical techniques or other technological changes. Research concerning the effects on health of group practice,[63, 64] intensive care units[65, 66] and special arrangements for neonatal surgery,[67] has yielded encouraging results with respect to these organizational innovations. In other cases, results have been disappointing, e.g., multiple screening,[68] periodic medical examination of school children[69] and cancer control programs differing in duration, intensity and cost.[70]

This very brief review indicates that no simple generalization is possible about the effect of health services on health. Although many health services definitely improve health, in other cases even the best known techniques may have no effect. This problem of relating input to output is one of the most difficult ones facing economists who try to do research on the health industry. They must gain the support and advice of doctors and public health specialists if they are to make progress in this area.

Environmental Factors and Health

One of the factors contributing to the difficulty in reaching firm conclusions about the relationship between health services and health is the importance of environmental factors. Some environmental changes are biological, involving the appearance and disappearance of bacteria, viruses and other sources of disease. Many environmental variables are related to economics in one way or another. Some are tied to the production process, e.g., the factors associated with occupation. Others are part of consumption, e.g., diet, recreation. Major attention has frequently been given to income, partly because many other environmental factors tend to be highly correlated with real income, both over time and cross-sectionally. Examples include housing, education, urbanization, drinking and the use of automobiles.

The prevailing assumption, in some cases with good evidence, has indicated that an increase in real per capita income has favorable implications for health, apart from the fact that it permits an increase in health services. This assumption for the United States at present, except for infant mortality, may reasonably be questioned. This country may have passed the peak with respect to the favorable impact of a rising level of living on health. This is not to say that some favorable elements are not still associated with a higher income, but the many unfavorable ones may outweigh them.

After a period of neglect of environmental factors by medical researchers, the tendency in recent years has been to overemphasize the favorable aspects of rising income levels. For example, the American Medical Association recently stated, "Medical science does not seek major credit for the improvements in the health levels during the past 25 years. Certainly, our standards of living and higher educational levels have contributed substantially to the betterment of the health level in the United States."[71] Although modesty is becoming, the Association provides no evidence to support this statement, and the chances are good that it is wrong.

Altenderfer[72] was able to show some slight negative association between age-adjusted death rates and income across cities in the United States in 1940, but the adjustment for the effect of color was crude, and no allowance was made for the correlation between health services and income. The question at issue here is the relation between income and health, not of the fact that higher income permits a higher rate of utilization of health services.

Some preliminary work suggests that education is indeed favorable to health, but by far the largest share of the credit for improvement in health levels over the past 25 years probably should go to what economists call improvements in technology—better drugs, better medical knowledge, better diagnostic techniques, etc. Cross-sectional regressions across states, for instance, reveal a positive relation between income and mortality for whites, except in the case of infant mortality.

Death rate patterns in countries where the level of income is far below that of the United States, should also cause one to question the level of living argument. In Table 2, death rates for five European countries in 1960 are compared with rates for the United States in 1960 and 1925. The latter date was included because, in 1960, these five countries were at a level of real per capita income roughly comparable to that of the United States in 1925.[73]

The table shows that the over-all age-adjusted death rates for the European countries are very similar to those for the United States, and far below the level of the United States in 1925. The European crude rates tend to be higher because of the larger proportion of older people in Europe. Despite this bias, the crude rates for tuberculosis and influenza and pneumonia (two causes where the rise in income levels has been alleged to be particularly important) are

TABLE 2. COMPARISON OF DEATH RATES OF UNITED STATES IN 1925 AND 1960 WITH EUROPEAN COUNTRIES 1960

	Age-Adjusted Death Rate All Causes*	Crude Death Rate All Causes	Crude Death Rate Tuberculosis (all forms)	Crude Death Rate Influenza and Pneumonia†
1925				
United States	1683.3	1170.0	84.8	121.7
1960				
United States	945.7	945.7	5.9	32.9
England and Wales	926.8	1150.2	7.5	70.1
France	926.8	1136.2	22.1	48.1
West Germany (excluding Berlin)	983.5	1136.8	16.2	43.8
Netherlands	766.0	762.1	2.8	26.6
Belgium	1002.4	1244.7	17.1	36.5

* Age-adjustment is by the "indirect" method. For each country the United States age-specific death rates in 1960 were applied to the actual population distribution and the result was divided into the actual number of deaths to obtain the age-adjusted death rate index. This was multiplied by the United States crude death rate in 1960, to obtain the age-adjusted death rate.

† 1959–61 average used instead of 1960 rates because of influenza epidemic in 1960.

Sources: United States in 1925: United States Bureau of the Census, HISTORICAL STATISTICS OF THE UNITED STATES series B114–128, B129–142, A22–33. European countries 1960 population distribution, influenza and pneumonia deaths 1959–61, total populations 1959–61, and total deaths 1960 in West Germany and Belgium: World Health Organization, ANNUAL EPIDEMIOLOGICAL AND VITAL STATISTICS, 1959, 1960, 1961, Table 4. Other crude death rates in 1960: United Nations, DEMOGRAPHIC YEARBOOK, 1961, Table 17. United States age-specific death rates in 1960: United States Department of Health, Education and Welfare, Public Health Service, National Vital Statistics Division, VITAL STATISTICS OF THE UNITED STATES, 1960, Vol. II, Part A, Table 1-C.

also much closer to the United States in 1960, than to the United States in 1925. One explanation worth investigating is that the European countries enjoy a medical technology that is similar to that of the United States in 1960, and that changes in medical technology have been the principal cause of the decrease in the United States death rate from 1925 to 1960.

One possible reason for the effect of income levels on health having been overestimated is that investigators often find a very high correlation between income and the health status of individuals. The tendency has been to assume that the latter was the result of the former, but some recent studies of schizophrenia[74] and bronchitis[75] suggest that the causal relationship may run the other way. Evidence shows that illness causes a deterioration in occupational status (from a skilled job to an unskilled job and from an unskilled job into unemployment.) The evidence relates to the decline in occupational status from father to son (where the latter is a victim of the disease) and also within the patient's own history.

Even though research on the relation between health services and health would seem to be primarily the responsibility of those with training in medicine and public health, the long experience that economists have had with the environmental variables, such as income, education and urbanization, suggests that a multidisciplinary approach would be most fruitful.

OTHER CONTRIBUTIONS OF HEALTH SERVICES

The effect of health services on health probably represents their most important contribution. However, two other types of output are worth noting—validation services and other consumer services.

Validation Services

One type of output that is not directly related to improvements in health can be traced to the fact that only a physician can provide judgments concerning a person's health status that will be widely accepted by third parties. This type of output is designated "validation services" in Figure 1. One familiar example is the life insurance examination. This examination may have some favorable impact on the health of the examinee, but it need not do so and is not undertaken primarily for that purpose. The insurance company simply wants to know about the health status of the person concerned. In

75

FIGURE I. SCHEMATIC OUTLINE OF THE PAPER.

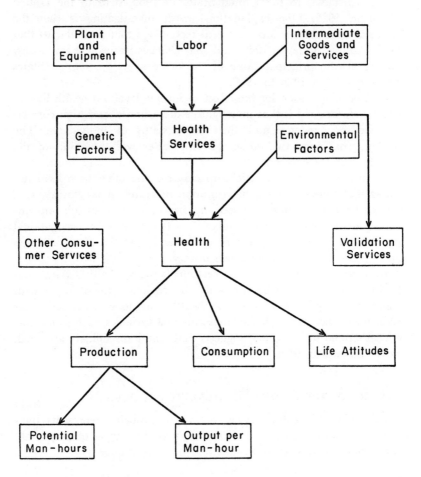

obtaining and providing that information, the physician is producing something of value, but it is not health.

Other examples include a physician's testifying in court, providing information in a workmen's compensation case, or executing a death certificate.

The validation role of physicians is probably much broader than in these sharply defined cases. Consider the following situation: a

76

person feels ill; he has various aches, pains and other symptoms. He complains and looks for sympathy from family, friends, neighbors and co-workers. He may seek to be relieved from certain responsibilities or to be excused from certain tasks. Doubts may arise in the minds of persons around him. Questions may be asked. Is he really ill? Is he doing all that he can to get well? A visit, or a series of visits, to one or more doctors is indicated. The patient may not have the slightest hope that these visits will help his health, and, indeed, he may be correct. Nevertheless, the service rendered by the physician cannot be said to result in no output. The visit to the doctor is a socially or culturally necessary act. The examination, the diagnosis and the prognosis are desired by the patient to provide confirmation to those who have doubts about him. Only the professional judgment of a physician can still the doubts and answer the questions.

The validation service type of output should not be confused with another type of problem that arises in measuring the output of health services; namely, that advance knowledge about the effect of health services on health is sometimes difficult to obtain. This problem is similar to the "dry hole" situation in drilling for oil. That is not to say that the work done in drilling dry holes results in no output. Rather, when the drilling operation is viewed in its entirety, some successes will be noted as well as some failures. All those who participate in the drilling operation are considered to be sources of the output. Similarly, if a surgeon operates on ten people and only six are helped, one should not say that no output occurred in the other four cases, if one could not determine in advance which cases could be helped and which could not. The output consisted of improving the health of six people, but this output was the result of a production process which encompassed the ten operations.

Other Consumer Services

The outstanding example of other consumer services produced by the health industry is the so-called "hotel" services of hospitals. Those hospital activities that directly affect health are difficult to separate from those that are equivalent to hotel services, but the latter clearly are not insignificant. One way of getting some insight into this question would be to study the occupational distribution of health industry employment. A very significant fraction consists of cooks, chambermaids, porters and others who are probably producing "other consumer services."[11]

77

In mental hospitals and other hospitals providing long-term care a major proportion of all costs are probably associated with producing consumer services other than health. The fact that these other consumer services would have to be provided somehow, either publicly or privately, if the patients were not in the hospital, is often neglected in discussions of how total hospital costs are inflated by the presence of people who are not really ill. Possibly some of these consumer services are actually produced more inexpensively in a hospital than on the outside. This point comes to the fore in New York City, now grappling with the problem of housing and feeding patients who have been discharged from mental hospitals, not because they are cured, but because the new drugs mean they no longer need to be confined to an institution.

Some of the services rendered by nurses outside hospitals also bear little relation to health, but nevertheless they may have considerable value to consumers. This type of service is likely to grow in importance with the increase in the number of elderly people with income who are seeking companionship and help with their daily chores.

The failure of mortality indexes to decline with increased expenditures for health services in recent years has led some people to conclude that mortality no longer measures health levels properly. But if most of these increased expenditures have gone for health services that largely produce "other consumer services" rather than health, a great deal of the mystery is removed.

HEALTH AND THE ECONOMY

An increase in health has two potential values for individuals—consumption and production. Good health is clearly something consumers desire for itself. (That they do not put an overriding value on health is also abundantly clear from the figures on smoking, drinking, overeating, fast driving, etc.) To the extent that health services lead to better health, they make a contribution to the economy comparable to that of any industry producing a good or service wanted by consumers.

In addition, better health may contribute to the productive capacity of the economy. It may do this, first, by increasing the supply of potential man-hours through a reduction in mortality and decrease in time lost because of illness and disability. Second, better health may in-

78

crease production by improving productivity, that is, increasing output per man-hour.

Beyond its potential direct contribution to production and consumption, better health probably has important indirect effects on the economy. These indirect effects occur through the changes in life attitudes which may accompany changes in health. When the average life expectancy in a country is only 30 or 35 years, attitudes toward work and saving, for instance, may be different from those in countries where life expectancy is 50 or 75 years. When infant mortality rates are very high, attitudes toward birth control are likely to be different from those in countries where mortality rates are low. Indeed, the idea of progress itself may be intimately bound up with the health levels of the population and the rate of change of these levels.

Health and Production

A substantial literature is now available which attempts to measure the impact of changes of health levels on the productive capacity of the economy.[76] The principal approach is to ask how many more people are available for work as a result of a decrease in death rates, and what potential or actual production can be attributed to this in-increased supply of manpower. The capitalized value of the increase at a given point in time can be obtained by summing the value of future potential production represented by the lives saved. Current earnings patterns are usually used with or without adjustment for future increases in earnings per man, and with future earnings discounted at some appropriate interest rate.

The details of calculating the value of lives saved vary greatly from one investigator to another, but one result is common to all: the value of a man (in terms of future production potential) is very different at different ages. Table 3 shows some calculated values for United States males at three different discount rates based on average patterns of earnings and labor force participation rates in 1960.

The principal implication of the age-value profile is that the economic return (in production terms) from saving a life is not the same at all ages. Different kinds of health programs and different kinds of medical research are likely to affect various age groups differently; therefore, wise planning should give some consideration to these matters. For example, accidents accounted for only 6.6 per cent of all male deaths in the United States in 1960, but accounted for 12.8 per cent

TABLE 3. AGE-VALUE PROFILE OF UNITED STATES MALES IN 1960
ESTIMATED FROM DISCOUNTED FUTURE EARNINGS

	Discount Rate		
Age	4.0 Per Cent Per Annum (A)	7.2 Per Cent Per Annum (B)	10.0 Per Cent Per Annum (C)
0	$32,518	$14,680	$ 8,114
10	48,133	29,361	21,047
20	68,363	52,717	45,023
30	81,300	70,515	64,697
40	73,057	67,365	64,012
50	54,132	52,406	51,363
60	30,285	29,853	29,570
70	9,395	9,395	9,395
80	2,465	2,465	2,465
90	0	0	0

Note: The indicated discount rates were applied to the following earnings:

Age	Annual Earnings
0–14	$ 0
15–24	1,201
25–34	4,582
35–44	5,569
45–54	5,327
55–64	4,338
65–74	1,386
75–84	493
85 and over	0

No discounting was applied within ten-year age groups. No allowance was made for future increases in real earnings or for life expectancy.

No deduction was made for additional consumption attributable to decreased mortality. No earnings were imputed for males not in the labor force.

Source: United States Bureau of the Census, 1960 CENSUS OF POPULATION. Occupational Characteristics, Table 34.

of the economic cost of these deaths as measured by age-value profile B in Table 3. On the other hand, vascular lesions accounted for 9.5 per cent of all male deaths, but only 5.7 per cent of the economic cost of these deaths.

Table 4 shows how the age-value profile can be used to calculate the economic value (in production terms only) of the United States, using the 1960 death rate instead of the 1929 rate, or of lowering the United States rate in 1960 to the Swedish rate in 1960. In the former comparison, the greatest savings in number of lives were for infants and ages 75–84, but the greatest gain from a production point of view was from the reduction in the mortality rate for men 35–44. The United States-Swedish comparison highlights the current importance and potential of the 45–54 age group.

Most studies that attempt to place a value on a life saved (or on the cost of premature death) discuss the question of whether some deduction from discounted future earnings should be made for the future

TABLE 4. LIVES SAVED AND ECONOMIC VALUE OF REDUCED UNITED
STATES DEATH RATE, 1929 AND 1960 AND OF REDUCTION OF UNITED
STATES DEATH RATE TO SWEDISH DEATH RATE, 1960

| | United States Male Population 1960 (Thousands) | Death Rate* | | 1960 United States Rate Compared with 1929 United States Rate | | | Economic Value of Lives Saved (Millions) |
Age		1929	1960	Number of Deaths At 1929 Rate (Thousands)	At 1960 Rate (Thousands)	Number of Lives Saved (Thousands)	
Under 1	2,090	79.8	30.1	166.8	62.9	103.9	$1,525
1–4	8,240	6.5	1.2	53.6	9.9	43.7	834
5–14	18,029	2.0	.6	36.1	10.8	25.3	743
15–24	11,906	3.7	1.5	44.1	17.9	26.2	1,381
25–34	11,179	5.1	1.9	57.0	21.2	35.8	2,524
35–44	11,755	7.8	3.7	91.7	43.5	48.2	3,247
45–54	10,093	13.9	9.7	140.3	97.9	42.4	2,222
55–64	7,537	26.7	22.7	201.2	171.1	30.1	899
65–74	5,116	57.6	48.3	294.7	247.1	47.6	447
75–84	2,025	126.8	99.6	256.8	201.7	55.1	136
85 and over	362	256.0	208.4	92.7	75.4	17.3	0
Total	88,331	16.2	10.8	1,435.0	959.4	475.6	13,958

TABLE 4. (CONCLUDED)

| | Death Rate* Sweden 1960 | Swedish Death Rate Compared with United States Death Rate | | Economic Value of Lives Saved (Millions) |
Age		Number of Deaths at Swedish Rate (Thousands)	Lives Saved If U.S. Rate Lowered to Swedish Rate (Thousands)	
Under 1	19.1	39.9	23.6	$ 347
1–4	1.0	7.8	2.1	39
5–14	.5	9.0	1.8	53
15–24	1.0	11.9	5.9	314
25–34	1.2	13.4	7.8	552
35–44	2.0	23.5	19.9	1,346
45–54	5.1	51.5	46.4	2,433
55–64	14.1	106.3	65.6	1,958
65–74	38.2	195.4	51.2	481
75–84	98.2	198.9	4.5	11
85 and over	236.0	85.4	−9.3	0
Total	8.4	743.1	219.5	7,533

* Three-year average centered on year indicated.

Sources: United States Death Rates: 1929: United States Bureau of the Census, HISTORICAL STATISTICS OF THE UNITED STATES, series B123–154. 1960: United States Public Health Service, VITAL STATISTICS OF THE UNITED STATES, 1960, 1961, Table 1C. United States Population: United States Bureau of the Census, 1960 CENSUS OF POPULATION, United States Summary, General Characteristics, PC(1) 1B, Tables 45 and 46. Swedish death rates: ANNUAL EPIDEMIOLOGICAL AND VITAL STATISTICS, 1959, 1960 and 1961, Table 4.

consumption of the individuals whose lives are saved. The arguments for and against are usually framed in terms of whether the value being measured is the value to society including the individual or excluding him. A slightly different way of looking at this problem could be suggested. Consider someone contemplating whether a certain expenditure for health services is worthwhile for him in terms of its expected benefits. He is highly unlikely to think that his own future consumption must be subtracted to calculate the benefits. Many collective decisions might be listed concerning the allocation of resources to health in the same way. Who will be the beneficiary of these additional services is not known. Each person, therefore, will tend to evaluate the potential benefits in much the same way that he would a decision concerning his own expenditures for health; i.e., he will see no reason for deducting consumption, since he may be the one who will benefit from the expenditure. *Ex post* he may reason that saving someone else's life did not do him any good, but in advance of the event and in the absence of knowledge concerning who the beneficiary will be, the full value of the discounted earnings seems the appropriate basis for valuation.

Better health can increase the number of potential man-hours for production by reducing morbidity and disability, as well as by reducing mortality. Some estimate of the potential gains to the economy from this source can be obtained from data collected periodically as part of the National Health Survey. In 1964, approximately 5.5 workdays per person were lost for health reasons by those currently employed.[77] Additional loss was contributed by those persons who would have been employed except for reasons of health.

Health and Productivity

Common sense suggests that better health should result in more production per man, as well as more men available for work. Unfortunately, very little research has been done to provide a basis for estimating the magnitude of this effect. Company sponsored health programs would seem to offer an excellent opportunity for the study of this question, but not much has been done. In one investigation of what executives *thought* were the results of their company's health program, "less absenteeism" was mentioned by 55 per cent of the respondents, "improved employee health" was mentioned by 50 per cent, but "improved productivity on the job" was mentioned by only 12 per cent of the respondents.[78]

A number of studies have examined company health programs,[79-82]

82

but their emphasis is on turnover rates, accident rates, absenteeism and Workmen's Compensation insurance premiums, rather than on output per man-hour. Whether this is because the latter effect is small, or because it is difficult to measure, is not clear. Many of the studies suffer from failure to consider other relevant variables along with the presence or absence of a company health program. Also, these studies do not clarify whether the benefits of company health programs should be attributed to improvements in health. For example, absenteeism and medical expenses may be lowered because of better controls rather than because of any change in health.

One special aspect of company health programs is the periodic health examination, much favored by those interested in preventive medicine. The basic notion is that if diseases or other injurious conditions are discovered early enough the chances for arrest or cure are greatly enhanced. An extensive literature exists on this subject, reviewed by Roberts,[83] but, unfortunately, the studies do not clearly establish the economic value of such examinations. Roberts lists several values served by such examinations but concludes that both public health service activities and personal health practices have much more effect on health than do periodic examinations.

A thorough economic analysis of the costs and benefits of company health programs and periodic health examinations is needed. Such an analysis should pay special attention to all the real costs of these programs including, for example, the time demanded of the examinees. It should attempt also to distinguish between those benefits which are realized through improvements in health and those which are unrelated to health.

Health and Consumption

In contrast to the substantial number of studies that look at the economic value of health in terms of production, very little information is available concerning its value as an end in itself (consumption). Klarman has suggested that one way of approaching the problem would be to observe the expenditures that people are willing to incur for the elimination of nondisabling diseases or the expenditures incurred by those not in the labor force.[84]

Many people in the public health field greatly overestimate the value that the consumer places on health. The health literature frequently seems to read as if no price is too great to pay for good health, but the behavior of consumers indicates that they are often unwilling to pay even a small price. For example, surveys have shown that many people do not brush their teeth regularly, even when they believe that brushing would significantly reduce tooth decay and gum trouble.[85, 86] Smokers who acknowledge the harmful effects of smoking refuse to stop,[87] and a group of executives whose obesity was called to their attention by their physicians took no action to correct a condition which is acknowledged to be injurious to health.[88] Some cases (mostly communicable diseases) may be noted where the social consumption value of health is greater than the private consumption value because of important external effects. The examples cited, however, do not fall into this category.

One of the problems that should be squarely faced in framing a social policy for health services is that people differ in the relative value that they place on health, just as they differ in the relative value that they place on other goods and services. Any system which attempts to force all people to buy the same amount of health services is likely to result in a significant misallocation of resources.

Health and Life Attitudes

This is another area where one can do little more than say that research would be desirable. Many people have speculated about the effect of changes in health levels on attitudes toward work, saving, birth control and other aspects of behavior, but not much evidence has been accumulated. One interesting question concerns the ability of various populations to perceive changes in health levels. A study of low income Negroes in Chicago revealed very little awareness that a significant decline in infant mortality had actually occurred.[89] This suggests that changes in life attitudes, if they are related to changes in health levels, probably occur only after a lag.

CONCLUSION

The principal line of argument in this paper may be stated briefly: health services represent the combined inputs of labor, capital and intermediate goods and services used by the health industry. Their contribution to the economy must be measured by the output of this industry, which takes three forms: health, validation services and other consumer services. Of the three, health is probably the most important. The problem of measuring changes in health levels was examined and followed by a discussion of the relationship between health services and health. Measure of the latter is greatly complicated by the fact that health depends upon environmental factors as well as health services. Most of the studies treat rising income as favorable to health, but some reasons are presented for questioning the validity of this assumption for the United States at present. The economic importance of changes in health levels flows first, from the importance of health as a consumption goal in itself, and, second, from the effect of health on production. This effect can take two forms—changes in potential man-hours and changes in output per man-hour. Changes in life attitudes attributable to changes in health levels also may indirectly affect the economy.

Throughout the paper the need for additional research on each of these concepts and relationships has been stressed. Many of the studies cited have also dealt at length with the question of needed research. The best stimulus to good research is a good example; exhortation is a poor substitute. Nevertheless, this paper will conclude with a few comments on possible points of departure for research.

One promising line of inquiry would be to capitalize on the fact that health services in this country and abroad are produced and financed under a bewildering array of institutional arrangements. Important differences may be found with respect to the ownership and control of facilities, the organization of medical practice, the pricing of health services, the remuneration of health personnel and many other aspects of industrial organization. A basic question to be asked in each case is, "What are the implications of these differences for health and for the economy?"

Another potentially fruitful area of work concerns the advances in medical technology which are the principal source of productivity gain for this industry. The American Medical Association has compiled a list of "significant advances and technological developments" for the period 1936–62, by specialty, based on the response of knowledgeable physicians to a mail survey.[90] The same source presents a list of 30 important therapeutic agents now in use that have been introduced since 1934.[91] Both could provide a useful departure for research on the costs and benefits of medical research as well as for studies of innovation and diffusion similar to those that Mansfield[92] and Griliches[93] have developed for other parts of the economy.

The introduction to this paper argued that one of the principal reasons for wanting to know something about the contribution of health services to the economy is to be able to make better decisions concerning the allocation of resources to health. These decisions are increasingly made by government and are implemented in the form of subsidies for hospital construction, medical education and even medical care. This suggests that one line of fruitful research might be developed as follows:

1. First, the question of health versus other goals must be considered. Although lip service is often paid to the notion that health is a goal to be desired above all else, the most casual inspection of human behavior provides ample refutation of this proposition. Viewed as a source of consumer satisfaction, good health is often shunted aside in favor of the pleasure to be derived from other objects of expenditure and other patterns of behavior. Although the path to better health is frequently portrayed in terms of more hospitals, more doctors and more drugs, most people have the potential of improving their own health by their own actions. Ignorance may be cited to explain the failure of people to take these actions, but this is manifestly untrue in many cases (e.g., doctors continue to smoke). Furthermore, "ignorance" frequently means nothing more than that people have not taken the time or trouble to obtain readily available information about health.

Health also contributes to the economy through production, but alternative ways of increasing output are available. To cite two important ones, resources allocated to increasing health could be allocated to increasing the stock of physical capital, or to increasing the rate of technological change through research and development. Anyone arguing for greater investment in health to increase production should be prepared to show that the return to investment in health is greater than the return to alternative forms of investment.

2. Once a decision has been made regarding the allocation of resources for health relative to other consumer goals and alternative forms of investment, a second allocation decision is required to divide resources among health services and alternative routes to better health. For instance, expectant mothers may benefit from frequent visits to a board-certified obstetrician, but they may also benefit from a better diet, or from not having to work during the last months of pregnancy, or from having someone to help them with their other children.

One can think of health problems where the environmental factors are of negligible importance and health services can make the difference between life and death. However, many situations also exist where both the environment and health services have a role to play and, given a fixed amount of resources to be used for health purposes, knowing the relative contributions (at the margin) of each is important so that resources may be allocated efficiently.

3. The third and most detailed level of decision-making concerns the allocation of resources among various types of health services. More doctors, more nurses, more hospitals, more dentists—in short, more of everything—is needed. Given the decision about resources available for health and the allocation of these resources among health services and other health factors, however, one must have some notion about the contribution (again at the margin), of various types of health services. The absence of such knowledge probably means that public decisions concerning increases of these services can be made on only an arbitrary basis. The argument that the various health resources must be increased in fixed proportion is refuted by the evidence from other countries where health systems are successfully using doctors, nurses, hospital facilities and other health inputs in proportions that differ strikingly from those used in the United States, as well as differing among themselves.

One final note of caution seems to be in order. Whatever research approach is pursued, and whatever questions are attacked, economists must become familiar with health institutions and technology. The practice of medicine is still more an art than a science. The intimate nature of the relationship between patient and doctor, the vital character of the service rendered, and the heavy responsibilities assumed by medical personnel suggest the dangers inherent in reducing health care to matters of balance sheets, or supply and demand curves. Economics has something to contribute to health problems, but it should proceed as the servant of health, not its master.

REFERENCES

[1] Klarman, Herbert E., THE ECONOMICS OF HEALTH, New York, Columbia University Press, 1965.

[2] Mushkin, Selma J., Health as an Investment, *Journal of Political Economy,* Supplement, 70, 129–157, October, 1962.

[3] Wolf, Bernard M., The Economics of Medical Research and Medical Care —From the Point of View of Economic Growth, Washington, D.C., Public Health Service, Resources Analysis Branch, 1964 (manuscript).

4 The University of Michigan Department of Economics and Bureau of Public Health Economics, THE ECONOMICS OF HEALTH AND MEDICAL CARE, Ann Arbor, The University of Michigan Press, 1964.

5 Arrow, Kenneth J., Uncertainty and the Welfare Economics of Medical Care, *American Economic Review,* 53, 941–973, December, 1963.

6 Klarman, *op. cit.*

7 Mushkin, Selma J., Why Health Economics?, *in* THE ECONOMICS OF HEALTH AND MEDICAL CARE, *op. cit.,* pp. 3–13.

8 American Medical Association, COMMISSION ON THE COST OF MEDICAL CARE REPORT, Chicago, The American Medical Association, 1963–64, Volume I, p. 19.

9 Anonymous, An Interview with J. Douglas Colman, *Hospitals,* 39, 45–49, April 16, 1965.

10 American Medical Association, *op. cit.,* p. 9.

11 Reed, Louis S. and Rice, Dorothy P., National Health Expenditures: Object of Expenditures and Source of Funds, 1962, *Social Security Bulletin,* 27, 11–21, August, 1964.

12 United States Department of Commerce, Office of Business Economics, NATIONAL INCOME, 1954 EDITION, A SUPPLEMENT TO THE SURVEY OF CURRENT BUSINESS, Washington, United States Government Printing Office, 1954.

13 ———, SURVEY OF CURRENT BUSINESS, Washington, United States Government Printing Office, annual July issues.

14 ———, U.S. INCOME AND OUTPUT, A SUPPLEMENT TO THE SURVEY OF CURRENT BUSINESS, Washington, United States Government Printing Office, 1958.

15 Merriam, Ida C., Social and Welfare Expenditures, 1963–64, *Social Security Bulletin,* 27, 3–14, October, 1964.

16 United States National Health Survey, PERSONAL HEALTH EXPENSES: DISTRIBUTION OF PERSONS BY AMOUNT AND TYPE OF EXPENSE, UNITED STATES JULY–DECEMBER 1962, Series 10, Washington, United States Government Printing Office, 1965.

17 ———, MEASUREMENT OF PERSONAL HEALTH EXPENDITURES, Series 2, Washington, United States Government Printing Office, 1963.

18 Anderson, Ronald and Anderson, Odin W., Trends in Personal Health Spending, *Progress in Health Services,* 14, November–December, 1965.

19 United States Bureau of Labor Statistics, STUDY OF CONSUMER EXPENDITURES, INCOMES AND SAVINGS, Volume VIII, SUMMARY OF FAMILY EXPENDITURES FOR MEDICAL CARE AND PERSONAL CARE, Philadelphia, University of Pennsylvania Press, 1956.

20 ———, STUDY OF CONSUMER EXPENDITURES, INCOMES AND SAVINGS, Volume XVIII, SUMMARY OF FAMILY INCOME, EXPENDITURES AND SAVINGS, ALL URBAN AREAS COMBINED, Philadelphia, University of Pennsylvania Press, 1957.

21 United States Department of Commerce, Bureau of the Census, CENSUS OF POPULATION, Washington, United States Government Printing Office, decennial.

[22] United States Department of Commerce, Bureau of the Census, U.S. CENSUSES OF POPULATION AND HOUSING: 1960, 1/1000, 1/10,000: TWO NATIONAL SAMPLES OF THE POPULATION OF THE UNITED STATES, Washington, United States Department of Commerce.

[23] United States Public Health Service, HEALTH MANPOWER SOURCE BOOK, Sections 1–19, Washington, United States Government Printing Office, 1952–64.

[24] American Hospital Association, HOSPITALS, Guide Issue, Part 2, 38, August 1, 1964 (annual).

[25] United States Treasury Department, Internal Revenue Service, STATISTICS OF INCOME . . . 1962: U.S. BUSINESS TAX RETURNS, Washington, United States Government Printing Office, 1965 (annual).

[26] United States Department of Commerce, Bureau of the Census, UNITED STATES CENSUS OF MANUFACTURERS, Washington, United States Government Printing Office, 1963 (currently every five years).

[27] Becker, Gary S., A Theory of the Allocation of Time, *The Economic Journal*, 75, 493–517, September, 1965.

[28] World Health Organization, Constitution of the World Health Organization, Annex I, *in* World Health Organization, THE FIRST TEN YEARS OF THE WORLD HEALTH ORGANIZATION, Geneva, The World Health Organization, 1958.

[29] Roberts, Ffrangcon, THE COST OF HEALTH, London, Turnstile Press, 1952.

[30] Johnson, R. H., The Health of Israel, *The Lancet*, 7417, 842–845, October 23, 1965.

[31] Morris, J. N., USES OF EPIDEMIOLOGY, Second Edition, Baltimore, The Williams & Wilkins Co., 1964, p. 14.

[32] Sullivan, D. F., Conceptual Problems in Developing an Index of Health, *in* VITAL AND HEALTH STATISTICS, DATA EVALUATION AND METHODS RESEARCH, Public Health Service Publication Number 1000, Series 2, Number 17, Washington, United States Government Printing Office, May, 1966.

[33] Sanders, B. S., Measuring Community Health Levels, *American Journal of Public Health*, 54, 1063–1070, July, 1964.

[34] Anderson, Alice L. and Altman, Isidore, Methodology in Evaluating the Quality of Medical Care, An Annotated Selected Bibliography 1955–61, Pittsburgh, University of Pittsburgh Press, 1962.

[35] Terris, Milton, The Relevance of Medical Care to the Public Health, paper delivered before American Public Health Association, November 13, 1963.

[36] Rosen, George, The Bacteriological, Immunologic and Chemotherapeutic Period 1875–1950, *Bulletin of the New York Academy of Medicine*, 40, 483–494, 1964.

[37] Long, A. P. and Sartwell, P. E., Tetanus in the U.S. Army in World War II, *Bulletin of the U.S. Army Medical Department*, 7, 371–385, April, 1947.

[38] Long, A. P., Immunization to Tetanus, *in* Army Medical Services Graduate School, RECENT ADVANCES IN MEDICINE AND SURGERY, Washington, Walter Reed Army Institute of Research, 1955, pp. 311–313.

[39] American Medical Association, *op. cit.*, Volume III, Chapter 4.

[40] ————, *op. cit.*, Volume III, Chapter 7.

[41] Lerner, Monroe and Anderson, Odin W., HEALTH PROGRESS IN THE UNITED STATES 1900–1960: A REPORT OF THE HEALTH INFORMATION FOUNDATION, Chicago, University of Chicago Press, 1963, p. 43.

[42] Marks, Herbert H., Longevity and Mortality of Diabetics, *American Journal of Public Health,* 55, 416–423, March, 1965.

[43] World Health Organization, EXPERT COMMITTEE ON WATER FLUORIDATION, FIRST REPORT, Technical Report Series, Number 146, Geneva, The World Health Organization, 1958.

[44] Schlesinger, E. R., Dietary Fluoride and Caries Prevention, *American Journal of Public Health,* 55, 1123–1129, August, 1965.

[45] Farmer, A. W. and Shandling, B. S., Review of Burn Admissions, 1956–1960—The Hospital for Sick Children, Toronto, *Journal of Trauma,* 3, 425–432, September, 1963.

[46] Kaiser, R. F., *et. al.,* Uterine Cytology, *Public Health Reports,* 75, 423–427, 1960.

[47] Dunn, John E., Jr., Cancer of the Cervix—End Results Report, *in* National Cancer Institute and American Cancer Society, FIFTH NATIONAL CANCER CONFERENCE PROCEEDINGS, Philadelphia, J. B. Lippincott Company, 1956, pp. 253–257.

[48] Krementz, Edward T., End Results in Skin Cancer, *in* National Cancer Institute and American Cancer Society, FOURTH NATIONAL CANCER CONFERENCE PROCEEDINGS, Philadelphia, J. B. Lippincott Co., 1961, pp. 629–637.

[49] Lewison, Edwin F., An Appraisal of Longterm Results in Surgical Treatment of Breast Cancer, *Journal of the American Medical Association,* 186, 975–978, December 14, 1963.

[50] Sutherland, Robert, CANCER: THE SIGNIFICANCE OF DELAY, London, Butterworth and Company (Publishers) Ltd., 1960, pp. 196–202.

[51] Stout, John, *et al.,* Status of Congenital Heart Disease Patients Ten to Fifteen Years After Surgery, *Public Health Reports,* 79, 377–382, May, 1964.

[52] Wilson, May G., *et al.,* The Decline of Rheumatic Fever—Recurrence Rates of Rheumatic Fever Among 782 Children for 21 Consecutive Calendar Years, *Journal of Chronic Diseases,* 7, 183–197, March, 1958.

[53] The Rheumatic Fever Working Party of the Medical Research Council of Great Britain and The Subcommittee of Principal Investigators of the American Council on Rheumatic Fever and Congenital Heart Disease, American Heart Association, Treatment of Acute Rheumatic Fever in Children: A Cooperative Clinical Trial of ACTH, Cortisone, and Aspirin, *British Medical Journal,* 1, 555–574, 1955.

[54] Kutner, Ann G., Current Status of Steroid Therapy in Rheumatic Fever, *American Heart Journal,* 70, 147–149, August, 1965.

[55] Brest, Albert N., Treatment of Coronary Occlusive Disease: Critical Review, *Diseases of the Chest,* 45, 40–45, January, 1964.

[56] Combined Staff Clinic, Recent Advances in Hypertension, *American Journal of Medicine,* 39, 634–638, October, 1965.

[57] Lindsay, Malcolm I., Jr. and Spiekerman, Ralph E., Re-evaluation of Therapy of Acute Myocardial Infarction, *American Heart Journal,* 67, 559–564, April, 1964.

[58] Lockwood, Howard J., *et al.,* Effects of Intensive Care on the Mortality Rate of Patients with Myocardial Infarctions, *Public Health Reports,* 78, 655–661, August, 1963.

[59] Cain, Harvey D., *et al.,* Current Therapy of Cardiovascular Disease, *Geriatrics,* 18, 507–518, July, 1963.

[60] Lowenthal, Milton, *et al.,* An Analysis of the Rehabilitation Needs and Prognoses of 232 Cases of Cerebral Vascular Accident, *Archives of Physical Medicine,* 40, 183–186, 1959.

[61] May, Philip R. A. and Tuma, A. Hussain, Schizophrenia—An Experimental Study of Five Treatment Methods, *British Journal of Psychiatry,* 111, 503–510, June, 1965.

[62] Schwartz, Samuel and Vinyard, John H., Prenatal Care and Prematurity, *Public Health Reports,* 80, 237–248, March, 1965.

[63] Shapiro, Sam, *et al.,* Comparisons of Prematurity and Prenatal Mortality in a General Population and in a Population of a Prepaid Group Practice, *American Journal of Public Health,* 48, 170–187, February, 1958.

[64] ————, Further Observations on Prematurity and Prenatal Mortality in a General Population and in the Population of a Prepaid Group Practice Medical Plan, *American Journal of Public Health,* 50, 1304–1317, September, 1960.

[65] Lockwood, *et al., op. cit.*

[66] United States Public Health Service, CORONARY CARE UNITS: SPECIALIZED INTENSIVE CARE UNITS FOR ACUTE MYOCARDIAL INFARCTION PATIENTS, Washington, United States Government Printing Office, October, 1964.

[67] Forshall, Isabella and Rickham, P. P., Experience of a Neonatal Surgical Unit—The First Six Years, *The Lancet,* 2, 751–754, October, 1960.

[68] Wylie, C. M., Participation in a Multiple Screening Clinic with Five Year Follow-Up, *Public Health Reports,* 76, 596–602, July, 1961.

[69] Yankauer, Alfred and Lawrence, Ruth A., A Study of Periodic School Medical Examinations, *American Journal of Public Health,* 45, 71–78, January, 1955.

[70] McKinnon, N. E., The Effects of Control Programs on Cancer Mortality, *Canadian Medical Association Journal,* 82, 1308–1312, June 25, 1960.

[71] American Medical Association, *op. cit.,* Volume III, p. ix.

[72] Altenderfer, Marion E., Relationship Between Per Capita Income and Mortality in the Cities of 100,000 or More Population, *Public Health Reports,* 62, 1681–1691, November 28, 1947.

[73] Denison, Edward F., Study of European Economic Growth, Washington, The Brookings Institution, unpublished.

91

[74] Morrison, S. L. and Goldberg, E. M., Schizophrenia and Social Class, *Journal of Mental Science,* 109, 785–802, 1963.

[75] Meadows Susan H., Social Class Migration and Chronic Bronchitis: A Study of Male Hospital Patients in the London Area, *British Journal of Preventive and Social Medicine,* 15, 171–175, 1961.

[76] Klarman, *op. cit.,* pp. 162–172.

[77] United States National Health Survey, DISABILITY DAYS: UNITED STATES JULY 1963–JUNE 1964, Series 10, Washington, United States Government Printing Office, 1965, p. 16.

[78] National Industrial Conference Board, COMPANY MEDICAL AND HEALTH PROGRAMS, Studies in Personnel Policy, Number 171, New York, National Industrial Conference Board, 1959, p. 12.

[79] Grant, Ellsworth S., The U.S. Concept of and Experience in Small-Plant Health Services, *in* PROCEEDINGS OF THIRTEENTH INTERNATIONAL CONGRESS ON OCCUPATIONAL HEALTH, New York City, 1960, pp. 118–120.

[80] National Health Forum, Are Occupational Health Programs Worthwhile?, *in* Maisel, Albert Q. (Editor), HEALTH OF PEOPLE WHO WORK, New York, National Health Council, 1960, pp. 11–28.

[81] Cipolla, J. A., The Occupational Health Experiences of Two American Hotels for 1955 and 1956, *in* PROCEEDINGS OF FOURTEENTH INTERNATIONAL CONGRESS ON OCCUPATIONAL HEALTH, Madrid, Spain, 1963, Volume II, pp. 290–291.

[82] Blankenship, Marilyn, Influenza Immunization and Industrial Absenteeism—A Seven Month Study, *in* PROCEEDINGS OF THE FOURTEENTH INTERNATIONAL CONGRESS ON OCCUPATIONAL HEALTH, *op. cit.,* pp. 294–295.

[83] Roberts, Norman J., The Values and Limitations of Periodic Health Examinations, *Journal of Chronic Diseases,* 9, 95–116, 1959.

[84] Klarman, *op. cit.,* p. 64.

[85] Kirscht, John P., A National Study of Health Beliefs, Ann Arbor, University of Michigan, 1965 (manuscript).

[86] Haefner, Don P., *et al.,* Preventive Actions Concerning Dental Disease, Tuberculosis and Cancer, paper delivered at the 22nd Annual Meeting of the Association of Teachers of Preventive Medicine, Chicago, October 17, 1965.

[87] Swinehart, James W. and Kirscht, John P., Smoking: A Panel Study of Beliefs and Behavior Following the PHS Report, paper delivered at the Annual Meeting of the American Psychological Association, Chicago, 1965.

[88] Wade, Leo, *et al.,* Are Periodic Health Examinations Worthwhile?, *Annals of Internal Medicine,* 56, 81–93, 1962.

[89] Bogue, Donald J., Inventory, Explanation, and Evaluation by Interview of Family Planning: Motives—Attitudes—Knowledge—Behavior: Fertility Measurement, document prepared for discussion at International Conference on Family Planning Programs, Geneva, Switzerland, August 23–27, 1965.

[90] American Medical Association, *op. cit.,* Volume III, pp. 4–12.

[91] ———, *op. cit.,* Volume III, pp. 13–14.

92

[92] Mansfield, Edwin, The Diffusion of Technological Change, National Science Foundation Reviews of Data on Research and Development, October, 1961.

[93] Griliches, Zvi, Hybrid Corn: An Exploration in the Economics of Technological Change, *Econometrica,* 25, 501–522, October, 1957.

ACKNOWLEDGMENTS

I am grateful to Deborah W. Sarachek for the preparation of the bibliography and tables and for numerous contributions to the text. I am also grateful to Dr. Richard H. Kessler for reading the section on medical care, and to Irving Leveson for several useful suggestions.

HEALTH CARE
AND THE UNITED STATES ECONOMIC SYSTEM
An Essay in Abnormal Physiology

VICTOR R. FUCHS

Health care affects and is affected by the economic system in so many ways as to preclude any attempt at complete enumeration or description. The objective of this paper is more modest. I shall assume that the reader is reasonably familiar with health care, its institutions, technology and personnel, but is less familiar with an "economic system" that is used by economists to describe and analyze economic behavior. Therefore, major emphasis will be given to indicating the place of health care in this system and showing how related economic concepts can contribute to an understanding of problems of health care in the United States. I shall also attempt to indicate some of the limitations of economics in dealing with such a complex area of human activity and concern.

INTRODUCTION
Definitions
Health care can be defined as those activities that are undertaken with the objective of restoring, preserving or enhancing the physical and mental well-being of people. These activities may be aimed at the relief of pain, the removal of disabilities, the restoration of functions, the prevention of illness and accidents or the postponement of death. Some health care is produced within the "household;" e.g., the triage, first-aid and

95

nursing services rendered to children by parents. Some is bought and sold in the "market"; e.g., physicians' services, hospital services. Most health care is applied to identifiable individuals but some may be aimed at a population; e.g., fluoridation of a water supply.

The *economic system* consists of the network of institutions, laws and rules created by society to answer the universal economic questions: (a) What goods and services shall be produced? (b) How shall they be produced? and (c) For whom shall they be produced?[1] Every society needs an economic system because *resources* (natural, human and manmade) are scarce relative to human wants. The resources have alternative uses and there is a multiplicity of competing wants. Thus, decisions must be made regarding the use of these resources in production and the distribution of the resulting output among the members of society.

Two Fallacies

Before turning to several important issues concerning health care in relation to the economic system it will be useful to dispose of two fallacies that have frequently obstructed clear thinking in this area.

1. Resources are no longer scarce. Some people seem to be so inspired, terrified or confused by automation and other technologic advances as to proclaim the end of scarcity. A decade ago it was not unusual to find writers prophesying that in ten years no one would have to work because machines would turn out all the goods and services needed. The falsity of such predictions becomes more apparent each year. That inefficiency and waste exist in the economy cannot be denied. That some resources are underutilized is clear every time the unemployment figures are announced. That the resources devoted to war could be used to satisfy other wants is self-evident. But the fundamental fact remains that even if all these imperfections were eliminated total output would still fall far short

of the amount people would like to have. Resources would still be scarce in the sense that choices would have to be made. An economic system would still be needed. Not only is this true now, but it will continue to be true in the foreseeable future. Some advances in technology make it possible to carry out current activities with fewer resources (e.g., automated laboratories), but others open up new demands (e.g., for renal dialysis or organ transplants) that put further strains on resources. Moreover, time, the ultimate scarce resource, becomes more valuable the more productive we become.[2,3]

2. Health is the most important goal. Some of those in the health field recognize that we cannot satisfy all wants, but they seem to believe that health is more important than all other goals and therefore questions of scarcity and allocation are not applicable in this area. It requires only a casual study of human behavior to reveal the fallacy of this position. Every day in manifold ways people make choices that affect health and it is clear that they frequently place a higher value on satisfying other wants; e.g., smoking, overeating, careless driving, failure to take medicine.

Criteria for an Economic System in Relation to Health Care

What is it that we want the economic system to do with respect to health care? Given the scarcity of resources and the existence of competing goals we want a system that will result in:

1. An optimum amount of resources devoted to health care;
2. These resources being combined in an optimal way;
3. An optimal distribution of health care;
4. An optimal allocation of resources between current provision of health care and investment for future health care through research, education and so forth.

The general rule for reaching such optima is "equality at the margin." For instance, the first criterion would be met if the last dollar's worth of resources devoted to health care increased human satisfaction by exactly the same amount as the last dollar's worth devoted to other goals.

The contrast between this view of a social optimum and the notion of "optimal care" as used in the health field can be appreciated with the aid of Figure 1. The relation between health and health care inputs can usually be described by a curve that may rise at an increasing rate at first, but then rises at a decreasing rate and eventually levels off or declines.[4] "Optimal care" in medicine would usually be defined as the point where no further increment in health is possible; i.e., point A.[5] The social optimum, however, requires that inputs of resources not exceed the point where the value of an additional increment to health is exactly equal to the cost of the

FIGURE I. DETERMINATION OF OPTIMUM LEVEL OF HEALTH CARE UTILIZATION

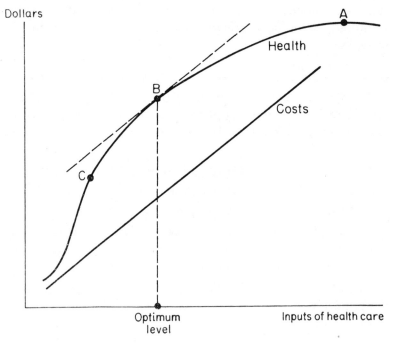

inputs required to obtain that increment (point B). It should be noted that point C, where the *ratio* of benefits to costs is at a maximum, is not the optimal point because additional inputs still add more to benefits than to costs. One of the problems with current health care policy is that it frequently fluctuates between trying to drive utilization to A, and then, in frenzied attempts to contain costs, cuts back some programs to point C or below.

Types of Economic Systems

Economists have identified three "pure types" of economic systems—traditional, centrally directed and market price. Every actual economy is a blend of types, but their relative importance can and does vary greatly. Most primitive and feudal societies rely heavily upon a traditional system; the process of decision-making is embedded in the total culture—its customs, traditions and religious rituals. In some ancient empires (Egypt, Babylonia) central direction played a major role. The basic decisions were made by one man or a small group of men who controlled the power apparatus of the society and were in a position to enforce their decisions concerning the allocation of resources and the distribution of output. This system has also been dominant in the Soviet Union since 1928 and in many other countries since World War II. The United States, Canada and most countries of Western Europe have relied heavily on a market system for the past century or two. Thus a discussion of health care and the United States economy requires a close look at the working of a market system. An additional reason for concentrating on this third type is for its normative value. Under certain specified conditions the results produced by the theoretical market system set a standard against which the performance of any real economy can be evaluated.[6]

The Elementary Model

The elementary model of a market system consists of a collection of decision-making units called *households* and another collection called *firms*. The households own all the productive resources in the society. They make these resources available to firms who transform them into goods and services, which are then distributed back to the households. The flow of resources and of goods and services is facilitated by a counterflow of money (see Figure 2) .[7] This is called a market system because the exchanges of resources and of goods and services for money take place in markets where *prices* and *quantities* are determined. These prices are the signals or controls that trigger changes in behavior as required by changes in technology or preferences. The market system is sometimes referred to as the "price" system.

In the markets for resources the households are the *suppliers* and the firms provide the *demand*. In the markets for goods and services the firms are the suppliers and the households are the source of demand. In each market the interaction between demand and supply determines the quantities and prices of the various resources and goods and services (see Figure 3) .

The income of each household depends upon the quantity and quality of resources available to it (including time) and their prices; the amount of income determines its share of the total flow of goods and services. The household is assumed to spend its income (and time) in such a way as to maximize *utility* (i.e., satisfaction) . It does this by following the principle of "equality at the margin;" i.e., it adjusts its purchases so that marginal utility (the satisfaction added by the last unit purchased) of each commodity is proportional to its price.

It is assumed that firms attempt to maximize *profits* (the difference between what they must pay the households for the use of resources and what they get from them for the goods and services they produce) . To maximize profits they too must follow the equality at the margin rule, adjusting their use of different types of resources so that the marginal products (the addition to output obtained from one additional unit of input) are proportional to price.

If the markets are perfectly competitive and if certain other

100

FIGURE 2. ELEMENTARY MODEL OF A MARKET SYSTEM

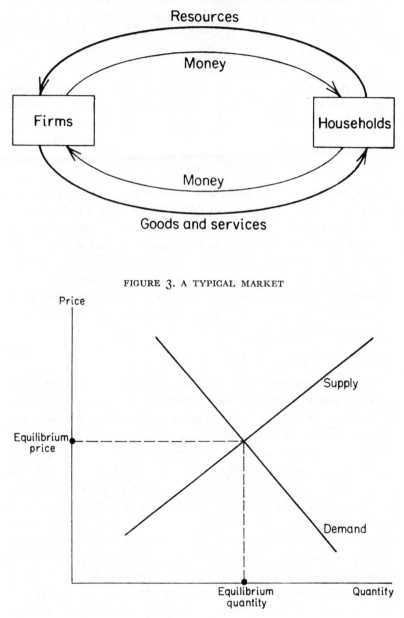

FIGURE 3. A TYPICAL MARKET

conditions are met, it can be shown that a market system produces an optimum allocation of resources, given the distribution of resources among households and given their "tastes" or preferences. The United States economy departs in many respects from the abstract perfectly competitive market system; this is particularly noticeable in the health care sector. The main body of this paper is devoted to a discussion of these departures and the problems they pose for health care policy.

IMPERFECTLY COMPETITIVE MARKETS

The essence of a competitive market is (1) that there are many well-informed buyers and sellers no one of whom is large enough to influence price; (2) that the buyers and sellers act independently (i.e., no collusion) ; and (3) that there is free entry for other buyers and sellers not currently in the market. Most health care markets depart substantially from competitive conditions, sometimes inevitably, and sometimes as the result of deliberate public or private policy. A discussion of some of the principal problems follows.

Fewness of Sellers

In most towns and even moderate size cities the market is too small to support enough hospitals or enough practitioners in each speciality to fulfill the requirements of a workably competitive market. For instance, most students of hospital costs believe there are significant economies of scale in general hospitals up to a size of 200 or 300 beds, and some believe that economies are to be realized in even larger hospitals. Assuming a ratio of four beds per 1,000 population, a city of 60,000 could support just one 240 bed hospital. Thus, it would be extremely uneconomical to require numerous competitive hospitals except in large, densely populated markets. These constraints are even more significant when specialty care is considered. It is doubtful that even a population of one million would justify enough independent maternity, open heart surgery and transplant services and the like to approximate competitive conditions.[8]

In such a condition of "natural monopoly" the traditional United States response has been to introduce public utility regulation (e.g., electricity, telephone, transportation). The results, however, have not always been satisfactory, partly because the regulators often tend to serve the regulated rather than the public and partly because it is inherently difficult to set standards of performance without competitive yardsticks. Many other countries rely on government ownership and control, but the United States experience with government hospitals has not, on balance, been favorable. Another possible solution is the development of what J. K. Galbraith has termed "countervailing power" and what the economics textbooks describe as bilateral monopoly. If, for instance, in a one-hospital town all the consumers were organized into a single body for purposes of bargaining with the hospital, at least some of the disadvantages of monopoly would be lessened.

The typical "solution" in the hospital field has been to emphasize the "nonprofit" character of the hospitals and to assume that therefore the hospital will not abuse its monopoly power. Two criticisms of this "solution" are (a) the absence of a profit incentive may lead to waste, inefficiency and unnecessary duplication, and (2) the hospitals may be run for the benefit of the physicians.[9]

Cooperation (Collusion) Among Sellers

Even when numerous sellers of the same health service are in the same market there may be significant advantages to society if they do not maintain a completely arms-length competitive posture vis-à-vis one another. The free exchange of information, cooperative efforts to meet crisis situations and reciprocal backup arrangements may help to reduce costs and increase patient satisfaction. Unfortunately, the intimacy and trust developed through such activities may spill over in less desirable directions such as price fixing, exclusion of would-be rivals and other restrictions on competition. For 200 years economists have been impressed with the wisdom of Adam Smith's observation that "people of the same trade seldom meet together, even for merriment and diversion, but the conversation ends in a conspiracy against the public, or in some contrivance to raise prices." Pathologists have been found guilty of price-fixing, and price discrimination by physicians is not uncommon. The latter practice, which physicians view benevolently as a way of reducing inequality of access to medical care, is viewed by some economists as evidence of the use of monopoly power to maximize profits.[10]

Restrictions on Entry

Probably the most obvious and most deliberate interference with competition in the market for physicians' services is the barrier to entry imposed by compulsory licensure. The case for licensure presumably rests on the proposition that the consumer is a poor judge of the quality of medical care and therefore needs guidance concerning the qualifications of those proposing to sell such care. Assuming this to be true the need for guidance could be met by voluntary *certification,* rather than compulsory licensure. Indeed, the need could probably be better met through certification because there could be several grades or categories and periodic recertification would be more practicable (and less threatening) than periodic relicensure. Under a certification system patients would be free to choose the level of expertise that they wanted, including uncertified practitioners.

The principal objections that could be raised against such a system are that some patients might receive bad treatment at the hands of uncertified practitioners, and that it might result in an expansion of unnecessary care. The obvious advantages of such a system are greater availability of care and lower prices. For certain health care needs, practitioners with lesser qualifications than present physicians have would clearly be adequate. The existing system results in some persons receiving no care,

104

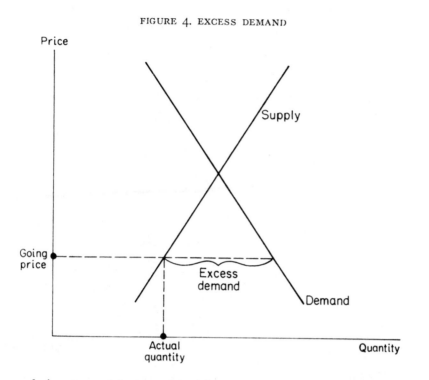

FIGURE 4. EXCESS DEMAND

or being treated by persons without any medical training (e.g., family members, neighbors, friends) .

Another example of entry restrictions is the system of limiting hospital privileges to certain physicians. This has been justified in terms of the desire to insure quality of care (in the institution) and as a way of obtaining free services from the physicians. However, it can also be viewed in an economic context as a way of limiting competition.

In general, the codes of professional ethics that physicians have evolved undoubtedly serve many useful social purposes. But it is well to recall Kenneth Arrow's observation that "codes of professional ethics, which arise out of the principal-agent relation and afford protection to the principals, can serve also as a cloak for monopoly by the agents."[11]

105

FIGURE 5. EXCESS SUPPLY

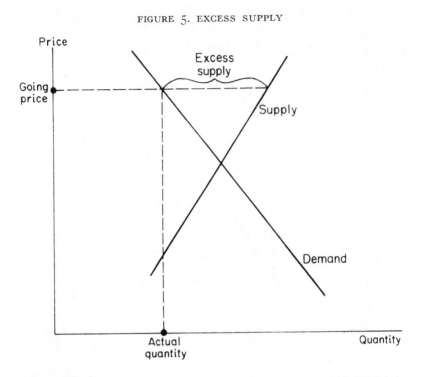

Disequilibrium

One disturbing characteristic of some health care markets is the failure of price to reach an equilibrium level (the level where the quantity demanded and the quantity supplied are equal). For instance, the market for house calls seems to be characterized by excess demand (see Figure 4). The "going price," about $20 per visit, is not high enough to bring supply and demand into balance. The quantity (number of house calls) that patients are willing and able to pay for at that price is much greater than the quantity physicians are willing to supply. Some observers, notably Martin Feldstein,[12] believe that the market for physicians' services in general is characterized by excess demand.

The market for general surgery, however, can best be described as an example of excess supply (see Figure 5).[13] At the

106

going price for most general surgical procedures, $300 for a herniorrhaphy, the quantity that surgeons are willing and able to do is much greater than the quantity demanded. A condition of excess supply is also probably present for many types of specialty surgery (ophthalmology, gynecology).

The persistence of a disequilibrium price is a clear indication that the market departs substantially from the competitive norm. In the case of excess demand, physicians are apparently reluctant to let the price of house calls rise to their equilibrium level; they introduce a form of rationing instead. This may yield certain psychic satisfactions in lieu of the higher income that is clearly possible. In the excess supply example, the price fails to fall either because the individual surgeon does not think it would be to his advantage to cut price or because surgeons have collectively reached this decision. A contributing factor is the option that most surgeons have of using their nonsurgical time for general practice or other income-producing activities.

The alleged shortage of nurses indicates another potentially troublesome health care market. If what is meant by "shortage" is that it would be nice to have more nurses, no analytical problem arises and the point is trivial. In that sense there is a shortage of every type of good or service. If, however, the allegation refers to a shortage in the sense shown in Figure 4 (i.e., an excess demand for nurses), the failure of nurses' salaries to rise to their equilibrium level must be explained. Some investigators[14,15] claim that it is monopsonistic behavior on the part of hospitals that keeps nurses' salaries from rising to the point where supply and demand would be equal.

Costs of Information

The elementary competitive model assumes that all information relevant to decision-making is known by the households and firms—prices, production possibilities, utility to be derived from different commodities. In the real world, of course, such information may be difficult or even impossible to obtain. High information costs are characteristic of many health care markets; frequently the only way a person can know whether he needs to see a physician is to see a physician. The incorporation of information costs into economic analysis is relatively recent,[16] and the theory is far from complete. Many health care markets function poorly because of imperfect information but there is considerable disagreement as to how to make them function better. One point might have general validity. Where the costs of information are increased as a result of public or private policy, reversal of that policy would probably be desirable. For instance, restrictions on the right of physicians to advertise and on the right of pharmacies to advertise prices of prescription drugs ought to be reexamined in the light of the consumer's need to know more about physicians and drugs to make intelligent choices. A study of variations in restrictions on advertising by optometrists and opticians found that prices were substantially lower in states that permitted advertising.[17]

EXTERNALITIES

An externality exists when the actions taken by an individual household or firm will impose costs or confer benefits on other households or firms, and where no feasible way exists of arranging direct compensation for these costs or benefits. The presence of externalities indicates that the individual household or firm, in attempting to maximize its own utility or profit, will not make socially optimal decisions.[18] A classic example of an externality is the costs of air pollution imposed on others by the smoke emanating from a factory. Another classic example is the benefit to society that results when an individual decides to be vaccinated or treated for a communicable disease.

One way to deal with externalities is for the state to prohibit or require certain actions. Another is to attempt to modify the prices facing individual firms or households (through taxes or subsidies) so that the price properly reflects the social costs or benefits. In principle, use of the price mechanism will permit a much closer approximation to a social optimum, but practical difficulties may preclude the price approach in some situations.

Externalities are very important to health care in the broadest sense of the term. Consider, for instance, the effects of automobiles on health. The decisions of individual households involving the purchase and use of an automobile, the speed and manner of driving, the amount of maintenance and repair and even the choice of gasoline have potentially important implications for the health of others, but these implications are not reflected in the prices facing the household. Similar problems arise in connection with many other consumption or production activities that create environmental health hazards.

In seeking to reduce such hazards a few central points should be kept in mind. First, costs (resources used or wants unsatisfied) are usually associated with the reduction of hazards, and these costs frequently increase at an accelerating rate, the greater the reduction desired. It follows, therefore, that the social goal should rarely be the complete elimination of the hazard, but rather its reduction to the point where the value of a further reduction is less than the cost of achieving it. A major problem for health care policy is to identify these externalities, estimate their effects and impose appropriate taxes or subsidies so that individual households and firms, in seeking to maximize their own utility or profits, will make socially appropriate decisions.

Medical research is a good example of an activity with large external benefits, and, therefore, in the absence of specific public policy, too little will be undertaken. One solution is to permit the discoverer of new knowledge to appropriate the benefits (e.g., through patent protection), but with regard to much health research this solution will frequently not be feasible or acceptable. The alternative is for the government to subsidize research. It has done this to a considerable degree; the question is how much health research is socially desirable? The answer, in principle, is the same as for any other decision regarding the use of scarce resources—the optimum level of research is reached when the incremental value of the prospective benefits is equal to the incremental cost. The more basic the research the more

109

likely it is to give rise to external benefits, but the more difficult it is to estimate their value or incidence.

In contrast to environmental programs and medical research, medical care today frequently does not involve significant external benefits. For instance, the benefits of most surgery accrue primarily to the patient and his family. This is equally true for treatment of most major diseases such as heart disease and cancer.[19] The best known examples of externalities arising from medical care involve the prevention of and treatment for communicable diseases. Another potentially important source of externalities is the treatment of mental illness, but lack of knowledge concerning causes or cures makes it difficult to reach firm policy conclusions in this area.

One important application of the externality idea is with respect to the problem of inequality of access to care. A frequent criticism of the market system is that it results in an unequal and "unfair" distribution of income.[20] Households that are poorly endowed with resources will earn relatively little and will command only a small share of the nation's output.

Many people would like to see a reduction of inequality, either in general or with respect to a particular commodity (medical care). To the extent that they are prepared to back their demand for less inequality through voluntary redistribution (philanthropy), no modification of the elementary model is required. We simply note that some households derive utility from giving money to others or from knowing that other households are receiving medical care. They are, therefore, willing to devote a part of their income (or part of their time) for that purpose. The purchase of a good or service for someone else is no different analytically from the purchase of a good or service for one's own household.

The externality problem arises because a philanthropic act by one household confers benefits on all other households that derive utility from observing a decrease in inequality. If each potential philanthropist considers only the psychic benefits *he* derives from reducing inequality, the total volume of philanthropy will be less than warranted by the collective desires of the group.[21]

One solution is compulsory redistribution. Society, working through government, may decide that the distribution of income resulting from the market system is inequitable or otherwise unsatisfactory and may seek to change it through taxation. This requires only a slight modification of the elementary model. The simplest way to do this is to take money away from some households and give it to others. Each household is then free to allocate its income as it pleases.

For any given amount of redistribution the utility of households is presumably maximized by a general tax on the income of some households and grants of income to others rather than by taxing particular forms of spending or by subsidizing particular types of consumption. Mathematical proofs of this proposition are available and its plausibility is obvious. If a household is offered a choice of either $100 or $100 worth of health care, it will prefer the former because it can use the additional income to buy more health care (if that is what it wants), but usually utility will be maximized by increasing consumption of many other commodities as well. Similarly, if a household is offered a choice between giving up $100 and giving up $100 worth of health care, its utility will be diminished less by the general tax on income.

Despite the obvious logic of the foregoing many nonpoor seem more inclined toward a reduction in inequality in the consumption of particular commodities (medical care is a conspicuous example) than toward a general redistribution of income.[22] Two reasons may explain this behavior. First, the nonpoor may believe that significant externalities are associated with medical care (in addition to the psychic benefits of observing a reduction in inequality) that are not associated with other commodities. The earlier discussion indicated some grounds for skepticism concerning this belief.[23] A second reason may be that the nonpoor think they know better what will maximize the utility of the poor than do the poor themselves.

111

A special aspect of the problem arises when the emphasis is put on reducing inequality of access to medical care *per se* rather than raising the consumption of medical care by the poor. This goal may require rationing the amount available to the nonpoor as well as subsidizing the poor. One economist has argued that the British approach to health care through a national health service can best be understood in these terms.[24]

Compulsory Insurance

At the extreme, the demand for reductions in inequality takes the form of an assertion that "health care is a right;" that if someone needs health care society has an obligation to provide it. To the extent that society honors that obligation, the incentive for households to provide for their own health care (as through voluntary insurance) is diminished. Those without insurance and especially those individuals who prior to their illness could have afforded the normal premium, become, in effect, "freeloaders" on the rest of society.

If this behavior is widespread, the only solutions are to make insurance compulsory or to modify the ethical imperative. Thus far the United States has opted for a little of each. Insurance is virtually compulsory for many through their employment contract; on the other hand, free care is made less attractive by means tests, long waiting lines, unpleasant surroundings and similar inconveniences.

Another argument advanced in favor of compulsory insurance is that it overcomes the problem of adverse selection. If insurance is completely voluntary it may be impractical to adjust each household's premium to its expected utilization. To the extent that uniform premiums are charged, however, households with lower than average expected utilization have an incentive to drop out and this process can continue until the plan collapses.

It seems likely that the United States will move further in the direction of compulsory insurance, but this development is likely to create new problems even as it solves others. It increases the incentive to reduce health care in the home and throws more of the burden on collectively provided care. If the money price of market-provided care goes to zero, people will tend to use more than the amount they would like to use if they were free to shift resources to satisfy other wants.

SOME LIMITATIONS OF THE MODEL

The "Taste" for Health

It is becoming increasingly evident that many health problems are related to individual behavior. In the absence of dramatic breakthroughs in medical science the greatest potential for improving health is through changes in what people do and do not do to and for themselves. Household decisions concerning diet, exercise, smoking, drinking, work and recreation are of critical importance.

It is useful to distinguish between two different classes of decisions. The first consists of those that affect health, but without the decision maker's awareness of these effects. In such instances, public policies are needed to increase information. The question of how much of this activity can be justified can be answered (in principle) along the familiar lines of weighing incremental costs and benefits.

A more difficult problem is posed by those decisions that are made with full information available, and that, according to economists, reflect the household's "tastes." Tastes is a catchall term given by economists to the underlying preference patterns that determine demand at any given structure of income and prices. The overeater, the heavy smoker, the steady drinker are all presumably maximizing their utility, given their tastes. They may be knowingly shortening their lives. Should it be an object of public policy to try to change their tastes—to try to increase people's tastes for health? Economics can provide very little guidance in this area because economists have no way, even in principle, of saying what has happened to utility once tastes have changed. Economists are not, of course, alone in this

113

dilemma. None of the other social sciences has a well-developed theory of preference formation or the capacity to make judgments about the relative merits of different social goals.

The issues involved are extremely complex. Tastes are not acquired at birth or formed in a vacuum. It seems that economists should make an effort to determine how the working of the economic system itself influences tastes. They should study the impact of advertising and other sales efforts on demand, and try to determine whether taxation or subsidies of such efforts and counter efforts are justified. Tastes are also undoubtedly influenced by the information and entertainment media, by the schools, by religious institutions and by other organizations that are either tax supported, subsidized through tax exemptions or regulated by government to some degree.

Another way of thinking about this problem has been proposed by Gary Becker and Robert Michael.[25] In their approach, all households have the same basic wants or "tastes." They try to satisfy these basic wants by producing "commodities" with the aid of purchased goods and services plus inputs of their own time. Households differ greatly in their ability to produce different "commodities" and these differences explain much of the observed differences in purchases of goods and services in the market.

This approach has been developed and applied to health by Michael Grossman.[26] In his model it is the household, not the physician or the hospital, that produces health. Health care and other goods and services (food, shelter) are used in the production of health and some goods (e.g., cigarettes) may have negative effects.

If one pursues this approach, it could be a legitimate aim of public policy to help households become more efficient producers of health.[27] The chief ways of doing this would be through health education and by providing more information about the health care that is purchased in the market. It is of some interest to note that the United States government cur-

114

rently assumes more responsibility for informing consumers about the quality of steaks they buy than about the quality of hospitals or physicians they use.

Behavior Within Households and Firms

A significant shortcoming of the elementary model in analyzing health care is its treatment of the firm and the household as the basic elements of analysis. In recent years some economists have directed their attention to decision-making within the firm[28-30] and within the household.[2,31]

Attention to decision-making and allocation within the firm is particularly important if we are to try to understand one of the major institutions in health care, the nonprofit, voluntary hospital. It is relatively easy to identify several significant interest groups within the hospital—the board of directors, the management, the full-time medical staff, the attending staff—but it is more difficult to weigh their impact to formulate a predictive theory of hospital behavior. When the goals of the various interest groups are similar, the simple theory of the profit-maximizing firm may be adequate, but when they conflict, (e.g., the selection of cases for admission) such a theory is obviously incomplete.

Decision-making and allocation within the household also pose problems that have special relevance to health care. The quantity and quality of health care provided to children by parents differ greatly among households, even among households with equal incomes. The ability of parents to "produce" health for themselves and for their children seems to vary considerably. Society feels an obligation to protect the health rights of minors, but has found this difficult to do. The health care provided elderly parents by their children also varies greatly. The decline of family ties tends to shift some production of health care from households to firms, and part of the observed rising cost of health care in recent decades is undoubtedly attributable to such a shift; e.g., the growth of nursing homes.

115

This paper has discussed health care in relation to the economic system. The conference, however, is primarily concerned with technologic change, so it is appropriate to conclude with an attempt to relate the preceding discussion to technology.

Certainly the most important point to be made is that the basic economic principles concerning resource allocation and utility maximization apply in a world of technologic change as well as in a static one. Neither blanket endorsement nor condemnation of technology is rational; every change in technology involves costs and benefits and wise social policy depends upon an accurate assessment of their relative magnitudes.

There is a widespread belief that the health care sector harbors many wonderful technologic changes that have not been diffused widely and rapidly enough. An opposing view has been advanced by Richard Nelson of Yale, one of the nation's leading students of the economics of technologic change. He has written, "In both defense and health there has been a lot of R and D, and technical change has been extremely rapid; but it also has been extremely expensive and poorly screened . . . In health one has the strong impression that one of the reasons for rising health costs has been the proclivity of doctors and hospitals to adopt almost any plausible new thing—drugs, surgical methods, equipment—that increases capability in any dimension (and some for which even that isn't clear) without regard to cost."[32]

Nelson's view has considerable validity. The tendency toward rapid and indiscriminate adoption of innovations in the medical care field can be attributed in part to efforts of suppliers of the innovation, especially drug companies. Possibly the most important reason is the technologic imperative that influences medical choices.[33] This is instilled in physicians by their training, and reinforced by present systems of financing health care. It produces the attitude that if something can be done it should be done. Most medical decision-makers, be they physicians or hospital administrators, are not trained to weigh marginal benefits against marginal costs. Moreover, present methods of third party payment and provider reimbursement do not give them any inducement to acquire that ability. To be sure, patient pressure and the ethical imperative to do everything possible for the patient make this a complex problem. But a more rational approach could result in saving more lives and providing greater overall patient satisfaction.

Another popular misconception is that any change in health care technology that reduces labor requirements must be desirable. No such a priori assumption is warranted. A change in technology that is capital saving and labor intensive may be more valuable than the reverse, and a change that permits the substitution of two relatively unskilled workers for one highly skilled one may be more valuable than either.

The nature of technologic change can have profound effects on resource requirements, and some attention should be paid to this matter in granting funds for research and development. In choosing between two projects, for instance, it is not sufficient to consider only the importance of the problem and the probability of success. The granting agency should also consider what resources will be required to implement the solution if the project is successful.[34] Some technologic advances, such as the antibiotic drugs, greatly reduced the demand for physicians' services. Others, such as organ transplants, greatly increased demand.[35]

Traditional societies resist or inhibit technologic change. Society probably errs in the opposite direction. We seem to be fascinated by technology and often look to it to solve problems when less expensive solutions lie elsewhere. This may be particularly true of health care. It is to be hoped that this conference, with its emphasis on technology, will not serve to divert attention from other fundamental questions concerning the organization and financing of health care and personal responsibility for health.

Consider the problem of hospital costs. Hundreds of millions are being spent to make hospitals more efficient through new

117

technology, but the return is likely to be small compared to the savings possible now with existing technology through reductions in utilization. Most informed observers believe that on any given day approximately 20 per cent of the patients in the average general hospital do not need to be there. Research probably will prove this to be a conservative estimate because it still assumes customary medical interventions, conventional lengths of stay and so forth.

What, for instance, is the appropriate length of stay after hernia surgery? A British team, in a carefully controlled study, showed that patients discharged one day after surgery did as well as those discharged after six days. Another British team compared surgical repair of varicose veins with injection compression sclerotherapy. The former method involves expensive hospitalization; the latter is done on an outpatient basis at minimum cost. Outcomes seem to be similar, (except that surgical patients lost four times as many days from work) and patients seem to prefer the injection/compression technique.[36]

No reasonable person would want to inhibit the development of new technologies or their application to health problems. But everyone concerned with American health care should realize that the most pressing problems are not centered around technology and their solutions will probably be found in other directions. As this paper has suggested, we need to make health care markets work better; we need to quantify and control the externalities that affect health; and we need to recognize the importance of individual behavior and personal responsibility for health. Substantial alterations in organization, financing and education are required to achieve these objectives.

These are the realities. Tomorrow's technology may help to bring about these changes, but let us not underestimate what is possible today if we have the will to do it. Let us not oversell technology. Let us not divert attention and misdirect energies that could be devoted to the complex task of creating a more equitable, more effective and more efficient health care system.

REFERENCES

[1] Samuelson, P., ECONOMICS, New York, McGraw-Hill Book Company.

[2] Becker, G. S., A Theory of the Allocation of Time, *Economic Journal*, 75, September, 1965.

[3] Linder, S. B., THE HARRIED LEISURE CLASS, New York, Columbia University Press, 1970.

[4] Health might be measured by life expectancy, absence of disabilities, speed of recovery after surgery and so forth. Health care inputs might refer to the size of a health care program, or the total amount of care given to a particular patient or a particular aspect of care such as number of tests or number of days in the hospital.

[5] This assumes that some input—e.g., the state of technology—is fixed at any given point in time.

[6] This point is well recognized in the theoretical literature on socialist planning (cf., Lange, O., On the Economic Theory of Socialism, in Lippincott, B. E. (Editor), ON THE ECONOMIC THEORY OF SOCIALISM, Minneapolis, University of Minnesota Press, 1956) and in the attempts of the Soviet government and other East European governments to make greater use of the market mechanism.

[7] The flow of resources (and the reciprocal flow of goods and services) in the United States is currently at a rate of approximately one trillion dollars per annum. About seven per cent of these resources flow to "firms" producing health care. Fifteen years ago only about 4.5 per cent of such smaller resource flow went in that direction. The resource flow, measured in dollars, depends upon the quantities of various resources and their prices. Over long periods of time prices of equivalent resources usually change at about the same rate in all sectors of the economy. Thus the increased share in dollar terms reflects a substantial increase in the share of real resources as well. This large shift of resources over a relatively short period of time is the most important element in the present "health care crisis."

[8] The fact that these services proliferate contrary to what economies of scale would indicate is the result of other problems such as the absence of appropriate incentives and constraints for physicians and hospital administrators.

[9] Pauly, M. V. and Redisch, M., The Not-for-Profit Hospital as a Physicians' Cooperative, Northwestern University, 1969, mimeographed.

[10] Kessel, R. A., Price Discrimination in Medicine, *Journal of Law and Economics*, 1, October, 1958.

[11] Arrow, K. J., The Organization of Economic Activity: Issues Pertinent to the Choice of Market vs. Non-Market Allocations, in THE ANALYSIS AND EVALUATION OF PUBLIC EXPENDITURES: THE P.P.B. SYSTEM, Subcommittee on Economy in Government of the Joint Economic Committee, 91st Congress of the United States, First Session, Volume 1, p. 62.

[12] Feldstein, M. S., The Rising Price of Physicians' Services, *The Review of Economics and Statistics*, 52, 121–133, May, 1970.

[13] Hughes, E. F. X., Fuchs, V. R., Jacoby, J. and Lewit, E., Surgical Workloads in a Community Practice, *Surgery*, 71, 315–327, March, 1972.

119

[14] Altman, S. H., The Structure of Nursing Education and Its Impact on Supply, in Klarman, H. E. (Editor), EMPIRICAL STUDIES IN HEALTH ECONOMICS, Baltimore, The Johns Hopkins Press, 1970.

[15] Yett, D. E., The Chronic Shortage of Nurses: A Public Policy Dilemma, in Klarman, *op. cit.*

[16] For a pioneering article see Stigler, G., The Economics of Information, *Journal of Political Economy,* 69, 213–225, June, 1961.

[17] Benham, L., The Effect of Advertising on Prices, Chicago, Graduate School of Business, 1971, mimeographed.

[18] The firm or household will presumably equate *its* marginal cost and *its* marginal benefit. The social optimum requires taking into account the costs or benefits imposed on others.

[19] When medical care keeps an employed head of family alive and well, a type of external benefit is created because society does not have to provide for his or her dependents. Much medical care, however, goes to the young or the aged or to keeping people alive but not well enough to work so it is doubtful if on balance a positive externality exists in this sense.

[20] What would constitute a "fair" distribution of income has never been satisfactorily answered by economists or anyone else. One feature of the market system that makes it attractive to some is that a household's share of goods and services will be roughly proportional to its contribution to total output as evaluated by all households collectively.

[21] Note the analogy with the individual household's decision regarding vaccination.

[22] Pauly, M. V., MEDICAL CARE AT PUBLIC EXPENSE: A STUDY IN APPLIED WELFARE ECONOMICS, New York, Praeger Publishers, Inc., 1971.

[23] However, where medical care for the poor is tied to using them for teaching and research purposes, significant externalities are probably present.

[24] Lindsay, C. M., Medical Care and the Economics of Sharing, *Economica,* 36, November, 1969.

[25] Becker, G. S. and Michael, R. T., On the Theory of Consumer Demand, 1970, mimeographed.

[26] Grossman, M., THE DEMAND FOR HEALTH: A THEORETICAL AND EMPIRICAL INVESTIGATION, New York, National Bureau of Economic Research, in press.

[27] But there would be no a priori case for favoring health over other commodities. The choice should depend upon relative costs and benefits.

[28] Cyert, R. M. and March, J. G., The Behavioral Theory of the Firm: A Behavioral Science-Economics Amalgam, in Cooper, W. W. (Editor), NEW PERSPECTIVES IN ORGANIZATION RESEARCH, New York, John Wiley & Sons, Inc., 1964.

[29] Simon, H. A. New Developments in the Theory of the Firm, *American Economic Review,* 52, 1–15, May, 1962.

[30] Williamson, O. E., CORPORATE CONTROL AND BUSINESS BEHAVIOR, Englewood-Cliffs, New Jersey, Prentice-Hall, Inc., 1970.

120

[31] Gronau, R., The Intrafamily Allocation of Time: The Value of the Housewives' Time, paper presented at the National Bureau of Economic Research Conference on Research in Income and Wealth, 1971.

[32] Nelson, R. R., Issues and Suggestions for the Study of Industrial Organizations in a Regime of Rapid Technical Change, in Fuchs, V. R. (Editor), POLICY ISSUES AND RESEARCH OPPORTUNITIES IN INDUSTRIAL ORGANIZATION, New York, National Bureau of Economic Research, 1972.

[33] Fuchs, V. R., The Growing Demand for Medical Care, *New England Journal of Medicine*, 279, July 25, 1968.

[34] Weisbrod, B. A., Costs and Benefits of Medical Research: A Case Study of Poliomyelitis, *Journal of Political Economy*, 79, 527–544, May–June, 1971.

[35] Fuchs, V. R. and Kramer, M. J., The Market for Physicians' Services in the United States, 1948–68, 1971.

[36] Ford, G. R., Innovations in Care: Treatment of Hernia and Varicose Veins, in McLachlan, G .(Editor), PORTFOLIO FOR HEALTH, London, Oxford University Press for Nuffield Provincial Hospitals Trust, 1971.

ACKNOWLEDGMENTS

I am grateful to Barry Chiswick, Michael Grossman, Edward F. X. Hughes, Ben Klein, Marcia Kramer and Robert Michael for comments on an earlier version of this paper.

This article was prepared for a conference on Technology and Health Care Systems in the 1980's, sponsored by the National Center for Health Services Research and Development and held at San Francisco, California, January 19, 1972. It will also be published in the Proceedings of that conference.

RESEARCH ON THE DEMAND FOR HEALTH SERVICES

PAUL J. FELDSTEIN

INTRODUCTION

A Framework for Analysis

The sharp rise in the prices of medical care services and expenditures on medical care over the past 20 years has been the
major cause for concern over the adequate provision and financing
of health services.[1] If each person's consumption of medical care services were small and the prices charged for these services were low,
the welfare aspects of the problem would diminish as would the costs
of misallocation of medical care resources. Time could then be spent
analyzing other problems of concern to society. Unfortunately, the
converse is largely true. Therefore, to avoid costly errors in planning
and to minimize the hardships of any unmet needs, the factors
that influence prices and utlization in the medical care market must
be understood.

Interpreting the trend in health service usage and explaining variations in usage during any one year are difficult tasks. This paper
approaches these difficulties by dividing them into two areas: the
first is one of definition; the second is the development of an analytical
framework. Part of the observed variation in the utilization of
health services can be explained by changes in how services have been
defined and how their use has been measured over time. Adjusting
for changes in the product definition will not, however, explain
all the variations in use of health services. Therefore, a framework
must be developed to explain such variations.

123

This paper will describe an economic framework for explaining variations in the demand for health services. Lack of such a framework hinders, or even prevents a survey of the literature and research in this field to show where it fits in, on what parts of the framework knowledge is available and also where future research is needed. The framework should also serve as an aid in evaluating the findings of present research to the extent that such research does or does not incorporate into its analyses relevant parts of the framework.

A demand analysis is only one-half of the analysis needed to explain variations in the use of medical care services. If private expenditures for medical care services were plotted on a chart, using a series of points for the years, each point would be higher than the previous one. The height of a given point, or the magnitude of expenditures in any one year, is the result of many factors which the economist classifies according to those that affect the demand for care and those that affect the supply of care. To understand why the price of medical care is at a certain level or why the utilization of medical care is what it is, both the demand and supply factors must be known. A change in the quantity of medical care used between any two periods could result from a change in the demand for care, a change in the supply of care or, more likely, a change in both conditions. For example, if the number of persons covered by hospital insurance were to increase from one period to the next while all other factors remained constant, an increase in the demand for hospital care would be expected (assuming a positive causal relationship exists). If, however, along with this increase in insurance coverage changes occurred also in the costs of providing care, in the number and type of facilities and personnel, etc., then utilization in the next period would be difficult to predict. Changes are always occurring in the conditions affecting both the supply of care and the demand for care. The interaction of these sets of conditions determines the level of care provided in any period. Examining the factors affecting the demand for care, which this paper will do, is only one part of the problem of determining the health service utilization level and will not, by itself, enable a prediction of actual use to be made. A more complete study to explain the trends in utilization over the past 20 years would have to examine the changes in both demand and supply.

The Uses of Demand Analysis

Studies of demand generally have two purposes. The first is explanation; the ability to specify and estimate the relationship between use of a product or service and the factors influencing this use increases understanding of usage variations. Furthermore, identification and measurement of the "explanatory variables" are useful when formulating policies aimed at increasing or decreasing the use of services and also when assessments are being made on probable effects of public policy measures aimed at any of the explanatory factors.

The other important application of this kind of study is prediction of future demand. Forecasting utilization of medical care services depends essentially upon finding relationships between the variables to be forecasted and the other factors which determine the variables' magnitude. Projections are then made for the explanatory factors. These projections, when related to utilization, make possible an estimate of the demand for a future period. Such estimates can serve, for example, as guides for determining the number and types of personnel and the number of hospital beds or other medical care facilities needed in the future.

Demand and need for care are not necessarily the same. Need is the amount of care believed necessary by medical authorities while demand is the actual use of medical care services. Several factors account for discrepancies between the need and the demand for care. For instance, an individual may demand more care than is medically required. Conversely, he could be unaware of the value of medical care, or specialized facilities and services could be unavailable to him or he could be without the financial resources for the medical care he needs. Therefore, to plan for future use of a community's health facilities and personnel, the demand rather than the need for such resources must be projected. The need may be very great, but if it is not reflected in usage, facilities based on need will remain empty.

Private and "Public" Demand for Medical Care

The demand framework to be described does not cover a community's total demand for medical care. Excluded are aspects of demand involving externalities and indivisibilities. For example, certain services which can only be provided in large units, e.g., water fluoridation, are difficult, if not impossible, to purchase on an individual basis.

Moreover, the purchase of some services provides benefits to persons other than the purchasers, e.g., knowledge derived from medical research. Services of external or indivisible characteristics have traditionally been provided by governments through public health programs since, if left to the market, a smaller than optimal amount of such services might be provided. Although individual variations may occur in the demand for these services, the means by which they are provided and financed eliminate individual choice of usage. Hence, to incorporate this demand into the demand for personal health services would be incorrect. The role of the government should not be excluded completely from studies of the private demand for medical care, however. In addition to governmental provision of "public" goods, one may also find some public provision of what are normally considered private goods and services in medical care. Spending for personal health care by federal, state and local units of government totalled 6118.9 million dollars in the 1962–63 fiscal year. Of this amount, 4131.1 million, or 14 per cent, was allocated to programs which were not related to government employment.[2] Governmental provision of personal health care as a form of public assistance may be accomplished either through the existing medical care market, by means of subsidies, such as payments to a general hospital for welfare patients, or through the provision of such care outside the existing market, by the Veterans Administration, for example. Since the care being provided may be, to some extent, a substitute for care purchased by families and individuals, it should be included in the analysis of the demand for personal health services.

The way in which this care is provided—whether through subsidies or through direct provision of the services—will affect empirical estimates of the personal demand for health care. In either case, however, a complete model of the demand for medical care in the private sector should include the personal services aspects of public programs but exclude services, such as public health programs, which offer no individual choice other than the ballot box.

Expenditures on public health programs may be substituted to some extent for private health expenditures; e.g., the demand for private dental care is probably affected by water fluoridation. The decision to include public health programs in an analysis of the private demand for health services depends on the specific content and variety of public programs and on the study's level of aggregation. That is, a study of private demand for dental care in a community with water

126

fluoridation may exclude such a program. If, however, the study were being made in several communities, some with fluoridation and some without, the existence of fluoridation programs should be included in the analysis. (The choice in these situations is a collective choice.) Similarly, an analysis of private health services demand in different countries must allow for differences in expenditures on public programs when they may be substituted for private expenditures. This paper assumes that excluding public health programs that may be substituted for private expenditures has little or no effect on explaining variations in private demand.

THE PRODUCT—MEDICAL CARE

Until now, the general terms of supply and demand have been used for "health services." If the factors affecting the demand for health care are to be specified, a more precise definition of the "product" demanded must be found along with a better understanding of how the various components of care are used in its production. Furthermore, if empirical work on the estimation of demand is to be evaluated, more attention must be given to the interpretation of the various indices used to measure medical care demand.

Definition of the Product

Expenditures for medical care represent the purchase of a conglomeration of services. Drugs, hospital and physician care, for example, are all included. In empirical work, quality differences may not usually be distinguished in the same type of care or in differences in expenditures that reflect only differing amenities, such as private accommodations, that are not medically required. Medical care is not purchased merely for a hospital admission or a physician visit. Rather, it is purchased with the hope of receiving something more basic; good health. Good health, however, may also result from expenditures for food, clothing and housing. Thus, a more precise definition of "medical care" is needed.

One possible definition of the medical care product is that "medical care is the service consisting of the control and/or management of diseases (or other unwanted physical or mental conditions) be they actual or potential."[3] (Preventive care is included in this definition since it represents the management of a potential disease.) The different components of medical care services have traditionally been

127

analyzed separately without regard for the use of other components. According to the above definition, the components are used together when treating an illness and must therefore be considered both complementary and interchangeable. For example, hospital care may be used together with physician care in the treatment of an illness, and the two would thus be considered complementary. On the other hand, nursing home care and outpatient care may to some extent be substituted for hospital care.

Depending upon the degree to which components may be substituted for each other, analyses which examine the use of one care component without considering the extent to which the other components are used must be held incomplete for the purpose of explaining usage variations in medical care or in any one component of care. In many instances, the above definitional framework of the medical care product would have helped explain apparent differences in hospital use. Since a patient may be treated for an illness with different combinations of hospital care, physician visits, etc., different lengths of hospital stay may conceivably represent use of the other components of care in varying proportions. That is, higher hospitalization rates may reflect relatively less use of the other "inputs" in the production of a treatment. The reason for relatively greater use of some components will be discussed below. However, without consideration of all the components of care used in a particular treatment, conclusions cannot be drawn regarding the "proper" amount of care received from one component. To explain variations in that component's use would also be impossible if the factors influencing the relative mix of a treatment's components are not explicitly included in the analysis.[4]

Thus, to have as precise a definition of medical care as possible is important. In addition to using this definition to analyze the differential usage rates of any care component, the definition facilitates an explanation (and prediction) of what will happen when a change occurs in any of the factors affecting the demand for care. For example, if economic resources increase, are treatments of a different type demanded, or is an increase in the quality of treatment demanded? Which components will be used more? Although empirical problems are involved in holding the distribution of illness constant and measuring changes in treatment quality, a theoretical definition of medical care is still useful to see where current research fits in and whether any theoretical criticisms of the research can be made.

128

Measurement Problems

An empirical measure of medical care also becomes important when deriving estimates for the effect of the various factors that influence demand. Empirical measures of demand have generally been expressed as units of service such as hospital admissions, patient days, length of stay and physician visits. One writer has suggested that the appropriate dependent variable for medical care demand studies is the dollar amount a person spends, since for a given expenditure the physician will provide a set of components for treatment.[5] However, an empirical measure such as medical care expenditures may bias the effects of the factors believed to influence demand (prices and income), if it is not first adjusted for price changes and for changes in the product itself, e.g., quality changes. These problems, of developing a price index for medical care and adjusting for quality changes, are present in both time series and cross-section analyses.[6] For example, medical care expenditures are a combination of both the price charged for the treatment and the number of treatments purchased. If a rise in a patient's economic resources is accompanied by a rise in medical care expenditures, the latter may be merely the result of either an increase in the price to the patient or an increase in his consumption of comfort aspects. This would have different policy implications than an increased demand for treatments of higher quality or purchase of a different distribution of treatments.

The use of index number techniques in studies of medical care may help solve some problems. For instance, allowances might be made for the fact that the types of patients and the types of diseases being treated today are not the same as they were in the past. But a more important problem in arriving at an empirical measure of the product is eliminating differences in quality. For example, the results of a treatment for a particular illness today generally differ from the treatment results for that same illness ten or 15 years ago because the probability of recovery is greater, length of stay has been reduced or a lesser amount of other care is needed. An index of price changes over time, such as the medical care price index, that does not allow for these quality changes will greatly overestimate the price rise that has occurred and hence bias the estimates of the factors believed to affect demand. Measuring quality is not easy. A change in a person's chances of recovery from tuberculosis, for example, may take the form of a change in death rates from tuberculosis. Finer measurements would be desired, however, because some of those who would have died

129

from tuberculosis in the past may now contribute to an increase in the death rates from cardiovascular diseases. A change in death rates in one diagnostic category will generally affect the death rates in other categories.

Although measurement is difficult, a clear advantage may be gained by discussing the price of medical care in terms of treatment price, allowing for quality changes that have occurred, rather than by merely observing the changes in prices for the components of medical care.

Some research has been conducted on the measurement of medical care prices and on the estimation of quality changes. Scitovsky[7] has undertaken a study to price a treatment as a whole, rather than studying only one care component, such as room rates, as has been and still is the more usual approach. Griliches[8] has conducted a study in which he attempts to estimate the bias introduced in the automobile price index by an inadequate allowance for the changes in automobile quality over time. The estimation of quality change in medical care is a particularly difficult problem, but an attempt to estimate the extent to which the rise in medical care prices has been offset by changes in quality would be worthwhile. Several surveys of changes in the distribution of inputs for a treatment have been made. "Changing Patterns of Care"[9] was an attempt to measure the change in distribution of inputs for provision of hospital care over a 15-year period. Unfortunately, data on the other components of care (other than hospitals) were not available.

The purpose of this section has been to define more clearly the medical care product that is being demanded. When empirical demand studies are later described, attempts to explain variations in use of the components of care should be considered in terms of this definitional framework. When the theoretical definition, which may be difficult to measure empirically, is related to the various empirical measures presently being used, the definition itself may explain some of the observed variations in use and expenditures.

A FRAMEWORK FOR ANALYZING
DEMAND FOR HEALTH SERVICES

At any time innumerable factors may influence a person's decision to make an expenditure for medical care and the amount he spends. To investigate variations in utilization of medical care, the first step is to decide upon an approach. To gather data and analyze relationships in a meaningful way a "model," based on hypotheses about the expected relationships, could be constructed. Therefore, before discussing empirical research on factors affecting the demand for medical care, a framework will be described within which the empirical work may be placed. Assuming the framework to be an accurate skeletal model of the demand for medical care, a discussion of the work done to date should indicate the areas in which some knowledge exists of the underlying relationships and the area lacking information on the importance of certain relationships. To discuss research without reference to some such framework might result in placing too much emphasis on those areas in which more research has been conducted— not because that area is more important but because it is more easily subject to quantification or because particular disciplines were interested in it.

The economic framework to be developed does not exclude noneconomic factors, but it does attempt to distinguish between those factors that affect supply and those that affect demand. Both the demand and supply factors must be known to predict actual use, and a study of demand is a study of only one part of the complete model. With a knowledge of demand the net change in demand may be forecast if a change occurs in any one of the factors affecting demand while all else is unchanged. The value for all the demand and supply factors must be known to say what actual use will be.

The demand approach, simply stated, is that the demand for medical care is determined by several economic and cultural-demographic factors, prevailing medical practice, as well as the incidence of illness. Before developing this framework and all its interrelationships in greater detail, the "product" and the concept of "choice" in the medical care market should be discussed.

The demand for medical care is the demand for a treatment, and variations in demand are variations in either number of treatments or in their quality. Moreover, this demand is typically initiated by the patient. (For simplicity, those instances where a physician discovers new illnesses in a patient that has come for treatment of another condition are considered as patient-initiated.) The physician combines the "inputs"—his own services, hospital services, etc.—to provide a treatment of a given quality. The demand for these "inputs" then become "derived" demands; that is, they are determined largely by the initial demand for a treatment. For example, a patient does not demand prescription drugs; he demands treatment for an illness. In

131

treating this illness the physician is aware of the patient's financial resources and how much he can afford to spend, and this, in addition to the physician's medical knowledge (and other constraints to be discussed), influences the kinds of "inputs" he will prescribe. If the physician decides home care and drugs would be a better alternative than prolonged hospital care, he will then prescribe the necessary drugs.

Therefore, empirical demand studies should first describe the manner in which different factors affect the patient's demand for medical care, and secondly, how the physician then decides what care components to use in caring for the patient. (Although the patient and physician phase is discussed sequentially, they occur at the same time.) Once this general process or framework has been described, an estimate should then be made of the various relationships between these factors and utilization of medical care. For example, how important are the patient's financial resources as a factor in determining the components of care to be used in treatment, or what is the impact of the extent of the physician's knowledge of the efficiency of various forms of treatment on his choice of care components? The empirical research, then, is the estimation of the above theoretical relationships of the demand for care.

Assumptions Underlying an Economic Approach: the Role of Choice in the Medical Care Market

Implicit in studies of demand is the assumption of choice. In studies of the demand for medical care, the element of choice exists both in the amount of medical care purchased and in the way which the components of care are combined to produce a given treatment. If choice in these areas were not possible, much less variation would be expected in the use of medical care in relation to economic factors, e.g., income and prices, and less variation in the manner in which a treatment is provided.

The degree of choice, whether on the part of the patient or his physician, depends on two factors—knowledge and the availability of substitutes. If a person were cognizant of the benefits from annual checkups or good dental hygiene, for example, his utilization of these services would be different, other things being equal, than if he did not have the knowledge. (Similarly, he may incorrectly attribute too great a benefit to some forms of treatment; however, this would increase the observed variations in use, which is the interest of this

132

paper.) People often assume that no close substitutes for medical care exist. Even if this is true, families may still differ in their use of these services because they attach different values to the expected benefits of increased use and/or have varying knowledge of these benefits.

When discussing the degree of choice exhibited by the physician, remember that the physician, not the patient, combines the components of care into a treatment. In other markets the consumer, with varying degrees of knowledge selects the goods and services he desires from the available alternatives. In medical care, however, the patient does not usually make this choice directly. He does not usually decide, for example, which hospital he is to enter nor the form of treatment he is to receive; instead, he selects a physician who then makes these choices for him. Presumably, the physician has an element of choice available to him that produces observed variations in usage. Medical practice differs among doctors, as does their knowledge of the benefits of certain treatments. These differences, however, are not great enough in themselves to enable one to relate patient characteristics to variations in use. Another assumption is necessary, namely that the physician is cognizant of the patient's financial resources as well as of his medical needs, and thus acts in a manner consistent with the way the patient would behave if he were able to make the decisions. Evidence that this assumption is not wholly unrealistic may be seen from the numerous studies that relate hospital utilization to economic resources such as insurance coverage.

Implicit in the above assumption concerning the behavior of the physician is the belief that, in producing a form of treatment for the patient, he combines the components of care, depending upon their availability (closeness of substitutes) and their cost to the patient and to himself, to produce a treatment that is relatively low in cost to both the patient and himself. Also, the physician is assumed to be aware not only of the patient's needs and resources, but also of the various ways of combining the components of care to produce given treatments. Further, the physician presumably is cognizant of the increase in benefits that may be expected from an increase in use of any component, and he combines these components with regard to their relative cost to both the patient (insurance coverage, for example, would affect the relative prices to a patient) and to himself. (He would not combine components to result in the lowest cost to the patient if that combination increased his costs.)

133

In the studies that follow, these assumptions of choice in the medical care market need not be as clear-cut as described above each time a patient sees a physician and each time a physician treats a patient. However, to the extent that the above choices do exist and the physician acts with regard to the patient's financial resources, a greater empirical relationship should be observed between the patient's economic variables (financial resources) and utilization of medical care services. Further, a closer correlation may be expected between usage and economic variables if the following occurs: 1. knowledge of medical benefits to the patient and to the physician increases (the physician is able to combine the components of care differently with increased knowledge); 2. closer substitutes to be used in treatment are developed, e.g., the trend to use nursing homes as a partial substitute for hospital care.

Needless to say, much of the discussion of choice and the extent to which it exists is speculative. However, studies in this area would profitably increase understanding of the assumptions which are relevant to much empirical work and certainly to questions of public policy.[10]

The general framework of the demand for medical care within which the empirical research will be discussed is presented in Table 1.

TABLE 1. A MODEL OF DEMAND FOR MEDICAL CARE

Patient	Physician	Derived Demands for the Components of Care
Factors affecting a patient's demand for treatments	Factors affecting a physician's use of the components of care	hospital care physician care
Incidence of Illness Cultural-demographic factors Economic factors	Patient characteristics includes relative cost to the patient from using different components of care Institutional Arrangements Physician's knowledge Relative costs to the physician from using alternative sets of components of care	referrals to specialists nursing home care etc.

Briefly stated, the first phase is the patient's demand for care which is influenced by a number of factors, some of which imply an element of choice. The second phase involves the physician combining the inputs to produce a treatment. The way in which he uses these

134

components is also determined by several factors, some of which also imply an element of choice available to him. In arriving at the demand for any one of the components of care, therefore, both the patient and physician influences must be considered. As a means of further describing this multifaceted process that results in the demand for medical care and for each of its components, each facet will be discussed together with some research findings to indicate the influence of some of the factors involved.

Factors Affecting the Patient's Demand for Medical Care

The factors that affect a patient's demand for medical care may be generally categorized as incidence of illness, cultural-demographic characteristics and economic factors.

The first two of these factors may be considered to shape a family's "desire" for medical care, and depend primarily upon the family's perception of a health deficiency and belief in the efficacy of medical treatment. In translating this desire into expenditure, the family is limited by the extent of its financial resources, as care cannot generally be obtained free of charge. Determining the amount to be spent for personal health services, then, becomes a part of the problem of allocating scarce financial resources among alternative desires. The amount spent would thus partially depend on the amount of income and wealth available and also on the price of medical care relative to the prices of other goods and services.

Medical care has been said to be solely a "need" rather than a "want" and economic considerations such as income and price therefore have little or no influence in determining the amount used. For care which is expected to substantially improve well-being and which can be obtained at a cost which does not strain a family's financial resources, this may well be the case. Often, however, the type of illness present and its prognosis are uncertain. For example, the distinction between a severe cold and pneumonia is not clear-cut, at least to the untrained mind. Chest pains may indicate either indigestion or a serious heart condition. In these and similar instances, income and price would be expected to affect decisions involving the purchase of medical care. Also, even after treatment is initiated, economic considerations may influence its extent. The gain from palliating the discomfort associated with a chronic condition will not always be worth the cost.

135

Each of these general categories that affect demand are more fully discussed below.

The incidence of illness. Need is generated by the incidence of illness while demand is generated by the interrelationship of illness with other factors.

The onset of illness and the use of the hospital is to many people an unexpected occurrence. Thus, for individuals, illness may be considered as a random event. However, for the population as a whole, illness has a fair degree of predictability, given certain characteristics of the population such as age, sex, etc. (Since age and sex are also demographic factors, a discussion of them is postponed until the next section.)

The concept of illness being considered as random among individuals but having greater predictability for population groups has been the basis for planning medical care services through the use of mortality rates, bed/population ratios, and physician/population ratios as indications of need. The use of incidence rates together with standards of care were used for developing standard ratios of facilities to population, and these ratios were then prescribed throughout the country.[11]

The unexpected nature of illness to individuals and the fluctuating or random element in demand on a day-to-day basis with respect to individual hospitals have prompted a number of studies that deal with predicting demand. Persons with a knowledge of operations research have reasoned that if they could ascertain the underlying probability distribution of "need" that best fits the utilization data, they will have developed an explanatory model as well as an accurate predictive device. Some interesting work in this area has been done in both the United States and the United Kingdom. These studies have used essentially the same technique for examining utilization in a hospital department as for examining the utilization of the hospital itself or the use of all the hospitals in a community.[12]

A basic assumption underlying the use of these studies in predictions of hospitalization is that admission is based on incidence of illness and that length of stay in the hospital, except for scheduling problems, is also based on medical necessity. If these studies were based on other assumptions, a stochastic distribution should not be used to describe or simulate it.

In a lecture before the Research Seminar in Hospital and Medical

Systems, Long made several points about the use of the random component of demand for planning hospital facilities. If at any time utilization is random, having large facilities brings certain economies. This random component should also be used for determining the number of beds to be built, for if facilities are built according to the mean expected level of use, the cost is a penalty of not being able to satisfy demand in excess of that mean level. This penalty cost will vary according to the community—the existing level of facilities, available substitutes, etc.—and will depend upon what the unsatisfied demand consists of, e.g., emergency versus elective cases. The optimum number of beds in a community is the point where the penalty cost to a community of not having an additional bed is equal to the long-run costs of adding an additional bed.

To be able to estimate what amount of medical care is solely a "need," i.e., may be considered as either emergent or urgent care, is important. If this quantity is very large in relation to the total demand for medical care, variations in medical care demand with reference to cultural-demographic and economic factors cannot be explained even with the possibility of determining why some components of care are used more in treatment.

Some studies attempt to estimate the size of this random element. According to the admission records of one particular hospital studied, patients classified as "emergent" (admitted immediately) and "urgent" (admitted within 24–48 hours) consisted of less than 20 per cent of the total admissions each month, the rest being classified as "elective" patients.[13] Anderson, reporting on a study of Massachusetts hospitals, said that, excluding maternity cases, 32 per cent of admissions were same-day emergency ones and 33 per cent were for illnesses that had been present for more than a year.[14]

The studies conducted by the operations researchers described above estimate the probability distribution of this random component with regard to only one componet of care—namely, hospitals. These studies are generally confined to a moment in time, that is, the other factors affecting demand are unchanged. In addition to the cultural-demographic and economic factors being constant, the factors affecting the physician's use of any components should also be considered as being constant. If these factors were to change, i.e., if the demand for medical care or the demand for any one component were to be examined over a period of years, using stochastic distributions could not explain variation as well as a method that holds other factors, such as patient and physician factors, constant and then fits a stochastic distribution to the unexplained variation.

Assuming a large random component in medical care has been the basis for many policy and planning decisions concerned with such matters, for example, as the location and size of facilities. Hence, the determination must be made of whether the nature and extent of this random component are changing. The percentage of total demand considered to be random is probably decreasing. This would be expected as the discretionary amount spent on medical care increases. If this is the case, then limiting the size of the hospital for reasons of accessibility decreases in importance, and greater advantage may be taken of economies of scale. Also, the cost of maintaining peak-period facilities and the means by which they are financed, might be re-examined.

Cultural-demographic factors. Cultural-demographic factors affecting a patient's demand for medical care represent physiological condition, perception of illness and attitudes toward seeking medical care. Since these factors can seldom be measured directly, specific population characteristics are substituted as indicators. Some of the characteristics commonly used in demand studies are age, sex, marital status, family size, education and residence (urban or rural). Differences in utilization of medical care services according to these characteristics have been documented in a number of studies. The relationship between the characteristics and the utilization of the various components of care, however, has not necessarily been similar. For example, the relationship between age and utilization of hospital services is different from that between age and utilization of dental services. A difference also exists in the relationship of the various characteristics to hospital admissions and lengths of stay. Although these population characteristics may not affect each of the components of health services in the same way, they are important in explaining variations in use of these services.

As individuals age, incidence of illness increases and morbidity patterns change; accidental injuries and chronic diseases become more frequent causes of death.[15] In considering the average difference in utilization of health care services between men and women, both marital status and age must be taken into account. Medical care expenditures are approximately the same for both sexes in the early years of life. Later on, the expenditures incurred by women exceed those incurred by men, mainly because of obstetrical charges. The

138

difference persists, however, far beyond the normal child-bearing age. Also, the relationship between age and use of medical care services is not a simple linear one. Tables reproduced from the various surveys would show the relationship between all the cultural-demographic factors mentioned and the utilization of each component of care with the different measures used for each category. However, because, for instance, hospital care may be represented by expenditures on hospitals, number of admissions, patient days and length of stay, reproducing such tables would not be feasible. Instead, the interested reader is referred to the original sources for such information.[16]

Marital status is also considered to affect the consumption of certain components of medical care. For example, unmarried persons generally consume more total days of hospital care than married persons. The availability of persons in the home to care for married persons may account for their using the hospital less.

Together with marital status, the size of the family will be an important influence on demand. The increase in demand, however, is not expected to be proportional to the number of persons in the family. Also important in the use of the various components of care is the age distribution of the family members.

A direct correspondence does not necessarily exist between physiological condition and desire for medical care. An actual need for care may not be perceived in some instances, while a nonexistent or imaginary "need" may be perceived in others. Also, a recognized health deficiency may not be translated directly into expenditure because of variations in disposition toward risk-taking and differences in belief in the effectiveness of medical treatment. Variables which might explain these factors include education and area of residence. Whether the prompt translation of physiological need to medical care spending results in higher or lower ultimate demand for medical care is difficult to foretell. A person who is well aware of the dangers of ill health and is desirous of treatment is likely to incur relatively large expenditures for preventive services, but may incur lower expenditures for treatment of morbid physiological conditions because they have been prevented. On the other hand, one who tends to ignore the symptoms of disease will have low expenditures for preventive services and care of noncritical conditions, but may well spend more for treatment in the long run (unless he succeeds in avoiding medical care entirely).

The interest of this paper is not in developing a theoretical model

139

of demand that will explain variations in demand for each individual family. Innumerable factors determine whether or not a person seeks medical care, the type of medical care he selects and the amount of medical care he uses. Demand studies do not attempt to specify all the many factors that might be important in individual cases; rather, they attempt to relate only those factors that are considered on the average to be most important in influencing usage of medical care services. For this reason the above list of factors has been kept fairly short.

Much of the knowledge of the factors affecting the use of health services has come from survey data. These data are usually presented by classifying utilization of a component according to some population characteristics. The ability to cross-classify tables according to more than one population characteristic or to use one characteristic in greater detail, e.g., an age breakdown for both males and females, increases understanding of the net effect of a particular factor on utilization. However, gross relationships between variables are generally presented because detailed subclassifications are limited by the size of the page and the reader's ability to comprehend them. Only within the last few years has a statistical technique long in use in other fields been applied to the interpretation of utilization data. This technique, multivariate analysis, holds promise to enable the determination of the net effect of any one characteristic on utilization.

A number of studies have used this technique on survey data and derived estimates of the effects of some cultural-demographic variables on utilization. The purpose of these studies was to determine the effect of a particular variable on utilization while holding constant the effects of other variables. The studies have been conducted for total medical care expenditures for a particular component of care, as well as for subclassifications within a component, such as pediatric, obstetric or medical-surgical utilization in a hospital, and also for a finer breakdown such as hospital diagnosis.[17]

Multivariate studies have been few and have differed widely with regard to the variables included, the method by which the same variables were represented, the data used, the components of care studied, etc. Therefore, the results on the net effects of the variables studied cannot be used with any high degree of confidence. More multivariate studies, however, would be very worthwhile, and greater consensus on the effects of the particular variables might be reached in a few years.

140

Though determining the effect of cultural-demographic factors on use of health services is important to increase understanding, cultural-demographic factors are not usually subject to sudden changes. The age composition changes gradually, and abrupt changes in cultural-demographic factors are unlikely over short periods of time. Also, for policy purposes, affecting utilization by changing these variables is difficult. With regard to the next set of factors to be discussed, information on their net effects can have more immediate value for policy and prediction.

Economic factors. Prices and income theoretically affect not only a person's decision whether or not to seek medical care, but also the extent of the care once treatment is undertaken. For example, the effect of prices or of income may or may not have much effect on whether or not a maternity patient goes to the hospital (although it may influence the choice of hospital), but once she has been admitted, it may affect the length of her stay.

Economic theory hypothesizes that, other things being equal, the consumption of any commodity or service varies inversely with the price of the service. That is, as the price of the service is lowered, consumption increases. As applied to the discussion of the cultural-demographic factors, however, not only the direction but also the extent of the effect of a price change must be known. Economists use the term "elasticity" to indicate the responsiveness of changes in consumption to a change in one of the factors affecting consumption. An estimate of elasticity greater than one means that the percentage change in consumption will be greater than the percentage change in the factor that brought about this change. An estimate of zero elasticity means that consumption of a particular service is unaffected by changes in the factor being studied.

Those in the health field have generally assumed that changes in prices have little effect on the use of medical care services. That is, price elasticity is considered to be less than one because of the few substitutes for medical care. Adequate data to test this belief have been lacking. To estimate a price effect empirically a "net" price variable must be used, that is, the "out-of-pocket" price to the patient and not the stated price. To arrive at this estimate, the effect of health insurance, "free" care and the tax deductibility aspects would first have to be eliminated, for these factors actually reduce the price the patient pays for services. Some of the empirical demand studies have used a price variable in their analyses, and their findings show

141

that the price elasticity of the components of care studied is much less than one. However, these results may be criticized on the grounds that the price variable was either not a true "net" price to the patient,[18] or that the manner used for constructing a "net" price to the patient had biased the derived estimates.[19]

In theory, health insurance acts as a proxy price variable, i.e., it lowers the price the patient pays for the covered service. Insurance will therefore have two effects: 1. it reduces the over-all price of medical care to the patient with insurance, hence increasing his consumption of medical care services (this is an "income" effect), and 2. it causes components of care that are covered to be substituted for those that are not (this is the "price" effect). Both these effects are difficult to empirically measure.

A number of studies have related the existence of health insurance in one form or another to the use of health services, primarily hospitals. These studies have varied in their degree of sophistication from single cross-tabulations of how much persons with and persons without insurance use hospitals, to studies attempting to adjust insurance by its benefit structure and to hold constant the effects of other cultural-demographic and economic factors believed to have an effect on utilization. Generally these studies show that insurance is positively related to both medical care expenditures and hospital use, but that the elasticity of insurance with respect to both is less than one.

In some empirical studies in this area, economic and cultural-demographic variables have been related to the different components of care, and different measures, such as admissions, length of stay and total patient days, have been used to represent hospitalization. The effect of the factors representing patient characteristics will differ according to which variables are used to represent hospitalization. For example, Cardwell, Reid and Shain[20] found that the birth rate now largely determines the obstetrical admission rate, but that economic factors exert the most influence on how long women stay in the hospital after childbirth.[21]

A number of questions are still unanswered, and further research in this area would be fruitful. For example, is the relationship between insurance and utilization in fact a causal one, or do persons who expect to use health services buy health insurance? Also, since age, education, income, etc., are correlated with the holding of insurance, determining the net effect of insurance on utilization is difficult. Part of the so-called insurance effect may really be the effect of these other factors. Further, how large are the substitution effects between use of the components of care according to the range of insurance benefits?

In empirical studies of the demand for medical care, the price effect must be eliminated to derive accurate estimates of the effects of the other factors influencing demand, such as income. This is because of the relation between pricing practices and income in the provision of medical services. The use of the "sliding-scale" in setting fees, as well as other price-related factors such as "free" care, health insurance and tax deductibility of medical expenditures, are examples.[22]

If those in higher income groups pay higher prices for the same services, and if higher prices result in greater expenditures (and expenditures are used as a proxy measure for quantity), then estimates of the income effect based on expenditure data will be biased upward. Statistical evidence of the effect of the sliding scale on prices paid by those at different income levels is lacking, probably because differences in prices are difficult to separate from variations in the amount of service and amenity received. Medical care cannot easily be considered a service of homogeneous quality, and therefore, even with similar "quantities" of service, a person with a relatively high income paying a higher price may be receiving a somewhat different product. Because of this element of "trading-up," income elasticities calculated from expenditure data will result in higher estimates than elasticities based on quantities as they are usually measured, e.g., dental visits.

The relationship between family income and consumption of medical care services has been examined in a number of studies. In general, these studies indicate that families with higher incomes have higher expenditures—signifying higher consumption—for medical care, but the percentage of income spent on medical care decreases with higher levels of income. In other words, the consensus of these surveys and multivariate analyses is that the income elasticity is less than one.[23] The paper by Feldstein and Carr[24] contains a summary of the income-expenditure relationships derived from a number of surveys. For a number of such surveys, from 1917 to 1960, income elasticity was estimated by means of regression analysis and summarized in that paper. The calculated estimates from these surveys all indicate an income elasticity of less than one. A number of other studies have calculated the relation between income and medical care expenditures or between income and some component of care. Many of the studies, however, are not comparable with regard to the data used, components of care studied, technique used, etc.[25]

The manner in which family income is measured must be understood if the estimate of the effect of income derived from surveys and analyses in the health field is to be interpreted correctly. A family's income in any given year may be abnormally low or high because of temporary loss of employment, windfall gains or other unexpected events. Empirical evidence suggests that total consumption (that is, the use of products and services) is not generally raised or lowered to correspond with temporary changes in income. Rather, a family's level of consumption is determined primarily by its expected normal or "permanent" income.[26] Nearly all categories of consumption, including the total, probably exhibit this unresponsiveness to temporary fluctuations in income.

In general, then, transitory income is hypothesized to have little or no effect on the consumption level. Thus, if all income differences were transitory and people spent only according to their permanent incomes, no relationship between income and expenditures for medical care could be found. On the other hand, if incomes differed but contained no transitory components, the regression line would approximate the effect of normal income. Empirical observations of incomes of individual families are mixtures of normal and transitory components. Regression lines fitted to them will therefore lie somewhere between these two extremes. In terms of Figure 1, the slope of a line based on reported income (AA) would be less steep than the slope of a line based on normal income (BB), but steeper than the nearly horizontal line which would be derived from data containing only transitory income differences (CC).

Another way of looking at this is to consider the distribution of the transitory components of income. One postulate of the permanent-income theory is that transitory income is not correlated with normal income. Therefore, families with negative transitory incomes (e.g., people who are sick are likely to be below their "normal" income) are most likely to be found in the lower portion of the distribution of reported incomes, while those with positive transitory incomes most probably lie in the upper part. In terms of normal income, incomes in the lower portion of the distribution thus tend to be understated while those in the upper part are likely to be overstated. To this extent, a regression analysis of expenditures and total income will underestimate the effect of differences in normal income on medical care spending. (Random errors in the amount of income reported will also bias the income expenditure regression in the same direction as differences

144

FIGURE 1.

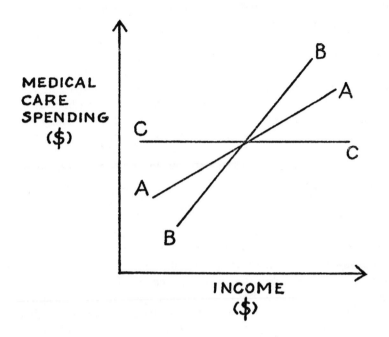

in transitory income because they affect the level of income reported but not the level of expenditure.)

The relationship presented by survey data and by multivariate analyses compares medical care expenditures with total income, which includes both permanent and transitory components. A more useful estimate would be based on the relationship between expenditures and normal (permanent) income alone. Since transitory income is included in the income variable, but presumably has little effect on the level of expenditure, the indicated relationships presented in the above mentioned analyses provide a biased estimate of the effect of normal income on medical care spending. Therefore, removing the effects of transitory income would considerably improve estimates of the effect of normal income.

Another important income-related consideration is that physiological condition may affect both expenditure and income. Illness may result in higher medical care spending and, at the same time, reduce family income by causing the disability of a wage earner. This may occur in either the permanent or transitory sense. In both cases, the result is to lower the measured effect of income on medical care spending. To the extent that physiological condition does not depend upon income, it should be held constant among income groups in calculating the income-expenditure relationship, or else income estimates based on family survey data will also be biased downward by this factor.

Another factor which must be taken into account in analyzing the income effect is that employer and other third-party contributions to health insurance premiums are not normally included in family expenditure data. To determine the over-all elasticity of private medical care spending, these expenditures must be included in the analysis. Although spending for group plans is probably fairly independent of individual families' incomes within a given plant or company, the average income of the group as a whole exhibits a strong influence on third-party expenditures for health insurance. In addition, tax considerations provide an incentive for increased employer contributions at higher average levels. Employers' contributions toward the payment of health insurance premiums do not constitute taxable income to the recipients. Thus, the higher the average income tax bracket, the larger the potential tax saving to the employee and the greater his incentive to have payments made by the employer. Rice has estimated that roughly one-half of total health insurance premiums are paid by third parties, and that the income elasticity of third-party payments must be much greater than one. To some extent, these employer contributions act as substitutes for family payments. Any estimate of the over-all income elasticity of medical care spending will therefore be biased downward if third-party payments of health insurance premiums are not included. The bias would be expected to be even greater in recent years because the percentage of private medical care expenditures accounted for by insurance rose from 12.8 in 1950, to 29.7 per cent in 1960.[27]

In the study by Feldstein and Carr, in which the effect of transitory income and the growth in health insurance enrollment were allowed for, the estimate of income elasticity increased to approximately one. In other words, the percentage of income spent on medical care is approximately constant at higher levels of income. These conclusions, which differ from those presented earlier, must still be considered tentative since the effect of prices and price-related factors correlated with income could not be completely eliminated.[28]

Additional research on the effect of economic factors on use of medi-

146

cal care should be in two general areas. First, continued effort should be made to estimate the net effects of each economic factor on use. As the above discussion shows, difficulty lies not only in separating the effects of the economic factors from each other, as with prices, but also in separating them from the cultural-demographic factors. However, this separation must be accomplished to understand the effects of either the economic or the cultural-demographic factors on the use of health services. Second, further studies in this area should attempt to examine utilization in terms of the illnesses being treated at different income levels and to classify them according to their discretionary aspects. A shift in the distribution of illnesses with increased family income will have important policy implications with regard to financing health care.[29]

Factors Affecting the Physician's Use of the Components of Care

Earlier the hypothesis was made that the physician knows the patient's needs and financial resources and that, other things being equal, he acts as a purchaser for the patient. Therefore, the patient characteristics, both economic and cultural-demographic, are expected to be related to the use of medical care services. In other words, the physician is making the decisions that the patient would make if he had the knowledge to do so. In this role, the physician can be thought of as a firm combining the inputs (components of care) for producing a treatment. When choosing the components of care to be used in treatment, he will be guided not only by their efficacy in treatment but also by their relative prices to the patient. For example, if care in a nursing home could be substituted for additional care in a hospital but the patient's insurance coverage provides only for hospital care, the physician would probably provide care in the hospital, not in the nursing home. (Providing the set of components of care least expensive to the patient but not to the community may cause the physician to act against the interests of the community, as in the above example.) Though this behavior of the physician will be limited by factors to be discussed later, this assumption has enough basis in fact to be useful in predicting use of the other components if other factors are unchanged. An example of the discretion a physician can exercise in choosing alternatives to hospitalization is the following:

> Surgical admissions accounted for 49 per cent of the total, medical for 35 per cent, admissions for diagnostic tests for 14 per cent, and other sorts of admissions for the remaining 2 per cent . . . Physicians were . . . asked to

147

choose among four alternatives in the handling of each patient in an attempt to determine the size of the area of discretion open to them . . . Physicians felt that there was much less leeway in performing surgery outside of the hospital than for appropriate handling of medical patients and those admitted for diagnostic purposes: for 76, 46 and 45 per cent, respectively, of three categories of patients, hospital admission was absolutely necessary according to the admitting physician.[30]

Other forces affecting the physician, however, may prevent his using the set of components that would result in lowest cost to the patient. He may be limited by institutional arrangements. For example, if two hospitals in a community provide about the same care to their obstetrics patients, but one hospital is more expensive than the other, unless the physician has a staff appointment at the lower-priced hospital, his obstetrics patient will be limited to the more expensive one.[31]

Another factor which will limit a physician in providing his patient with a set of components at lowest cost is the extent of his knowledge of different methods of treatment. For example, if recent developments suggest that patients should be ambulatory in shorter time, but the physician is not aware of these developments, he will probably keep his patient in the hospital longer than is necessary.[32]

Further, some hospitals have sanctions preventing the physician from prolonging a patient's stay unnecessarily when other forms of care are available, e.g., utilization committees reviewing admissions and length of stay for each of the physicians on the staff. If this occurs, little relationship could be observed between the patient's economic characteristics and the use of the components of care.[33]

Another factor not explicitly mentioned above greatly affects the manner in which the physician uses the components of care. Presumably, if certain institutional arrangements, the physician's knowledge, and possible sanctions were not present, the physician would combine the components of care in a manner to produce a treatment at lowest cost to the patient. Therefore, one would expect patient characteristics and the demand for medical care and its components to be closely related. However, in combining the components of care, the physician is acting not only in the patient's interest but also in his own. Since physician care is also a component of treatment, the extent to which this care is used depends not only on the patient characteristics and patient cost for this care relative to alternative combinations, but also on the cost (implicit or otherwise) to the physician of using relatively more or less of his care. For example, if hospitals were

148

to lower their weekend rates drastically to raise the occupancy over this period (assuming staff costs are similar for both weekend and weekday use), the physician could, in elective cases, reduce the patient's hospital bill by admitting him over the weekend. However, the cost to the physician must be considered in terms of loss of leisure time if he is required to work over the weekend to achieve a lower hospital bill to the patient. The result might actually be a higher *total* bill to the patient, if the physician charges him a higher rate for his own loss of leisure.[34]

Different forms of organizing medical care have their affect on the manner in which physicians use the components of care. To affect a lower total cost of care to the community, new forms of organization must first enable the physician to produce care of given quality with lower cost components, e.g., to substitute outpatient care for hospitalization when medically possible. At the same time, organization forms must allow the physician to act in the patient's interest, e.g., to substitute insured for uninsured services. Second, they must not change the relative cost to the physician for using a new set of components of care unless the change is downward, e.g., by requiring less of his time, increasing his convenience of performing his tasks, increasing his productivity, resulting in economies of scale, etc. The important point is that if a change in organization is to be accepted, it must result in a lower cost to the patient, the physician or both.

Therefore, the effect of both prepaid group practice plans, and also increases in the availability of facilities, is largely through their effect on the costs to either the patient or the physician. The use of specific components of care will be influenced by changes in their relative costs. Studies of the effect that prepaid group practice has had on hospital utilization and on the other components of care have been subject to varying interpretations because of the difficulty in examining organizational structure's net effect on use, while holding constant insurance coverage changes and the resultant additional case finding by physician.[35]

As for the availability of facilities, the question whether changes in the supply of beds affect the demand for them or whether beds are built essentially in response to changes in demand has been much discussed.[36] The author's opinion is that increases in bed supply affect the relative cost to the physician for providing care. For example, if other influences, such as the patient's financial resources, are constant, then an increase in the bed supply in an area with few physicians will probably

149

increase the physician's use of the hospital. The physician will substitute hospital beds for his own time in treating the patient because he can see more patients in a given time.

The point here is that patient characteristics, such as economic and cultural-demographic factors, influence the amount and type of medical care a physician will prescribe. The effects of these factors, however, are muted by institutional arrangements, the extent of the physician's knowledge and possible sanctions against him. An important factor which will also influence his behavior in use of the components of care is the relative costs to himself. Therefore, he will tend to substitute some components for others according to his own needs or convenience. In this latter context organizational arrangements may have, and accessibility of beds will have, their effect. (In addition to the above explanation on the effect changes in bed supply have on hospital use, beds also set an upper limit to use. Other increases in bed supply either are responses to an already present demand or would have resulted given the trend in demand over time. For these reasons bed supply was not included as a separate factor affecting demand, as some persons might suggest.)

CONCLUSION

This paper has presented a framework for analyzing the factors affecting people's demand for medical care and for its components. Within this framework, previous research has been surveyed to show where, in this writer's opinion, research fits into the over-all model and also to indicate the sections of the framework with little or no knowledge of the theoretical relationships.

Others may well suggest modifications in the proposed framework. Such suggestions are welcome, for unless a researcher has an understanding of the over-all set of relationships that are assumed to exist, his study may exclude relevant relationships, or he may concentrate on a relatively insignificant aspect of the problem. Apparently, in this age when computers and bountiful sums of money are available for data collection, less effort is spent on specifying in advance the theoretical relationships and their interrelationship. Because of this, studies of demand for health care are by themselves incomplete. To achieve a more complete understanding of why use of health services is at a certain level and why it is changing, all the demand relationships must be specified and a framework for explaining variations in the conditions affecting supply must be developed. Additional work will hopefully be directed toward developing a more complete general model of the market for medical care services and of the factors causing changes in both the amount of services provided and their prices. (In the framework presented, the economic factors have been emphasized. Economic incentives are strong even in medical care. Also, economic factors are relatively easier to affect, and they will respond much more quickly when changes are desired in the use or the provision of services.)

Once a set of hypotheses has been developed, the next step is to collect data on them and test them. One way to collect data to test the framework is presented here; namely, to study the entire treatment of an illness and not merely a hospital episode or the use of any particular component of care. Interest should be in the factors influencing the demand for treatments and, therefore, knowledge of what treatments are being demanded is necessary.

Unless the illness pattern and how it might shift with changes in income levels, for example, are known, whether future differences in expenditures between high- and low-income persons represent unfilled medical needs cannot be determined. Differences in expenditures on medical care may represent a shift from inelective to more discretionary utilization, or a shift to increased quality of care, or to more comfort, or differences may merely represent higher prices to the high-income family for essentially the same care.

Even a study of only one component of care should consider the factors affecting the use of the other components that could be or are being used for treatment. Changes in economic variables, such as a change in insurance coverage of previously uncovered illnesses, may change either the patterns of use or the relative prices to the patient of the alternative forms of care. Therefore, the substitutability and complementary nature of the components of care must be known along with the effect that changes in their relative prices have on component usage, and the factors influencing the physician in his use of these components.

Once data representing theoretical relationships have been collected, techniques of estimation should be used that will provide the net effects of any one factor on demand, while holding constant the effects of the other factors. The usual method of presenting survey data does not

151

accomplish this. When so many factors are interrelated, such as education, income, insurance coverage, etc., one cannot be certain which effect or combination of effects he is observing. Multivariate analyses are beginning to be used in health studies and the results look promising. A word of caution, however. Results derived by statistical techniques, no matter how highly sophisticated, cannot give substance to poorly formulated hypotheses and are no more reliable than the raw data. One further comment on the expected benefits from estimation techniques. Showing that a certain relationship exists is not enough. An estimate of the magnitude of the relationship is needed. For example, one must know, for policy and predictive purposes, not only that a given change in the insured population will cause a change in demand, but also how much the demand will change.

A final point in the discussion of the role and effect of information and knowledge on demand for health services: the demand for health services is dynamic. Progress in medical science increases the possible benefits from health care, while also changing the costs of providing services. Thus, empirical relationships may change drastically. One should know whether this information is transmitted to those making decisions on health care so that they may decide on the basis of the most complete knowledge possible. Consider this knowledge transmission in two areas. First, how informed is the practitioner of changes in medical practice and on the use of alternative forms of care in treatment? Rapid dissemination of information to the physician will enable him to produce better medical care at lowest cost to his patient and, hopefully, to the community. Also, to the extent that variations in use are a result of differences in information, increased information will decrease these variations. Second, what is the discrepancy between medical need and demand for care? To the extent that financial resources are not a constraint, an increase in information about the benefits of care would help reduce the difference between need and demand for medical treatment in circumstances in which the apparent benefits to the individual from undertaking such treatment greatly exceed the expected cost.

Further increases in medical knowledge and in its dissemination can only serve to increase the demand for health services in the future. Perhaps through greater use of preventive care and early diagnosis, the demand for certain forms of treatment will decrease; however, offsetting increases will probably occur in the demands for other treat-

152

ments, such as with chronic diseases and mental illness. New knowledge, however, and its widespread dissemination can help increase the choices available to the physician in providing care, and at least in this manner a given treatment may be provided at lowest cost.

REFERENCES

[1] Reed, Louis S., Private Consumer Expenditures for Medical Care and Voluntary Health Insurance, 1948–63, *Social Security Bulletin,* 27, 15, December, 1964.

[2] *See* Merriam, Ida C., Social Welfare Expenditures, 1963–64, *Social Security Bulletin,* 27, 10, October, 1964.

[3] Baer, D. V. T., The Economics of Medical Care, unpublished paper, March 20, 1963, p. 18.

[4] Another case in which failure to consider the components of care as being the inputs for a treatment, and hence substitutable, can lead to faulty reasoning is in interpretating the rise in hospital expenses per patient day. Part of this rise is merely a result of the fact that relatively more of the treatment is being provided in the hospital than formerly. If no other changes had occurred, a rise in the cost of the hospital component of care could be expected, while the total bill for the treatment remained the same.

[5] Friedman, M. and Kuznets, S., INCOME FROM INDEPENDENT PROFESSIONAL PRACTICE, New York, National Bureau of Economic Research, 1945, pp. 157–158.

[6] For a number of reasons time series analysis is of limited value for analyzing the demand for medical care. Historically, the trend reflects the influence of a multitude of factors which cannot be separated. A more promising approach for studies of medical care demand is cross-section analysis. By examining data for a cross-section of families in the same time period, the effect of factors influencing their expenditure over a wide range of values can be assessed while holding constant the state of technology and other conditions which change over time but cannot easily be quantified. The precision of the analysis is thereby increased and the complexities substantially reduced. The approach used in this paper is essentially cross-sectional.

[7] Scitovsky, Ann A., An Index on the Cost of Medical Care—A Proposed New Approach, *in* ECONOMICS OF HEALTH AND MEDICAL CARE, School of Public Health, Ann Arbor, The University of Michigan Press, 1964. *See also* the Comment by Margaret Reid in the same volume.

[8] Griliches, Zvi, Hedonic Price Indexes for Automobiles: An Econometric Analysis of Quality Change, *in* Joint Economic Committee hearings, Government Price Statistics, 87th Congress, May, 1961, pp. 173–196.

[9] Changing Patterns of Care, *in* REPORT OF THE COMMISSION ON COST OF MEDICAL CARE, Chicago, American Medical Association, Volume 4, 1964.

153

[10] The discussion of "choice," which is crucial to any economic analysis, may be criticized as being incomplete and an unrealistic approximation of behavior in medical care markets. Relevant to this is the following:

> A hypothesis is important if it "explains" much by little, that is, if it abstracts the common and crucial elements from the mass of complex and detailed circumstances surrounding the phenomena to be explained and permits valid predictions on the basis of this alone. . . . the relevant question to ask about the "assumptions" of a theory is not whether they are descriptively "realistic," for they never are, but whether they are sufficiently good approximations for the purposes at hand. And this question can be answered only by seeing whether the theory works, which means whether it yields sufficiently accurate predictions.

In Friedman, M., the Methodology of Positive Economics, in ESSAYS IN POSITIVE ECONOMICS, Chicago, The University of Chicago Press, 1953, pp. 14–15.

[11] Palmer, Jeanne, MEASURING BED NEEDS FOR GENERAL HOSPITALS: HISTORICAL REVIEW OF OPINIONS WITH ANNOTATED BIBLIOGRAPHY, Washington, United States Department of Health, Education and Welfare, Public Health Service, October, 1956, Mimeographed; Lee, R. I. and Jones, L. W., THE FUNDAMENTALS OF GOOD MEDICAL CARE, (Publication number 22 of the Committee on the Costs of Medical Care), Chicago, The University of Chicago Press, 1933; Lerner, Monroe, Mortality and Morbidity in the United States as Basic Indices of Health Needs, *Annals of the American Academy of Political and Social Science,* September, 1961.

[12] Thompson, John D. and Fetter, Robert B., Economics of the Maternity Service, *The Yale Journal of Biology and Medicine,* August, 1963; Newell, D. J., Statistical Aspects of the Demand for Maternity Beds, *Journal of the Royal Statistical Society,* 127, 1–40, 1964; Blumberg, Mark DPF Concept Helps Determine Bed Needs, *The Modern Hospital,* December, 1961; Young, John P., A Queuing Theory Approach to the Control of Hospital Inpatient Census, Johns Hopkins Hospital, Operations Research Division, July, 1962; Balintfy, Joseph L., Mathematical Models and Analysis of Certain Stochastic Processes in General Hospitals, Johns Hopkins University, Operations Research Division, 1962; ———, Outline of a Census-Predictor Model for General Hospitals, Tulane University, School of Business Administration, 1964 (unpublished); Bailey, Norman T. J., Calculating the Scale of Inpatient Accommodations, in the Nuffield Provincial Hospitals Trust, TOWARDS A MEASURE OF MEDICAL CARE, London, the Oxford University Press, 1962; Robinson, G. H., *et al.*, A Simulation Model for the Evaluation of Scheduling Decision Rules for Hospital Elective Admissions, The Human Factors in Technology Research Group, Berkeley, The University of California, February, 1964; As an aside, some other predictive techniques should be briefly mentioned at this point. These techniques are not explanatory approaches, but merely predictive devices. Fitting trends to utilization ratios has been suggested for use in planning health facilities and for estimating manpower requirements. The use of trend data for predictive purposes says little as to the underlying reasons for utilization. Examples of such methods may be found in: Division of Hospital and Medical Facilities, AREAWIDE PLANNING MANUAL FOR HOSPITALS AND RELATED HEALTH FACILITIES, Washington, United States Department of Health, Education and Welfare, Public Health Service, August, 1962; Cardwell, Rosson L., How to Measure Hospital Bed Needs, *The Modern Hospital,* 103, August, 1964; Some British Studies in this regard are: Forsyth, Gordon and Logan, Robert F. L., THE DEMAND FOR MEDICAL CARE, A STUDY OF THE CASE-LOAD IN THE BARROW AND FURNESS GROUP OF HOSPITALS, London, The Oxford University Press, 1960; Airth, A. D. and Newell, D. J., THE DEMAND FOR HOSPITAL BEDS, RESULTS OF AN ENQUIRY ON TEE-SIDE, Newcastle on Tyne, Kings College, 1961; Newell, David

J., Problems in Estimating the Demand for Hospital Beds, *Journal of Chronic Diseases*, 17, September, 1964; Brotherston, J. H. F., CONFERENCE ON RESEARCH IN HOSPITAL USE, Publication number 930-E-2, Washington, United States Department of Health, Education and Welfare, 1963.

[13] Feldstein, Paul, A Note on the Pricing of Hospital Services, *in* AN EMPIRICAL INVESTIGATION OF THE MARGINAL COST OF HOSPITAL SERVICES, Graduate Program in Hospital Administration, Chicago, University of Chicago Press, 1961, p. 67.

[14] Division of Hospital and Medical Facilities, CONFERENCE ON RESEARCH IN HOSPITAL USE, Publication number 930-E-2, Washington, United States Department of Health, Education and Welfare, Public Health Service, 1962.

[15] United States National Center for Health Statistics, THE CHANGE IN MORTALITY TREND IN THE UNITED STATES, Washington, United States Department of Health, Education and Welfare, Public Health Service, Publication number 1000, March, 1964, pp. 10–36.

[16] Falk, I. S., Klem, Margaret C. and Sinai, Nathan, THE INCIDENCE OF ILLNESS AND THE RECEIPT AND COSTS OF MEDICAL CARE AMONG REPRESENTATIVE FAMILIES: EXPERIENCES IN TWELVE CONSECUTIVE MONTHS DURING 1928–1931, Publication number 26 of the Committee on the Costs of Medical Care, Chicago, University of Chicago Press, 1933; Anderson, Odin W. and Feldman, Jacob J., FAMILY MEDICAL COSTS AND VOLUNTARY HEALTH INSURANCE: A NATIONWIDE SURVEY, New York, McGraw-Hill Book Company, 1956; Anderson, Odin W., Collette, Patricia and Feldman, Jacob, CHANGES IN FAMILY MEDICAL CARE EXPENDITURES: A FIVE-YEAR RESURVEY, Cambridge, Harvard University Press, 1963; United States Department of Health, Education and Welfare, National Health Survey, HOSPITAL DISCHARGES AND LENGTH OF STAY: SHORT-STAY HOSPITALS, UNITED STATES, 1958–1960, Washington, United States Department of Health, Education and Welfare, April, 1962; National Center for Health Statistics, MEDICAL CARE, HEALTH STATUS AND FAMILY INCOME, Series 10, number 9; Weeks, Ashley H., FAMILY SPENDING PATTERNS AND HEALTH CARE, Cambridge, Harvard University Press, 1961; In addition to the above, many local surveys have been taken. References for many of these may be found in Anderson and Feldman, *op. cit.*, pp. 1–2, footnote 3, and Anderson, Collette and Feldman, *op. cit.*, p. 3, footnote 6. Other articles of interest are: Kirk, Dudley, Anticipating the Health Needs of Americans: Some Demographic Projections, *Annals of the American Academy of Political and Social Science*, September, 1961; Odoroff, M. E. and Abbe, L. M., Use of General Hospitals: Demographic and Ecological Factors, *Public Health Reports*, 72, 397–403, May, 1957; Coe, Rodney M. and Wessen, Albert F., Social-Psychological Factors Influencing the Use of Community Health Resources, paper presented at the 92nd annual meeting of the American Public Health Association, New York City, October, 1964; An excellent review and description of the field and its problems is contained in Klarman, Herbert E., THE ECONOMICS OF HEALTH, New York, Columbia University Press, 1965. The chapters on Demand in this publication are particularly recommended.

[17] These studies have also included a number of economic factors in addition to cultural-demographic variables; these will be discussed in the next section of the paper; Wirick, Grover and Barlow, Robin, Social and Economic Determinants of the Demand for Health Services, *in* THE ECONOMICS OF HEALTH AND MEDICAL CARE, Ann Arbor, The University of Michigan Press, 1964; Feldstein, Paul, The Demand for Medical Care, *in* REPORT OF THE COMMISSION ON COST OF MEDICAL CARE, Chicago, The American Medical Association, June, 1964, volume 1; London, Morris, Variations in Post-Operative Study Among Appendectomy Patients, *Hospital Management*, 49–52, November, 1963 and 45–57, December, 1963; Rosenthal, Gerald, THE DEMAND FOR GENERAL HOSPITAL

FACILITIES, Chicago, The American Hospital Association, Monograph number 14, 1964; Cardwell, R., Reid, M. and Shain, M., HOSPITAL UTILIZATION IN A MAJOR METROPOLITAN AREA, Chicago, Hospital Planning Council for Metropolitan Chicago, 1964 (mimeographed); Berry, Charles, Family Medical Expense: Estimates and Projections, *in* VOLUNTARY MEDICAL INSURANCE AND PREPAYMENT, Ottawa, Royal Commission on Health Services, 1965; Riedel, Donald C. and Fitzpatrick, Thomas B., PATTERNS OF PATIENT CARE: A STUDY OF HOSPITAL USE IN SIX DIAGNOSES, Ann Arbor, The University of Michigan Press, 1964.

[18] Rosenthal, *op. cit.*

[19] Feldstein, *op. cit.*

[20] Cardwell, Reid and Shain, *op. cit.*, p. 130.

[21] Anderson, Collette and Feldman, *op. cit.*, p. 178; United States National Health Survey, PROPORTION OF HOSPITAL BILL PAID BY INSURANCE: PATIENTS DISCHARGED FROM SHORT-STAY HOSPITALS, Washington, United States Government Printing Office, 1961, pp. 1–40; Weisbrod, B. A. and Fiesler, R. J., Hospitalization Insurance and Hospital Utilization, *American Economic Review,* 51, 126–132, March, 1961; some studies that have used insurance in a multivariate analysis to derive its net effect are: Wirick and Barlow, *op. cit.*, 117–119; Feldstein, The Demand for Medical Care, *op. cit.*, pp. 73–74; Rosenthal, *op. cit.*, p. 35; Feldstein, Paul J. and Carr, W. John, The Effect of Income on Medical Care Spending, *Proceedings, American Statistical Association,* 38 and 42, 1964; some articles of interest in this regard are: Arrow, Kenneth, Uncertainty and the Welfare Economics of Medical Care, *American Economic Review,* December, 1963; Lees, D. S. and Rice, R. G., Uncertainty and the Welfare Economics of Medical Care: Comment, *American Economic Review,* 55, 140–154, March, 1965, and Arrow, Kenneth, Reply, in the same issue; Weisbrod, Burton, Anticipating the Health Needs of Americans: Some Economic Projections, *Annals of the American Academy of Political and Social Science,* September, 1961; Brewster, Agnes W., Voluntary and Health Insurance and Medical Care Expenditures, 1948–58, *Social Security Bulletin,* 22, 3–11, December 25, 1959; McNary, W. S., Controlling Hospital Use Through Prepayment Benefit Provisions and Reimbursement Formulas, *in* WHERE IS HOSPITAL USE HEADED, Proceedings of the Fifth Annual Symposium on Hospital Affairs, Chicago, University of Chicago Press, pp. 64–68; Roemer, M. and Shain, M., HOSPITAL UTILIZATION UNDER INSURANCE, Chicago, The American Hospital Association, 1959; Odoroff, Maurice E. and Abbe, Leslie M., Use of General Hospitals: Variations with Methods of Payment, *Public Health Reports,* 74, 316–24, April, 1959.

[22] Kessel, Reuben, Price Discrimination in Medicine, *Journal of Law and Economics,* October, 1958.

[23] A number of surveys have collected data on family income and expenditures on medical care. Examples of the income-expenditure relationship from a few of the better known surveys are Falk, Klem and Sinai, *op. cit.*, pp. 151 and 206; Anderson, Collette and Feldman, *op. cit.*, pp. 17–18; see also MEDICAL CARE, HEALTH STATUS AND FAMILY INCOME, National Center for Health Statistics, series 10, number 9; National Center for Health Statistics, LENGTH OF CONVALESCENCE AFTER SURGERY, Washington, United States Department of Health, Education and Welfare, Public Health Service, July, 1963.

[24] Feldstein and Carr, *op. cit.*

[25] Wirick and Barlow, *op. cit.*, p. 117; Cardwell, Reid and Shain, *op. cit.*, pp. 128–136; Friedman and Kuznets, *op. cit.*, pp. 163–169; Stigler, G., THE THEORY OF PRICE, New York, The Macmillan Company, 1952, pp. 50 and 52.

[26] The distinction between permanent and transitory components of income and their relationship to consumption is set out in Friedman's permanent-income theory of consumption. A statement of this theory, along with empirical evidence to support it, is contained in Friedman, Milton, A THEORY OF THE CONSUMPTION FUNCTION, Princeton, New Jersey, Princeton University Press, 1957.

[27] Reed and Rice, *op. cit.*, p. 4, Table 2.

[28] For a more complete review of this paper, see the comments by Rothenberg, J. and Klarman, H., PROCEEDINGS OF THE SOCIAL STATISTICS SECTION, American Statistical Association, 1964, pp. 106–112.

[29] Rothenberg, Jerome, Welfare Implications of Alternative Methods of Financing Medical Care, *American Economic Review, Papers and Proceedings*, 677, May, 1951.

[30] Physicians, Patients and the General Hospital: Patterns of Use in Massachusetts, *Progress in Health Services*, X15, 3, January–February, 1965.

[31] Multiple staff appointments would increase the availability of choice to the physician. This might be one method of achieving some of the benefits of competition among hospitals.

[32] One area where knowledge is incomplete, that of drugs, has resulted in the patient paying prices higher than necessary. Steele, after demonstrating that different firms sold the same drug at prices varying from $1.75 to $17.90 a bottle, commented: "In the absence of extremely imperfect market information, such great differences in prices would be impossible." Steele, Henry, Monopoly and Competition in the Ethical Drugs Market, *Journal of Law and Economics*, 5, October, 1962.

[33] For studies of "proper use" to be effective, an identity of interests must be arrived at to insure that the physician provides care at lowest cost to the patient and to the community; this might involve changes in insurance coverage.

[34] For a more complete discussion of peak and off-peak pricing of hospital services, *see* Feldstein, Paul J., A Note on the Pricing of Hospital Services, *in* AN EMPIRICAL INVESTIGATION OF THE MARGINAL COST OF HOSPITAL SERVICES, Graduate Program in Hospital Administration, Chicago, University of Chicago, 1961, Appendix C.

[35] For an excellent summary and discussion of studies of prepaid group practice and their conclusions, *see:* Klarman, Herbert E., Effect of Prepaid Group Practice on Hospital Use, *Public Health Reports*, 78, November, 1963; Densen, Paul M., Balamuth, Eve and Shapiro, Sam, PREPAID MEDICAL CARE AND HOSPITAL UTILIZATION, Chicago, The American Hospital Association, 1958; Densen, Paul M., *et al.*, Prepaid Medical Care and Hospital Utilization, *Hospitals*, 36, November 16, 1962; Roemer, Milton I., The Influence of Prepaid Physicians' Service on Hospital Utilization, *Hospitals*, October 16, 1958; Anderson, Odin W. and Sheatsley, Paul B., Comprehensive Medical Insurance; A. Study of Costs, Use and Attitudes Under Two Types of Plans, Research Series number 9, Health Information Foundation, 1959; Commission on the Cost of Medical Care, Solo and Group Practice, *in* THE REPORT OF THE COMMISSION ON THE COST OF MEDICAL CARE, Chicago, The American Medical Association, 1964, Volume I, Chapter 5.

[36] Shain, M. and Roemer, Milton, I., Hospital Costs Relate to the Supply of Beds, *Modern Hospital*, 92, April, 1959; Sigmond, Robert M., Does Supply of Beds Control Costs?, *Modern Hospital*, 93, August 2, 1959; Roemer, Milton I., Bed Supply and Hospital Utilization: A Natural Experiment, *Hospitals*, 35, November 1, 1961; Rosenthal, *op. cit.*, pp. 55–62.

ACKNOWLEDGMENTS

I wish to acknowledge the helpful comments of A. Alhadeff, J. Carr, J. German, M. Long and G. Rosenthal.

158

FINANCING FOR THE REORGANIZATION
OF MEDICAL CARE SERVICES AND THEIR DELIVERY

I. S. FALK

It is now generally recognized that the inadequate availability of medical care presents problems of crisis dimensions and intensities. It is also widely agreed that medical care services need reorganization for more adequate availability and more effective delivery to the population of the United States. Not the least of the causes of crisis is high and steeply escalating costs; and not the least among the needs is better financing of medical care. What then are the opportunities for the patterns of financing to contribute to better organization of the services and to better availability and delivery of care?

If we would deal realistically with financing for the future, we should be clear about current costs and prospective expenditures. If we would be understanding of current problems in meeting the costs, we must identify the satisfactions and dissatisfactions with medical care. If we would design financing to play a constructive role for good medical care, and if we would understand the current urgency of action, we must be mindful of all the major causes of crisis.

The costs of medical care do not stand alone or apart, though they have often been treated as though they could be measured and financed without reference to what brings them about. To whatever extent this was feasible before, it is impossible now when costs have reached levels that price essential services beyond the reach of millions—to even challenge the resources of the economy and to outrage the conscience of society.

Thus, even beyond an understanding of the current scene, decisions about the role of further financing depend upon our perspective of

159

what needs strengthening or reorganization, to what ends and with what promise of bringing satisfactions for the prices that are to be paid.

THE CAUSES OF CRISIS IN MEDICAL CARE

The medical care "industry" is one of the largest in the country, now (fiscal 1971–72) involving between 80 and 85 billion dollars a year, and accounting for about 7.6 per cent of a gross national product of about $1,100 billion. In many respects it is probably the most complex because of its "labor intensiveness," the almost indescribable intricacy of its technology and the pervasiveness of its human involvements. A hundred problems contribute to its crisis state, but they can be subsumed in a few categories—technically in four, constructively in five:

1. National shortages and maldistributions in various categories of health manpower and facilities, both old and new;
2. Steeply rising costs and their financing;
3. Inadequacies in the system for assuring availability and delivery of needed services;
4. Lack of sufficient and effective controls for the assurance of quality of care;
5. Interrelations among the preceding four.

The first four are, in a sense, the anatomic parts of the diagnosis; the fifth refers mainly to the lack of coordination that should hold the parts together and make them capable of functioning effectively.

All of these were foreseen as *potential* causes of crisis forty years ago.[1] But over the span of two generations we have launched attacks on the underlying problems through categorical rather than through comprehensive policies and programs, and with means that were in no single area proportioned to the magnitudes of the needs or the outlook for their enlargements. The result is crisis in the 1970s. The saving feature in the current scene is that now, at long last, there is a near-consensus that all four categories of cause must be attacked, and that they must be attacked simultaneously and adequately.[2]

There are some who challenge this conclusion. They counsel and advocate that we should deal with each categody separately and on its own convenient time schedule—essentially a continuation of the policies the nation has been following for decades. This is a counsel of caution but not of wisdom. Consider the consequences of further categorical pursuits. What will it avail us if we merely try to produce more manpower or facilities without assuring appropriate distributions in

160

relation to population, the availability of necessary funds and a better system for their utilization? Is it likely that we can contain the escalation of costs without a better system for the containment of unit costs of service and for the assurance of economy in volumes of utilization? Is it reasonable to expect that we can have or can afford either needed health manpower and facilities or assured and adequate financing without a better system of delivery? Can either the professions or the public go much longer without better assurances of quality and adequacy of care? Can the provision of more purchasing power for medical care be contemplated alone—without improvement in the system for delivery of care—inasmuch as an expansion of purchasing power, and thus of effective demand, would invite further strain on the resources for service and would increase the upward push of prices?

The near-consensus to which I refer—in favor of a broad and comprehensive program—extends in substantial measure to all major proposals before the Congress, excepting only "Medicredit" sponsored by the American Medical Association.[2] And it is reflected in testimony from a parade of witnesses before the Congressional committees, excepting only those individuals who speak for the contented hierarchies of the medical associations.

It is not difficult to understand reluctances to the needed massive commitments. Despite decades of national discussions, the United States still has no broad or unequivocal national policy for health care in general or for medical care in particular. It has no clear national program to implement national policy. *Per contra,* it has highly influential spokesmen who are defendants of interests, vested in the fragmented services of the *status quo,* and in financing methods that are imbedded in long-established practices and that provide handsome returns to the personal providers.

The difficulty to persuade is compounded by the difficulties inherent in implementing needed action. Since the constantly growing complexity of medical service long ago began to outrun the development of organization for the delivery of service—and the gap continuously widens—reorganization of organization and delivery is crucial. But because there is no substantial advocacy of national commitment to a national health service, reorganization must—as a practical matter—be effected on an evolutionary course. Consequently, sensible redesign of financing must be suited to the financial practices that prevail and to those that may be expected to support and encourage the desired evolutionary changes.

161

All the major causes of crisis have national characteristics and dimensions. Consequently, the problems and the needs they reflect cannot be substantially resolved at the local or the state level. Only national action, based on national authority and national resources, can be equal to the undertakings that are required.

"Crisis" is pejorative—depreciatory and disparaging. But it is applicable now to medical care because it reflects that circumstances worsen and will not become better spontaneously. The longer national action is delayed, the more heroic the needed remedies.

FINANCING FOR WHAT AND TO WHAT ENDS?

We have a near-consensus and we are approaching a clear and unequivocal social policy that in the United States good medical care should be available to everybody. But it is a consensus and a policy still in search of a program. Good financing to serve that policy should be designed not only to provide supports for the content of good medical care but, more, to provide leverage toward effective organization of the services for their availability and their delivery. What, then, should be the guidelines for the fiscal design?

If we agree that in the prospective "system" everybody should be eligible to seek and—as far as practical—to receive good medical care, obviously the financing should be national and based on the nation's resources. Financing for availability and delivery must start with the financial resources needed to support what we now have. It should, however, assure financial supports and incentives to encourage reorganization that provides an open door to the medical care system while retaining fiscal amplitudes for alternative patterns of both organization and delivery. And if we would avoid repeating mistakes of the past, the fiscal supports for the consequent evolutionary course should encourage only a single mainstream of medical care. Those supports should not be available, except on a temporary and transitional basis, for a separate and inevitably unequal system for the poor and near-poor based on the emergency room of the local hospital, the "ward" or "service" patient resource for the training of "house staff," the "charity" municipal or county hospital, or the neighborhood health center segregated by local geography of a means test. And those supports should not encourage another and separate system for all others in our national society. An accompanying corollary from the objective of good care is that if financing is effected from public sources it should be accompanied by standards of quality, and by requirements for the observance of such standards, to assure the worth of services supported by public funds.

These precepts lead, I believe, to a clear prescription for two categories of undertaking:

1. A nationally comprehensive system of financing to support good medical care for everybody, without means tests or contribution histories as prerequisites of eligibility.

2. An evolving national system for the availability and provision of services, with pluralistic patterns for organization and delivery.

THE COSTS TO BE FINANCED

When the problems of medical care costs first began to receive national attention the focus was on costs for the individual and the family. The concern was primarily with the variable, uncertain and—for the individual or family—the unbudgetable nature of the costs. Even the earliest studies demonstrated the need for group payment to substitute manageable averages for the unmanageable individual and variable costs.[1] This aspect of the costs faded into the background as private insurance expanded; and various studies showed that individual and family cost variations and distributions were being narrowed, especially among people of different income and expenditure levels.[3] Then, medical care costs escalated rapidly, and private insurance found itself unable to broaden its benefits adequately—in the face of higher and higher costs that had to be funded through marketable premiums. Millions of people were still without insurance protections or had only very limited coverage. Millions with insurance they had been led to expect would give them broad protections began to find that they were still being burdened by costs not covered by their private insurance. On the average, insurance was covering only about one-third of all private expenditures being incurred by the insured and the noninsured, and about two-thirds still had to be met through "out-of-pocket" expenditures. And, despite steeply rising insurance premiums, "exclusions" from insurance coverages and "deductibles," "co-payments" and "ceilings" on insured costs were leaving large numbers of families, though having some insurance, weighted down or even bankrupted by massive noninsured costs still to be incurred in increasing proportions of cases.

National Expenditures		1949–50	1964–65	1969–70	1970–71
			Expenditures in billions		
	Total	$ 12.1	$ 38.9	$ 67.8	$ 75.0
Private		9.0	29.4	42.8	46.5
Public		3.1	9.5	25.0	28.5
			Percentage distributions		
	Total	100	100	100	100
Private		74	76	63	62
Public		26	24	37	38
			Per capita expenditures		
	Total	$ 79	$198	$327	$ 358
Private		59	149	206	222
Public		20	49	121	136
GNP (in billions)		$263	$656	$953	$1,008
Percent for health care		4.6	5.9	7.1	7.4

Source: Rice, D. P. and Cooper, B. S., National Health Expenditures, 1929–71, *Social Security Bulletin*, 35, 3–18, Table 1, January, 1972.
Note: Does not include expenditures for medical education and training (from private and public services) or expenditures for air pollution and water pollution control, sanitation, water supplies and sewage treatment.

The outcries against the inadequacies of private insurance brought us back full circle to concern about the impacts of medical care costs on individuals and families.

What has been happening annually in millions of cases on the "micro" scale is readily understood from inspection of the national "macro" data, showing that while population was doubling between 1930 and 1970 (from 100 to 200 million persons), expenditures for all health care were multiplying from $3.6 billion to over $70 billion—about twentyfold—and the expenditures for personal health services from about $3.2 billion to about $64 billion—also about twentyfold.[4]

Since the end of World War II national health expenditures have been rising steeply from about $12 billion in 1949–50 to about $75 billion in 1970–71, and they are probably about $83 billion in fiscal 1971–72 (Tables 1 and 2). The increases extend to both private and governmental expenditures. The rise has been even steeper than the rapidly growing gross national product (GNP). Consequently the total expenditures of $12 billion for health care, which were 4.6 per cent of a GNP of $263 billion in 1949–50, have risen to $75 billion and 7.4 per cent of a GNP of slightly more than $1,000 billion in 1970–71. In 1971–72 health care expenditures had reached about $83 billion, which accounted for about 7.6 per cent of a GNP of nearly $1,100 billion.

For about twenty years the proportion of the expenditures for all health services derived from private sources had been about 75 per cent. Then, with the enactment of Medicare, Medicaid and other new governmental programs in 1965–67, the private share declined toward sixty per cent and the public expenditure portion rose toward forty per cent. In these years, a small proportion of the increase reflected growth of population; but most of the increase reflected prices and utilizations, witness that per capita expenditures that had been about $79 in 1949–50, were $198 in 1964–65, reached $327 in 1969–70, $358 in 1970–71 and were probably nearly $400 in 1971–72 (Table 1).[5]

Within these massive totals for all health care, personal health care expenditures have been responsible for about 90 per cent of the total. They were about $10.8 billion in 1949–50; they had risen to about $67.4 billion in 1970–71; and they are probably about $75 billion in the fiscal year that ended June 30, 1972. These, too, have been changing in composition, mainly reflecting a transfer from the private to the

TABLE 2. NATIONAL EXPENDITURES FOR ALL HEALTH CARE AND FOR PERSONAL HEALTH CARE SERVICES IN SELECTED FISCAL YEARS

National Expenditures	1949–50*	1964–65*	1969–70*	1970–71*
All	$12,130	$38,912	$67,770	$75,012
Personal health care**	10,841	34,739	60,856	67,428
Per cent of total	89.4	89.3	89.8	89.9
Other health care	1,289	4,173	6,914	7,584

*Personal Health Care Expenditures***

	1949–50	1964–65	1969–70	1970–71
Total	$10,841	$34,739	$60,856	$67,428
Private, total	8,721	27,763	39,740	43,441
Direct payments	7,146	17,590	22,929	24,262
Insurance benefits	879	8,281	14,406	16,615
Expenses for prepayment	274	1,212	1,515	1,600
Other	422	680	890	964
Public, total	$2,120	$ 6,976	$21,116	$23,987
Federal	996	2,858	14,040	15,803
State and local	1,124	4,118	7,076	8,184

* Millions of dollars.
** Personal health care services includes all expenditures for health services and supplies other than Government public health and related activities, expenditures of private voluntary agencies for other health services, medical research, and medical-facilities construction. The figures shown here exceed those for personal health care expenditures in the source document by inclusion here of expenses for prepayment in the private sector and expenses for administration in the (Federal) public sector.

Source: Rice, D. P. and Cooper, B. S., National Health Expenditures, 1929–71, Social Security Bulletin, 35, 3–18, Tables 2 and 5, January, 1972.

165

TABLE 3. PERCENTAGE DISTRIBUTIONS OF PERSONAL HEALTH CARE
EXPENDITURES, 1949–50 AND 1970–71

	1949–50		1970–71	
Total expenditures	100.0		100.0	
Private, total	80.4	100.0	64.4	100.0
Direct payments	65.9	81.9	36.0	55.9
Insurance benefits	8.1	10.1	24.6	38.2
Expenses for prepayment	2.5	3.1	2.4	3.7
Other	3.9	4.9	1.4	2.2
Public, total	19.6	100.0	35.6	100.0
Federal	9.2	47.0	23.4	65.9
State and local	10.4	53.0	12.2	34.1

Source: Rice, D. P. and Cooper, B. S., National Health Expenditures, 1929–71, Social Security Bulletin, 35, 3–18, Tables 2 and 5, January, 1972.

public sectors; and the public expenditures themselves have been changing because of a larger proportionate increase in federal than in state and local governmental financing (Tables 2 and 3).

The most critical aspect of these increases in expenditures has been the steepness of their escalation, increasing in recent years by ten to fifteen (or more) per cent a year when GNP and spendable personal income were increasing by about six to eight per cent.

Among the various categories of expenditure by type of service, hospital care, physicians' services and nursing home care have been the most steeply escalating and for diverse reasons (Tables 4 and 5). The increases have reflected rising expectations and demands for service, technologic developments, health manpower and facilities shortages, catch-up in some wage and salary levels and so forth. But they have also reflected inefficiencies in the ways in which the resources are made available and utilized. Not the least of the incentives for rising expenditures have been the guarantees of particular payments, and not of others, through the most widely sold patterns of private insurance, and the largely uncontrolled guarantees under public programs to pay charges determined by individual providers of care and to reimburse the full costs incurred by hospitals and other institutions.

If expenditures for health care continue to rise at rates experienced in recent years, they will attain frightening levels. Projections published by the Social Security Administration (SSA) in October 1970, and assuming substantially the continuance of recent trends, carry the national expenditures for *all* health care from $67 billion in fiscal 1969–70 and $75 billion in 1970–71 to $111–$120 billion in 1975, and to

166

TABLE 4. NATIONAL EXPENDITURES FOR PERSONAL HEALTH CARE SERVICES BY TYPE OF EXPENDITURE AND SOURCE OF FUNDS* FISCAL YEAR 1970–71

Object of Expenditure	Total**	Private	Source of Funds Public		
		Total**	Total**	Federal**	State and Local**
Total	$67,428	$43,441	$23,987	$15,672	$8,315
Hospital care	29,628	14,871	14,757	9,510	5,246
Physicians' services	14,245	10,700	3,545	2,522	1,022
Dentists' services	4,660	4,400	260	154	106
Other professional services	1,475	1,253	222	173	49
Drugs and drug sundries	7,470	6,930	540	271	269
Eyeglasses and appliances	1,915	1,849	66	37	30
Nursing home care	3,365	1,338	2,027	1,174	853
Other health services	2,375	500	1,875	1,266	609
Expenses for prepayment	1,600	1,600			
Expenses for administration	696		696	565	131

* Personal health services differs from total national health care expenditures by exclusion of government public health and related activities, expenditures of private voluntary agencies for other health services, medical research and medical facilities construction. The totals here exceed those in various tables published by the Social Security Administration because of inclusion here of expenses for prepayment and for administration.

** In Millions.

Source: Rice, D. P. and Cooper, B. S., National Health Expenditures, 1929–71, *Social Security Bulletin*, 35, 3–18, Tables 2 and 5, January 1972; and Cooper, B. S. and Worthington, N. L., Medical Care Spending for Three Age Groups, *Social Security Bulletin*, 35, 3–16, Table 1, May, 1972.

TABLE 5. DISTRIBUTIONS OF PERSONAL HEALTH CARE EXPENDITURES BY OBJECT OF EXPENDITURE, FISCAL YEARS 1969–70 AND 1970–71

Object of Expenditure	Composition (Billions) 1969–70	1970–71	Per Cent Increase in Dollar Amount 1969–70 to 1970–71
Total expenditures	$60.9	$67.4	11.1
Hospital care	26.1	29.6	11.4
Physicians' services	13.0	14.2	11.0
Dentists' services	4.2	4.7	11.0
Other professional services	1.4	1.5	10.7
Drugs and drug sundries	7.0	7.5	10.7
Eyeglasses and appliances	1.9	1.9	10.4
Nursing home care	2.9	3.4	11.7
Other health services	2.4	2.4	10.0
Expenses for prepayment and administration	2.1	2.3	11.0

Source: Rice, D. P. and Cooper, B. S., National Health Expenditures, 1929–71, *Social Security Bulletin*, 35, 3–18, Tables 2 and 5, January 1972; and Cooper, B. S. and Worthington, N. L., Medical Care Spending for Three Age Groups, *Social Security Bulletin*, 35, 3–16, Table 1, May, 1972.

TABLE 6. TYPE OF EXPENDITURE AND SOURCE OF FUNDS FOR PERSONAL HEALTH CARE SERVICES, 1970–71

Expenditure	Amount (Millions)	Per Cent
All expenditures	$67,428	100.0
Direct payments by patients	24,262	36.0
Private insurance, total	18,215	27.0
Insurance benefits	16,615	24.6
Expenses for insurance	1,600	2.4
Federal expenditures	15,803*	23.4
State and local gov't expenditures	8,184	12.2
All other	964	1.4

* Expenditures from federal general revenues for direct federal programs, federal-state programs, health insurance for the aged (Medicare) etc., from payroll taxes for Medicare, Part A, and from premium payments by or on behalf of subscribers for Supplementary Medical Insurance (Medicare, Part B).

Source: Rice, D. P. and Cooper, B. S., National Health Expenditures, 1929–71, *Social Security Bulletin*, 35, 3–18, Tables 2 and 5, January, 1972.

about forty to sixty per cent more in 1980; and those projections indicate increase of the national expenditures for *personal health care services* from $60 billion in 1969–70 or $67 billion in 1970–71 to $103–$111 billion in 1975, and to correspondingly higher figures in 1980 (Tables 2, 6 and 7). Those projections increase faster than the gross national product, thus health care would be absorbing larger and larger shares of the national economy.

The ssa projections, however validly reflecting the stated assumptions that accompany them, have seemed to me to race toward unacceptable expenditure levels, principally because—admittedly—they do not take into account countervailing measures to moderate the recent rates of escalation. Such measures have already been taken and more are in course of application. Therefore, in early 1971, I developed an "adjusted" model of projected expenditure levels to 1975, moderating somewhat the expected rates of annual increase in expenditures for hospital care and physicians' services.[7] In my model, expenditures for personal health care services would be expected to increase from $67 billion in fiscal 1971 to $85 billion in fiscal 1974 and to $93 billion in 1975 (Tables 8 and 9). Even this model emphasizes the urgency of instituting adequate program measures to further moderate—if not to contain—the escalation of medical care costs. It also emphasizes that the longer the needed improvements are delayed, the higher the expenditure level at which any new functional program would have to take over.

168

National Expenditures (In Billions)	Actual FY 1969–70	"SSA" Projections**			
		1975		1980	
		"Low"	"High"	"Low"	"High"
All (amount)	$ 67.2	$110.7	$120.1	$155.7	$189.2
Per capita	$324	$509	$552	$670	$814
Per cent of GNP	7.0	7.9	8.6	8.0	9.8
Health services and supplies	$ 61.9	$104.8	$113.5	$148.9	$180.6
Research	1.9	2.2	2.5	2.6	3.1
Construction of facilities	3.4	3.7	4.1	4.2	5.5
Personal Health Care Expenditures†					
Total (amount)	$ 60.1	$102.9	$111.4	$146.5	$178.0
Per cent of all expenditures	89.4	93.0	92.8	94.1	94.1
Per capita	$290	$473	$512	$630	$766
Per cent of GNP	6.3	7.4	8.0	7.6	9.2
Hospital care	$ 25.6	$ 48.2	$ 52.4	$ 76.4	$ 92.6
Physicians' services	12.9	22.1	24.0	29.2	36.5
Dentists' services	4.2	6.6	7.1	8.4	10.6
Other professional services	1.4	2.2	2.4	2.8	3.5
Drugs and drug sundries	6.7	9.3	9.9	11.3	13.2
Eyeglasses and appliances	1.8	2.9	3.0	3.9	4.4
Nursing home care	2.9	4.8	5.3	6.1	7.5
Other health services††	2.5	4.1	4.5	5.1	6.0
Prepayment and administration	2.1	2.7	2.8	3.3	3.7

* Table 1 and references in Table 4. Population: 207.3 million; gross national product (GNP): $956.2 billion. The figures in this column are slightly lower than for this year in other tables, the latter being based on subsequently revised estimates. The original figures are retained in this table.

** Social Security Administration projections by Rice and McGee, cited below. Populations 1975 and 1980: 217.6 and 232.4 millions; GNP 1975 and 1980: $1,398.4 and $1,935.0 billions.

† Includes all expenditures for health services and supplies other than government public health and related activities, expenditures of private voluntary agencies for other health services, medical research and medical facilities construction.

†† For the projections, the same proportion as in 1969–70 (86 per cent) of the estimated total for the category was included here as expenditures for personal health care services.

Sources: Rice, D. P. and Cooper, B. S., National Health Expenditures, 1929–71, *Social Security Bulletin*, 35, 3–18, Table 1, January, 1972; Rice, D. P. and McGee, M. F., Projections of National Health Expenditures, 1975 and 1980, *Research and Statistics Note*, No. 18, October 30, 1970.

I have made no further adjustments in the perspectives for the medical care costs of the near-time future in light of the price and cost control programs instituted by the Federal Administration in August 1971 and being conducted in 1972. We can only hope at this time that these newer undertakings will prove to be effective in moderating the medical care cost escalation to (or toward) the escalation rate of the

TABLE 8. ACTUAL EXPENDITURE IN 1970–71 AND ADJUSTED PROJECTIONS TO FISCAL YEARS 1974 AND 1975 FOR PERSONAL HEALTH CARE SERVICES

National Expenditures	Actual FY 1970–71*	Adjusted Projections** FY 1974	FY 1975
Total (amount)	$ 67.4	$ 85.1	$ 92.8
Per capita	$322	$397	$428
Per cent of GNP	6.7	6.7	6.9
Hospital care	$ 29.6	$ 36.9	$ 40.9
Physicians' services	14.2	18.6	20.3
Dentists' services	4.7	5.9	6.4
Other professional services	1.5	2.0	2.2
Drugs and drug sundries	7.5	8.6	9.0
Eyeglasses and appliances	1.9	2.6	2.8
Nursing home care	3.4	4.2	4.6
Other health services	2.4	3.8	4.0
Prepayment and administration	2.3	2.5	2.6

* From Table 4.
** Adjusted from the "SSA" projections in Table 7 (see the text).
Note: Corresponding further projections would give totals of $101.2 billions for FY 1976 and $110.4 billions for FY 1977.

TABLE 9. ACTUAL EXPENDITURES IN 1970–71 AND ADJUSTED PROJECTIONS TO FISCAL YEARS 1974 AND 1975 FOR PERSONAL HEALTH CARE SERVICES BY SOURCE OF FUNDS

National Expenditures by Source of Funds	Actual FY 1970–71*	Adjusted Projections** FY 1974	FY 1975
Total	$67.4	$85.1	$92.8
Private	43.4	54.8	59.8
Governmental	24.0	30.3	33.0
Federal	15.8	19.9	21.7
State and local	8.2	10.4	11.3

* From Table 2.
** Source of funds according to proportions in 1970–71.

economy as a whole. If they do, the problem of financing future medical care costs will not be further worsening. But whether the current programs are or are not successful, the urgency or major interventions with respect to medical care costs and the organization for better availability and delivery of care will still persist.

170

Three lessons stand out most prominently and most clearly from the financial experiences, and they are obviously interrelated.

1. The dynamics of the market place are no longer—if they ever were in modern times—adequate for the system of medical care.

2. The system must have an end to the near-total dominance of the provider of medical care and his control of the system's determinants.

3. The needed remedies for the system are fundamental and massive, not to be satisfied by applying adhesive, prescribing aspirin or relying on the healing effects of nature, time and nonintervention.

The marketplace relies heavily on the consumer's ability to determine need and to judge value; and, except for circumscribed interventions, it is guided by the rule of *caveat emptor* with an overlay from administered prices. In medical care, however, the consumer has only limited capacity to determine need, he has even less ability to judge the correctness or the value of what he purchases and he has too few protections where the provider exercises monopoly.

The dominance of the provider arises from the exclusivities of public licensure and registration, rooted in the intention to protect the general welfare against those not qualified to practice in the healing arts professions. It has been implemented in a measure by policies or decisions of the licensed professions that lead to shortages of health manpower. It has been implemented further by the methods of payment of services that have given almost monopolistic control of fees to the personal provider and of charges (or cost-reimbursements) to the institutional provider. Because utilization of service is also largely determined by decisions of the provider, he has had a large role in determining the costs of medical care—the product of price and utilization.

The costs of medical care have been, and still are, largely open-end and without societal controls; escalation of costs, therefore, has to be ascribed to the provider—except as constituents of his costs have to be purchased in the marketplace or are truly compelled by technology. Where demand is substantially affected by human need for relief from disease, disability and mental insecurity and by the pervasive desire to avoid morbidity and to postpone mortality, individual ability to pay provides no ordinary or adequate restraint on effective demand. In

171

these many respects the economics of the medical marketplace have been indifferent to the usual dynamics of the common marketplace; and the freedoms from that indifference have been drawing the medical marketplace toward fiscal disaster.

The needed remedies are obvious: The methods of paying for services need adaptation to the social purposes of medical care. Provider-determined fee-for-service, with its inherent elements of conflict of interest, if not abolished altogether needs at least to be restrained by social and fiscal controls; institutional costs and thus their charges, which have no inherent ceilings, have to be bounded by socially and fiscally determined prospective budget limitations. And because the method of payment, prices, charges and utilization rates, all affect and are affected by the arrangements under which services are made available and are provided, the patterns of financing must bear on organization itself.

The elements of financial need or control are not disparate. For example, the physician provides his own services and directs hospitalization and other supporting services. He receives only about twenty per cent of the personal-health-care dollar, but he determines and, in large measure, controls about sixty per cent more. The hospital responds to the physician's needs and orders, though typically he is not an officer or employee of the institution and is not responsible for the financing of its costs or for its legal obligations to society. And all this operates in a framework that gives medical care as a whole an open-end lien on the fiscal resources of society.

There was little appreciation of what was being done when this system was recently sanctioned in the Congressional enactments of Medicare, Medicaid and other public programs—enactments that included public guarantees to pay, without ceilings, substantially whatever is charged by personal providers and to reimburse institutional providers their self-determined production costs. The anguish now associated with cost levels and escalations in those public programs might have been anticipated, even if rapid extension of the consequences to the whole medical care system might not.

It is not difficult to see that guidelines for better fiscal management of medical care cannot suffice if limited to fiscal aspects alone, having also to deal with the reordering of many major elements of the system itself. Implementation of the guidelines must extend to the provision of incentives to halt the overemphasis on expensive institutional care, especially by orienting the availability of service to less expensive pri-

172

mary care, ambulatory and preventive. Implementation must also undertake to eliminate distortions in the spectrum of service and the consequent cost that results from patterns of private insurance that encourage and support what is convenient or feasible for insurance carriers, whether or not in the interest of good care or of economy in its cost.

The guidelines must also be concerned with quality of care and the worth of the services to the patient and to society as a whole. They must not be concerned merely with the size of the physician's fee, the cost of an inpatient hospital day or the price of a laboratory service.

At the risk of undue repetition, it may be said that the lessons evident from the financial experiences lead to guidelines that extend to all the major causes of the present crisis. In short, *fiscal guidelines* should assure that *fiscal measures* will provide what leverage they can toward dealing with the problems of health manpower and facilities, better organization for availability and delivery of health care and better assurance of quality, while effecting containment of cost at socially acceptable and feasible levels.

There was a time, extending over decades, when many who were exercised about the current medical care scene and who wanted improvements engaged in a "hen and egg" debate.[8] Some argued that if national insurance financing preceded improvement in the organization of the services, the financing system would have to accept undesirable current practices and might embed and support them, and thus delay needed reform; and they concluded that national insurance should therefore wait on organizational change. Others argued that inasmuch as organizational change comes slowly, financing should not wait but should be instituted as quickly as feasible and should provide fiscal supports to stimulate and accelerate organizational change; and they concluded that national insurance should not be postponed. The former view prevailed; and national financing was not instituted, leaving a clear field for the rapid expansion of private insurance. Then, while organizational improvements proceeded at a snail's pace, private insurance provided more and more powerful bulwarks for solo practice, fractionated specialty practice supported by fee-for-service payments, and injected strong stimuli for excessive and excessively expensive inpatient care. In short, private insurance effected precisely what had been feared from national insurance and what had been used as an argument when advising against the institution of national financing.

That debate is now ended, because neither the financing nor the

173

reorganization objective can any longer wait on the other. Even more important, there is now a near-consensus that national financing and system improvement are inseparable needs, each for its own objectives and each a necessity for the other.

Finally, it should be clear that the objectives fixed by these lessons and guidelines are attainable only through strong and directed measures of social policy and public law. The magnitudes of the expenditures involved compel that the financing of an adequate system of medical care for the whole population must have its base in the national economy. The needed redirections *of the national expenditures* require the authority of public law to allocate the impacts of the costs *according to the individual's ability to contribute to the national funding, independent of the individual's ability to buy needed care.* The needed redirections in the *organization of the services* demand financial resources sufficient to assure *adequate operational support funds for the system as a whole and sufficient to provide incentive support for the needed changes.* These prescriptions lead to the conclusion that the adequate financing of medical care can be effected only through national funding from the national resources.

SOME MAJOR SPECIFICATIONS FOR A NATIONAL PROGRAM

From these perspectives for the goals, the needs and the social policies that should guide action, a series of specifications emerges, and it provides the framework for the "Health Security" program developed by the Technical Subcommittee of the Committee for National Health Insurance.[9] The primary social goal is the availability of all needed services for health maintenance and medical care to everybody in the nation, as far as this is practical initially, and with increasing comprehensiveness as expansion of resources and services becomes feasible. Obviously, because the intent is to start with the resources that we have and to move toward greater adequacy, the progression would be on an evolutionary course.

1. The whole population should be eligible for all the benefits of the program, according to the need for health care, without financial tests or barriers—i.e., with no required insurance contributions history, no means tests and with no payments to be made by the patient at the time service is received.

2. As a corollary of national eligibility for services, the financing of the program should be national, with as equitable allocation of

the costs as may be feasible, and with built-in provisions for national cost controls on budget bases and geared to trends in the national economy as a whole.

3. Whereas the financing and fiscal management should be national, indeed "monolithic" as in our national social insurance, the availability and provision of the medical services should be private and "pluralistic" through self-elected diversities among providers of service as to their location, organization and selection of professional activities, subject however, to requirements to assure the worth of the services supported by the public funds.

4. Alternative patterns of organization for the provision of services should not only be permitted but even encouraged, especially toward the development of organized provisions for the availability of comprehensive care on a prepayment basis.

5. The financial resources should include special provisions of adequate dimensions to support improvements in the availability of medical care, especially with respect to shortages and maldistributions of health manpower and of facilities for primary and ambulatory services, and in organization for the delivery of care.

6. Administration of the public program should involve not only the public authority but also representatives of consumers as well as of providers of the services at all levels from policy making to ombudsman, with mandatory provisions to assure periodic public accounting of program operations, performances and evaluations.

Obviously, these specifications do not encompass all that is required for a legislative proposal or for an administrative design. Those would involve a long array of details that are not necessarily germane to our discussions here.

It will be noted that I have included no explicit provision with respect to the role of private insurance carriers. A system whose financing can be adequate through budgeted national funding abolishes the fiscal "risks" that are the usual basis for insurance or reinsurance. Whether a place exists in this pattern for the insurance industry—to serve certainly not as carriers of risk but even as claims takers or fiscal intermediaries—is not a question of logic or necessity but of political feasibility. Massive national experience shows that the insurance industry adds billions in cost through charges for prepayment and by distorting sensible patterns of service and expenditure, while contributing little in administration and less in quality and cost control. The job

Object of Expenditure	Private Expenditures Per Cent	Expenditures Under Public Programs** Per Cent	All Expenditures Per Cent
Total	69	57	66
Hospital care	92***	58	76
Physicians' services	95	77	90
Dentists' services	20	71	23
Other professional services	80	79	80
Drugs and drug sundries	27	75	30
Eyeglasses and appliances	40	38	40
Nursing home care	25	33	30
Other health services	15	25	24
Expenses for prepayment			
Expenses for administration	100†	96	100††
Resources development			†††

* Based on estimates derived from actual expenditures in the Fiscal Year 1969–70.
** Includes federal and state-local public programs.
*** Including: for general hospitals 95 per cent, and for psychiatric hospitals 10 per cent.
† Five per cent of aggregate expenditures for potentially included amounts.
†† Equal to 4.4 per cent of aggregate expenditures for potentially included amounts.
††† Two per cent of the amount available for obligation during the year.
Source: Falk, I. S., The Costs of a National Health Security Program and Their Fi-
nancing, Washington, Committee for National Health Insurance September 1971.

could be done at least as well and probably better by public administration.

The "Health Security" program to which these specifications apply
could extend on a budget basis initially to about 66 per cent of current
expenditures for personal health services (Table 10), and to perhaps
80 to 90 per cent later on as manpower and other needed resources are
developed for dental and other services not feasible without arbitrary
limitations at the outset. At the higher coverage level, the program
would be about as extensive as it should be—having regard for some
current expenditures that are wastes and unwarranted, and others that
are incurred for goods and services that are repugnant to standards
of good care.

I have developed estimates for the program that indicate that in
an initial operating year at the 1973–74 or at the 1974–75 level, it
would involve expenditures of about $57 or $63 billion, respectively,
when total expenditures for personal health services without such a
program may be expected to be about $85 or $93 billion a year; and

the program's costs on the proposed budget basis would escalate less than is to be expected without it. I have also documented why the estimates indicate that increases in the program's costs from the feasible expansions of services would be offset by the savings and economies the design makes possible.[7]

In short, the "Health Security" program does not contemplate or require increase in total expenditures for the personal health services. It requires mainly a rerouting of expenditures through the proposed system of national public financing, especially from private insurance and from noninsured private individual payments, and from local, state and federal expenditures being incurred for various categorical public programs like Medicaid and Medicare. And it requires organizational improvements of the kinds indicated here.[10]

It is no oversight that no specific consideration is given here to the details of tax structure or trust fund operations that would be required to support the financing of the proposed "Health Security" program, including the allocations of the costs so as to achieve equity as well as progressivity in their impacts. These important details are endlessly arguable and, being secondary to our discussion, are omitted.[12]

FINANCING FOR THE CRUCIAL GPPPS OR HMOS

The objective of a better system of financing is better financing of a better system of medical care, not merely of the present system with all its weaknesses as well as its strengths. It seems to me that there are two critical elements. The first is assured adequate global funding for the better system as a whole, with provisions to assure that cost levels will be reasonably related to the levels of the national economy, and that the impacts of the costs will be reasonably equitable among those who have to receive them. The second is leverage from financing to provide for expeditious movement from fractionated practices and services to organized practices and comprehensive services.

There are few quarrels about the first except with respect to the restraints that would have to be accepted by those who now profit from absence of financial controls. The second raises even more hackles because it demands basic changes in organization—from solo or quasi-solo practice to comprehensive organized practice, and from fee-for-service payment after services are provided to budgeted prepayment in advance of the occasions when the services are received. This aspect of the second is, in the main, the guideline to move toward prepaid

177

comprehensive group practice as rapidly as feasible, wherever it is practical and sustainable.

Group Practice Prepayment Plans

The reason for the second prescription is that the organized and comprehensive group practice prepayment plan (GPPP), first formally recommended for national development by the Committee on the Costs of Medical Care in 1932,[1] is the only pattern yet devised that has the promise for the medical care system to meet modern and currently prospective needs.[13] Technologic progress toward more and more unavoidable specialization compels this for its coordinating function to offset the inevitable fractionating effects of specialty practices. Health manpower shortages and steeply escalating costs require the efficiencies and economies that have been demonstrated, and continue to be expected, within the potentials of the organized practicing comprehensive group. Urgently needed restraints on the liberal or excessive use of inpatient facilities, inherently expensive and with steeply escalating costs, are readily available and are almost startlingly effective in well-documented GPPP experiences. And quality protections and assurances of the kinds that are well known, and widely applied within *inpatient* settings, become applicable or adaptable to the field of *ambulatory care within the organized group practice* as they have not been in the prevalent solo or single specialty practice. Thus, the GPPP has the potential of striking simultaneously at all major aspects of the current causes of crisis. Therefore, it deserves systematic and pervasive financial support through the national program that the nation needs.

Even if the development of GPPPs is generously supported financially, they cannot be produced overnight, but rather could come into being only over a span of years. Thus, GPPPs have to be encouraged on an evolutionary course, to become available for free-choice participation by the providers of care and for free-choice selection by the people to be served.

The fiscal support for such development would be clearly an investment in the future of the medical care system, and not merely a current expenditure. This is because of the substantial efficiencies GPPPs can affect. They can accomplish these through emphasis on primary and ambulatory care, leading to vast savings in the current extravagant practices of inpatient care, through more efficient utilization of scarce and expensive health manpower, and through restraints on unbridled surgical care and on laboratory and other ancillary ser-

178

vices. This is patently evident from various indexes, most notably from two. One physician per 1,000 persons (or per 1,100, 1,200 or even 1,300) suffices for good care in the mature comprehensive group practice setting, whereas one per 900, 800 or even 700 is insufficient in the prevailing system generally, which, for the most part, is in the non-group practice pattern. All needed inpatient care can be provided by the group practice with as much as 25 to 50 per cent fewer inpatient days than with non-group practice. Then, by substitution, such economies provide the fiscal support for a broadening of services that can be made available by the comprehensive group practice without increase in per capita cost.

An evolutionary course for the development of GPPPS is desirable, so that it can occur in a pluralistic environment by the strength of its attractions. Such a course is also unavoidable by reason of the complexities inherent in the GPPPS' gestation. In addition, I think that opportunities should be preserved for the testing of various designs of the GPPPS themselves—whether community or hospital based, whether wholly comprehensive and having their own inpatient resources, or ambulatory-based with supplementary reliance on associated or affiliated community hospitals, or whether and how they become related to the resources of the health manpower education and training system. There should also be opportunities for the evolution and testing of diverse patterns and practices within GPPPS with respect to their general organization, the composition and functions of their policy controlling boards, the structure of their staffs and the relation of the professional components to each other and to the plans as a whole.

The inherent complexity in the development of GPPPS in a competitive pluralistic system results basically from the fact that they are not merely group payment or insurance organizations but instead are direct service-providing organizations linked with group payment or prepayment. The usual insurance plan is not unlike a "hunting license" for people to find where to get needed services, and then to learn whether and to what extent the insurance carrier will pay the costs. The group practice prepayment plan undertakes to organize the availability of service—substantially all needed services, at all hours and on all days; and it undertakes to make the services available through a prepayment charge that has to be competitive with the premiums for insurance related to independent and disparate availability of the services.

The inherent complexity makes a long listing, whatever the detailed design. It reflects many factors:

179

Needs with respect to legal authorizations in the states;

Resources for planning, and the study of community characteristics, needs, interests and potential sponsorship;

Determination of intended scope of services and expected costs, geared to the needs of the population to be served and compatible with their ability to pay;

Availability of facilities in the community, and of capital funds if new construction is to be required;

Staff recruitment and preparation;

Decisions about self-insurance or reinsurance;

The prospects and advance provisions for the availability of a population to be enrolled for the contemplated services and the expected costs, and formulation of definitive marketing plans and procedures, especially through "dual choice" clauses in collective bargaining agreements;

Resources to fund expected initial operating deficits while enrollment and prepayment income are below the "breakeven" level, and so on.

Not the least of the problems is the availability of knowledgeable consultants to assist in such undertakings by local area groups.

Such a listing of inherent complexities in the development of direct service plans must, unfortunately, be lengthened by artifactual hurdles such as legal obstructions and professional interferences and discouragements injected by vested interests in the *status quo* that are not friendly to the development of a proposed GPPP in the community.[14]

The group practice prepayment plans have thus far been principally designed for urban and suburban populations. How and to what extent they may be adapted through regional designs for people in semirural and rural areas waits on newer undertakings.

The costs of GPPP development are highly diverse, depending on the pattern being considered and the local circumstances and resources. At the one extreme, a large existing medical center or hospital may be able to proceed with little financial help from external sources; at the other, a community group may need some hundreds of thousands of dollars for each of several years in its planning and initial development stages. Capital needs may range from little or nothing to $1 to $4 million for the ambulatory facilities required by a program of sufficient size to be viable, even apart from requirements with respect to construction and equipment of inpatient resources.[15] Initial operational

180

years could conceivably have assurances of sufficient enrollment, pre-payment income and working funds to be without need for subsidy; or a program to be community sponsored could be stillborn unless assured of amounts equal to (say) 25 to 50 per cent or more of the operating costs expected for its first two or three years when enrollment and prepayment income may be low.

Obviously, inasmuch as GPPPS are needed, national policy should recognize and accept that their development is in the public interest. And this position of public policy should lead to the provision of financial and technical support from public funds to the stage at which new GPPPS may reasonably be expected to be self-maintaining and viable. In my view, such public developmental support should be provided only to nonprofit organizations, leaving proprietary undertakings to their own resources.

Medical Foundation Plans

The intensified national concern for improvement of organization for the availability and delivery of medical care has led to crystallization of a consensus for an evolutionary course (I know of no substantial group that advocates a national governmental takeover toward creation of a national health service). Such a course may be supported by organizational developments that are intermediate between the prevailing fee-for-service solo practice of the present and the globally budgeted or per capita funded comprehensive group practice of the future.

A model for such potential intermediate planning is available in the so-called medical "foundation" pattern, sponsored by medical provider groups and associations. In such a plan, physicians in independent individual or specialty group practice agree to make their services available, as needed, to an enrolled population. The enrollees are to be served in the physicians' own offices rather than in a nuclear health center facility and are to make—or to have employers or others make on their behalf—fixed prepayments to the plan as a whole. The income to the foundation, less administrative costs, becomes available for payments to the participating physicians on any of several agreed patterns, whether by fees for services rendered according to an adopted fee-schedule, by specification of maximum fees that may be charged by the physicians, by global retainer amounts, combinations and so forth. Such a plan may be self insured (as in the older "medical service bureaus" developed by medical societies in Washington and

Oregon or in the "open-panel" prepayment plans that were forerunners of the Blue Shield type plans in the United States and Canada) ; or it may be insured or reinsured by an insurance carrier (as in some of the newer "foundation" plans of California), subject to specifications of inclusions, exclusions, deductibles, co-payments and limitations on covered services.[16]

Obviously, a foundation plan has the potential of augmenting the availability of medical care for its enrollees. It may be capable of improving the comprehensiveness and delivery of care. Its need to market the plan, at a predetermined cost in a competitive environment, and to remain solvent could lead to controls of service utilization, to economies and to peer reviews of performances to give some assurances of quality of care. It could thus contribute to containment of cost escalations without sacrifice of quality. In these respects, the foundation pattern could have promise of becoming a better resource for medical care than fee-for-service solo or specialty group practice. How much it could make of such contributions and how well it could do so, remains, of course, to be learned. The pattern has had only limited recent experience, and in a few places, and has provided extremely little in the nature of objective data on performances for comprehensive prepaid care. In saying this, I dismiss the generally unacceptable Blue Shield plans with their limitations on scope of services and primary emphases on surgical and inpatient attendances, their deductibles and co-payments, and other respects in which they may (or may not) differ from the proposed foundation pattern.

Too much must not be claimed for, or expected from, the medical foundation design. Obviously, it cannot provide for the close association among professional and technical personnel, inherent in comprehensive group practice, and important for quantity, quality and economy of care. It may not be able, in most communities, to aggregate the availability of services for the maximum efficiency of the providers or for the convenience of the consumers. It may not be able to affect sufficiently for its own success the diverse practice patterns of its associated but not group-integrated physician participants. It may not be able to contribute substantially to encouragement of ambulatory care and the concomitant control of inpatient care. And it certainly would have great difficulty in making available to its physicians, economically, the resources of supporting personnel and facilities now increasingly common in the health center facilities of GPPPs. Moreover, it remains yet to be seen whether—how many—physicians in inde-

182

pendent practice will be prepared to surrender the freedoms of their solo practices for the cooperative restraints of the foundation pattern.

In short, the foundation plan for medical care is not to be considered as an alternative to the comprehensive group practice prepayment plan. It may, however, properly be regarded as an intermediate step between fee-for-service solo practice and prepaid group practice. Many solo practitioners, who may be strongly reluctant to join group practice and thereby surrender what they esteem as the advantages and benefits of their solo pattern, may nevertheless be prepared to join in a foundation plan. This may, therefore, serve as a useful transitional step in the evolutionary course between what we now have and the system pattern to which I believe we should and will go.

The medical foundation plan, therefore, has some good promise, and its further development deserves legal, financial and technical public support. This pattern does not require health center facilities as the GPPP does and its planning and design are simpler; therefore, its needs for developmental or capital funds are much less. If it has broad professional support in a community, it can be organized and become clinically functional rapidly. It has to market its program and effect adequate supporting enrollment, and thus needs working and underwriting funds; but because its associated physicians do not need to become full-time participants until enrollment and utilization load warrant this step, the foundation plan would not ordinarily require more than token or very limited initial operating subsidy. In these respects, development of the foundation pattern involves much smaller public financial investment than the group practice pattern, a reasonable conformity to its more limited potential contribution to the national need.

Financing of HMOs in General

Viewed in proper perspective, there is no inherent quarrel between proposals for development of group practice plans and of nongroup practice ("open-panel") plans. Each prototype—and others that may be intermediate in design—may serve useful ends. It is therefore sensible that both are embraced within the recommendations that are now widely heralded under the name of "Health Maintenance Organizations" (HMOs) Both are included, though under somewhat diverse names, in various broad legislative submittals to the Congress; and both are being actively considered in specific bills before both the House (Roy, Rogers, *et al.*) and the Senate (Kennedy, *et al.*).[17]

Legislative proposals to support the development of HMOs toward

183

better organization of medical care deserve vigorous and widespread support. It is to be hoped they will have such support—to the point of speedy enactment and the appropriation of implementing funds. However, even though these may be desirable developments, they should not be mistaken for sufficient steps. HMOs can contribute to the restructuring and improvement of the system for delivery of health maintenance and medical care services. They cannot, however, go much further than this unless they are integral elements in a broader program of health care provisions that extend to the financing of the system as a whole. Moreover, if supported through the customary pattern of legislative authorization and annual appropriation, they are likely to suffer from the difficulties and shortcomings of outlook, foresight, planning and assured financing that result from the agonies of the annual appropriation process.

A far better, more sensible and more promising pattern is that built into the design of the Health Security program developed by the Committee for National Health Insurance and spelled out in bills before the Congress (S.3, Kennedy, *et al.;* and H.R. 22, Griffiths, Corman, *et al.*).[9] The availability of operating supports for the effective utilization of "comprehensive health service organizations" (group practice plans), "professional foundations" (open-panel plans) and "other health service organizations" are incorporated in the guarantees for payments on behalf of everybody who elects to be served by such agencies. The support for their development would be assured through the automatic (formula) assignment to a "health resources development account" of fixed percentages (starting at two per cent and rising to five per cent a year) from the amounts to be available for annual obligation in a permanent trust fund. This special fund account would have an estimated $1.1 billion available in an initial year (at the two per cent rate) and about $4.0 billion a year in the seventh operational year (at the five per cent rate). These special account funds are intended to serve other purposes as well (e.g., support to develop selected types of health manpower production, to improve the distribution of health service personnel and the location of facilities, to support system operational practices), but a major share could be available each year for development and underpinning of what are now being called HMOs.

This provision in the Health Security program and these figures are cited to indicate the nature and the magnitude of what is really required to meet an urgent national need. Only by being prepared to annually spend amounts to be measured initially in hundreds of millions of dollars and subsequently by some billions of dollars can the national need be met. For what is involved is the movement of the national system of medical care from a long-obsolescent structure to one that will be capable of supporting the availability and delivery of good medical care for large proportions of over 200 million persons.

Those who are troubled about unmet needs are only being soothed—and perhaps are being deluded—if they are led to believe that the objective so ardently desired by so many can be attained by a token fiscal commitment. Here I refer to the proposed authorization of $57 million for fiscal 1972 and $60 million for fiscal 1973 in the Administration's budget, toward the development of HMOs for an initial target of availability to ten million persons.[18] Several times as much should be profitably available at once, and—as the annual commitments cumulate and the needed program can grow—ten to fifty times as much is required.[19] If we continue as a nation to commit ourselves to less-than-adequate financial programs and persist in engaging in "demonstrations" instead of in adequate substantive programs, we will be accepting continuance of the crisis scene.

The crucially needed GPPPS and HMOs of other design will not appear in sufficient numbers, capacities and locations without federal financial support. And if we would overcome the medical care problems that plague our society, that financial support has to be what is both necessary and sufficient to provide the resources. Without such support, our circumstances can be expected to worsen and then demand even more heroic measures later on.

CONCLUSIONS

At the outset of this discussion on the role of financing for the reorganization of medical care services and their delivery I focused on the current crisis in medical care, on the causes of the crisis, and on financing toward explicit objectives and goals.

Unless efforts being made now to bring medical care costs and expenditures into more effective relation with national needs are even more successful than we dare hope they will be, we have to expect that the crisis circumstances will not lessen and that they may worsen. Many new undertakings are needed, and more rational and more adequate financing of the medical care system has to be the starting point. Such financing has to serve two main purposes: it has to assure adequate and sensible ongoing support for a better system of personal health services; and it has to assure the leverage for moving from where we are toward that better system.

The better system, compatible with national aspirations and needs, and with emerging national policy, requires the availability to everybody of as good medical care as is feasible, utilizing all current and prospective resources. In my opinion, the desirable system design is spelled out in the "Health Security" program, proposing a national governmental system of financing in the social security pattern to support private provision of the services. Its most important element is the development—on an adequate national scale—of organized arrangements for the availability and delivery of medical care through comprehensive group practice plans linked with prepayment of the costs. Other forms of organized preparations for the better availability of prepaid comprehensive care, like the professionally sponsored open-panel (non-group practice) "foundation" plans, which are also embraced within the proposals for Health Maintenance Organizations (HMOS), have some promise of being useful. Their role, however, should be expected to be transitional between the prevailing non-group-practice and the desirable eventual group-practice programs.

The financing of the needed prospective system is feasible for our economy, because what is involved is primarily a rerouting of expenditures we are and will be making, rather than commitment to new and larger financial obligations. Indeed, the "Health Security" program proposes containment of future cost escalations steeper than those of the national economy, thus having the promise of reducing the increase in future fiscal commitments we are otherwise likely to have to make.

There are serious disagreements about the strengths and weaknesses of the various national proposals that are already before the Congress. The disagreements center on two main issues: the extent of governmental intervention and assumption of responsibility for the financing of the future system of medical care; and continuing reliance on the insurance industry and the marketplace as the media for group payment and fiscal management of the system. The two are obviously interrelated.

Fortunately, there are also agreements. There is a near consensus for national action and that in the first instance it has to be federal action; there is widespread agreement on keeping the provision of medical care services within the private sector of our society; and there is nearly complete agreement that the system of financing, whatever that should be, must include commitments to improve the organization of the services.

Congressional decisions about the major national commitments will not be made this year; perhaps they will be in 1973 or 1974. It is not unlikely, however, that decisions will be made and enactments completed within 1972 for federal commitments to encourage and fund a substantial beginning for development of organizational improvements of various kinds. We have to hope that if this comes about—whether in 1972 or soon thereafter—the design of the commitments will be compatible with more extensive enactments in succeeding years. If the more extensive enactments do not come soon after such initial commitments, the latter may have only limited growth and could even prove to have been an expensive exercise in futility.

The near-consensus to which I referred earlier extends, I believe, to recognition that the medical care scene needs massive public interventions—massive because the present system is massive and complex and is in serious trouble. In view of the nonagreements about the specific nature of the interventions that are needed and are desirable, we are frequently advised to explore compromises among proposals. I hope we will not see the nation much longer burdened with inadequate medical care services by reason of compromises in the interest of avoiding decisions on clear-purposed objectives for the national health.

REFERENCES

[1] MEDICAL CARE FOR THE AMERICAN PEOPLE: THE FINAL REPORT OF THE COMMITTEE ON THE COSTS OF MEDICAL CARE, Publication No. 28, Chicago, University of Chicago Press, 1932. See also: Falk, I. S., Klem, M. C. and Sinai, N., THE INCIDENCE OF ILLNESS AND THE RECEIPT AND COSTS OF MEDICAL CARE AMONG REPRESENTATIVE FAMILY GROUPS, Committee on the Costs of Medical Care, Publication No. 26, Chicago, University of Chicago Press, 1933; Falk, I. S., Rorem, C. R. and Ring, M. D., THE COSTS OF MEDICAL CARE: A SUMMARY OF INVESTIGATIONS ON THE ECONOMIC ASPECTS OF THE PREVENTION AND CARE OF ILLNESS, Committee on the Costs of Medical Care, Publication No. 27, Chicago, University of Chicago Press, 1933.

[2] Falk, I. S., National Health Insurance: A Review of Policies and Proposals, *Law and Contemporary Problems*, 35, 669–696, Autumn, 1970.

[3] Anderson, O. W., Collette, P. and Feldman, J. J., CHANGES IN FAMILY MEDICAL CARE EXPENDITURES AND VOLUNTARY HEALTH INSURANCE, Boston, Harvard University Press, 1963; National Center for Health Statistics, CURRENT ESTIMATES FROM THE HEALTH INTERVIEW SURVEY: UNITED STATES—1970, Washington, Department of Health, Education, and Welfare, Series 10, No. 63, 1972; Bice, T. W., Eichhorn, R. L. and Fox, P. D., Socioeconomic Status and Use of Physician Services: A Reconsideration, *Medical Care,* 10, 261–271, May–June, 1972.

[4] Rice, P. and Cooper, B. S., National Health Expenditures, 1929–71, *Social Security Bulletin,* 35, 3–18, January, 1972. See also: Klarman H., Rice, D. P., Cooper, B. S. and Stettler, H. L., Accounting for the Rise in Selected Medical Care Expenditures, 1929–1969, *American Journal of Public Health,* 60, 1023–1039, June, 1970; Cooper, B. S. and Worthington, N. L., Medical Care Spending for Three Age Groups, *Social Security Bulletin,* 35, 3–16, May, 1972.

[5] It may be noted that these national expenditures for all health care understate the totals by exclusion of expenditures for the education and training of personnel for the healing arts professions.

[6] Rice, D. P. and McGee, M. F., Projections of National Health Expenditures, 1975 and 1980, *Research and Statistics Note,* No. 18, Washington, D. C., Social Security Administration, October 30, 1970.

[7] Falk, I. S., The Costs of a National Health Security Program and Their Financing, Prepared for the Committee for National Health Insurance, Washington, September, 1971. Also in Hearings on National Health Insurance Proposals, Committee on Ways and Means, HR, Part 3, 524–586, Washington, U.S. Government Printing Office, October 28, 1971.

[8] Sydenstricker, E., Group Medicine or Health Insurance: Which Comes First? *American Labor Legislation Review,* pp. 79–86, June, 1934.

[9] The Health Security Act, Senate Bill No. 3, 92-1st, Senators Kennedy, *et al.;* and House of Representatives Bill No. 22, Representatives Griffiths, Corman, *et al.,* January 25, 1971.

[10] The Actuary of the Department of Health, Education, and Welfare, making comparative studies of the expected costs for various national health insurance proposals, concluded that the "Health Security" program might need about $8.4 billion more for Fiscal 1974 than the $105.4 billion his model indicated would be expended in that year if no major new program were enacted. And that result reflects generous assumptions on his part of expected categorical increases in services and costs and ungenerous allowances for savings and economies that could be affected by the program. (His corresponding finding for the Administration's program was + $1.8 to 2.6 billion, with his generosities reversed.) Also, he gave no weight to the value of the unique and essential contribution of the Health Security program to prospective control of cost escalation.[11]

[11] Analysis of Health Insurance Proposals Introduced in the 92d Congress, Department of Health, Education, and Welfare, Committee Print, Committee on Ways and Means, 92nd-1st, August, 1971.

[12] These details are available in the document cited in reference 7.

[13] Falk, I. S., Group Practice Is (the) Pattern of the Future, *Modern Hospital,* 101, 117–120, 203–206, September, 1963. See also: Williamson, J. W. and Tenney, J. B., Health Services Research Bibliography 1971–72, Department of Health, Education, and Welfare Publication No. (HSM) 72-3034, February, 1972. Kosco, P. and Bloom, A., Selected Notated Bibliography on

188

Health Maintenance Organizations (HMOS) with Special Reference to Prepaid Group Practice, Department of Health, Education, and Welfare Publication No. (HSM) 71-6202, May, 1972.

[14] Greenberg, I. G. and Rodburg, M. L., The Role of Prepaid Group Practice in Relieving the Medical Care Crisis, *Harvard Law Review*, 84, 887–1001, February, 1971; Holley, R. and Carlson, R. J., The Legal Context for the Development of Health Maintenance Organizations, Minneapolis, Health Services Research Center of the Institute for Interdisciplinary Studies, December, 1971.

[15] The Kaiser Foundation Health Plans have indicated that, in their experience of recent years, the capital needs per 1,000 enrollees to be served have been about $100,000 for two beds for inpatient care, about $75,000 per physician to be utilized and about $25,000 for other supporting facilities, equivalent to about $200 per person to be enrolled (or about $100 per person exclusive of inpatient facilities).

[16] Steinwald, C., AN INTRODUCTION TO FOUNDATIONS FOR MEDICAL CARE, Chicago, Blue Cross Association, 1971.

[17] The Health Maintenance Organization Act of 1971, HR 11728, (92-1st) Representatives Roy, Rogers, *et al.*, November 11, 1971; The Health Maintenance Organization and Resources Development Act of 1972, S.3327 (92-2nd), Senators Kennedy, *et. al.*, March 13, 1972. See also: The Proposed Health Maintenance Organization Act of 1972, Congressman Roy, W. R., The Science and Health Communications Group, Washington, D. C., 1972.

[18] I ignore, at this point, the proposal for $300 million of loan guarantee because the value of this provision is uncertain and indeterminate at this time.

[19] A somewhat more comprehensive program was outlined by the Administration in its White Paper,"[20] and, more recently by Administration spokesmen for the development of HMOS over the next eight years toward serving an additional 32 million enrollees through the provision of about $1.1 billion over that period. It remains yet to be seen whether even this limited program will be supported by budget requests.[21]

[20] Towards a Comprehensive Health Policy for the 1970's: A White Paper, Washington, Department of Health, Education, and Welfare, May, 1971.

[21] Valiante, J. D., Start-Up Problems of Health Maintenance Organizations, in HEALTH MAINTENANCE ORGANIZATIONS: RECONFIGURATION OF THE HEALTH SERVICES SYSTEM, Proceedings of the Thirteenth Annual Symposium on Hospital Affairs, Chicago, University of Chicago Graduate School of Business, pp. 39–68, May, 1971. See also: Riso, G., Riso Foresees 40 Million Enrolled in HMOS by 1980, *Group and Welfare News*, 13, June 1972, p. 3.

RATIONALIZING THE MIX OF PUBLIC
AND PRIVATE EXPENDITURES IN HEALTH

NORA PIORE

The more one struggles to foresee the characteristics of the post-July, 1966, American health care economy, to classify the data that will measure those characteristics, and to speculate about future trends, the more one is troubled by the terms "public and private sectors," "public and private expenditures," as they have customarily been used. These over-simplifications do not quite seem to fit the new facts nor quite convey an accurate sense of the shift that is occurring in the public philosophy. Also, they may not provide the disciplines represented at this seminar quite the right rubrics for classifying empirical observations nor the right insights for devising useful analytical tools.

Nevertheless, these phrases are accepted shorthand in this community and the issues implied in the assigned topic of this paper, regardless of its exact wording, are central to the inquiry of this Public Policy Seminar: What trends can be expected to occur? What issues will new and future developments raise? What goals are envisaged? What means will be available, and which should be selected for achieving these goals? What choices will be open, and perhaps most important, what machinery will be available, should be available, for making the choices, selecting the means?

All of these hinge not only on what will be the role of government expenditures from tax funds in a mixed medical care economy, but also on the role and management of a broader definition of public funds and public resources—one that would include nonprofit insurance, voluntary hospitals, and other forms of community investment. Perhaps even

191

more importantly they hinge on what will be the role, the capability and the composition of public authority, administrative as well as legislative, local as well as federal.

Under these circumstances the ideological connotations—pro and con—that have come to be attached to the term "the public sector" are no longer either quite realistic or quite useful. A much broader starting point is now needed. Perhaps the more appropriate term is "the public interest." To break out the critical choices and to assess the alternatives, it is necessary to ask, not the single question, "What is public, what is private?," but rather a series of questions about the nation's health resources: "Who has access and who utilizes?" "Who pays, when, and by what means?" "Who rations?" "Who manages?"

The first two of these questions relate to the distribution of the benefits of medical knowledge, and of the costs of these benefits, among the entire population.

The third question involves the proportion of total national resources to be allocated to personal health care, and the distribution within this allocation as between various types of care—prevention, treatment, rehabilitation and so forth. It encompasses such decisions as, for example, whether an intensive battery of tests will be provided selected populations at high risk or with symptomology, or whether a less intensive, but more extensive array of screening procedures will be administered a much larger segment of the population (annual physical examinations for everyone, for example).

The fourth question relates to the locus and quality of decision-making in regard to all of these.

Finally, underlying all of these is a fifth and basic question—from where will come the leadership, the initiative, the incentive, to improve the management of medical care resources, so that rising health care expectations can be met, the new public promise honored?

Within the broad limits already stipulated or to be added by the federal government, the answers to these questions for a long time to come will largely be determined by the states and the localities, and within these by the capability of the professional community to respond to the internal dynamics of the medical care establishment itself and to the pressures on this establishment that will be generated by the great new waves of effective medical care demand consequent upon the appropriation of large sums by the federal government.

Starting, then, with that general view of the world, this paper attempts to set forth some general observations and considerations

192

about the national framework that has been and is being constructed to govern medical care arrangements, and to consider, against this background, what may occur as the diverse localities of the nation put their particular imprint on what comes out of federal fiscal pipelines.

The full scope of the historic shift in public policy that was accomplished in the last Congress, as well as the full measure of what has been left to be resolved, comes into clearer focus when viewed against the following quotation from a fifteenth-century seminarian, Geiler von Keisersberg:

> A physician should have compassion with everybody, especially the poor who has not much to give. He should not only help such a one from compassion and for God's sake, but he should also be at his service everyday. Afterwards he may take all the more from the rich who could afford to pay.

In writing on the statute books the goal of universal access to the benefits of medical knowledge, the country has completed a long, historical process of shifting from the individual physician to the entire body politic the responsibility for compassion—and for making the decisions as to how much shall be taken from whom, and by what mechanism, to carry out that responsibility.

What that mechanism will be—how the costs of care will be distributed over the economy and among the people—is a question that this Congress has only opened up: it will be at the center of public deliberations for a long time to come. So also will be the pace at which the notion of compassion is translated into the idea of entitlement.

It is a long time since the decision regarding who should pay for compassion was solely in the hands of the physician. Institutionalization—the process of socializing—of both compassion and the decision as to who should pay for it goes back to the beginning of organized charity and to the Elizabethan poor laws. It underlies the Welfare medical care program in the United States, the Hill-Burton program, federal support of research and medical education. What is more important and less frequently recognized is the extent to which that important social decision is involved in routine hospital bookkeeping. It takes place every time a hospital's charge for an appendectomy or a maternity delivery includes some part of the cost of that hospital's cobalt machine or equipment for open-heart surgery. Every debate over community-versus-experience rating involves precisely that issue. That process, of shifting or spreading or transferring medical care costs and "loading" medical charges, occurs throughout the medical care economy. It is one part of the reasonable costs problem in Medicare. It is part of the issue raised at an earlier seminar in regard to the costs of nursing education.

In the past, these decisions have been made by individual practitioners, by institutions, sometimes by government, but chiefly on an ad hoc basis, and nearly always without relating such decisions in one sector of medical care to similar decisions in other sectors.

Having staked out the goal which, for short, will be called "universal access," having in effect accepted the responsibility of reallocating income to improve the distribution of medical purchasing power as a public responsibility, the nation is far from through with the thorny issues of equity and feasibility in financing medical care, even that limited portion of medical care that is now on the federal statute books. Indeed, having made these issues now for the first time not just visible but very conspicuous, Congress has only begun to cope with them.

For it is impossible to attain compassion with everybody simply by "taking all the more from the rich who can afford to pay." As Irving Kristol put it in a recent article in *The New Leader* magazine: ". . . there are alas not enough rich and they don't have enough money to affect the economics of the matter in any substantial way. . . ."

"The economics of the matter" will not be examined here in detail. But two observations, juxtaposed, will suffice to underscore the constraints:

1. American families with incomes below $7,500 spend only one-third as much on medical care as do families with incomes above $7,500.

2. Of all tax receipts from American families, an estimated 46 per cent came from families with incomes below $8,000—30 per cent from families with incomes below $6,000.

Even such fragmentary figures suggest that, although a health program financed from general taxes can indeed modify the distribution of health care costs and health care benefits as between income classes, it provides very limited magic to relieve the substantial burden of these costs that fall on the middle income slice of the population. It does insure that the burden is leveled out over time, rather than falling catastrophically when illness strikes. But it is possible to argue, as Kristol does argue, that what Medicare will do in effect is to

. . . wisely compel [those who are already the main beneficiaries of our expanding economy] to insure themselves against . . . medical disasters . . .

194

insure themselves because, in effect, what they receive in benefits is pretty much what they have paid out in taxes. . . .

These figures are cited here to make an additional and a slightly different point. With the present quite primitive information too little is known about how the costs—social as well as individual—of medical care and the costs of medical neglect are distributed in society.

Perhaps the most far-reaching consequences of the new order will be an entirely new capability to measure, analyze and understand—as well as to manage—the medical care economy, as systematic data accumulate from experience under the new legislation. Not only will society for the first time have the ability to get at economic costs, rather than making do, as is now the case, with arbitrary cost allocations reflected in charges and prices, but will also be in a position to really measure how and on whom the costs fall and who receives the benefits.

As real tools develop with which to examine these questions, the area of technical judgment, in regard to many of the thorny issues of public policy, will broaden and the ideological gap will be substantially, though perhaps not correspondingly, narrowed.

Observing the history of Congressional performance in regard to atomic energy and federal science policy in general, one concludes that even in these highly technical areas, lay members of Congress specializing in these aspects of public policy have developed a remarkable capability of dealing with highly complex technical matters. Once the data and the analytical tools become available, the entire quality of the public decision-making process is likely to be enormously different from that which has characterized the public debate in the medical care field in the past 25 years. Needless to say, that will not occur immediately, and the public policy fabric of the future will continue to be woven with threads that reach back into history.

Clearly the economy, already quite mixed, will become more so. The extent of government intervention, including but not limited to, the chaneling of funds to directly underwrite the medical care of individual patients, will increase. That will not occur in any tidy fashion or according to any single blueprint, but will continue as in the past to reflect a variety of public purposes and be accomplished by a variety of devices. A good deal of the sorting out that will have to be done to make rational order out of this variety will be left to the localities. The federal government can be expected to set in motion certain additional forces that will press the localities to accelerate the sorting out, and will also prescribe certain additional boundaries within which this process can occur.

Among these boundary conditions are likely to be an expanded and increasingly systematic floor of entitlement for the least affluent and the most vulnerable. Also to be expected is fiscal support for the most expensive and for the least commonly used medical care resources and conditions. Those moves will, in turn, increasingly lift the burden of costs off of user charges at the time of service and off of the voluntary insurance system. In still another area, new federal legislation can certainly be expected, in the future as in the past, to channel the flow of resources in selected directions—to improve the capacity and underwrite the cost of care for particular disease entities; to encourage the construction of certain types of facilities, or the training of certain types of manpower, or the development of particular patterns of service, or the emphasis on certain aspects of care such as multiphasic screening, or to give priority to certain groups in the population—perhaps the poor, the minorities, the children, perhaps geographic areas with concentrated local needs whose origins are basically national rather than local in character.

All of these together will undoubtedly expand the fiscal dimensions of what is now called the public sector, though it is not at all certain that its proportionate role will increase by an equal amount, since quite possibly direct consumer expenditures may also expand.

If anything like this is what really lies in the crystal ball, then the administration proposals introduced in the 89th Congress, which give new support and impetus to local and regional planning and to the systematic and rational management of health care services and health care resources, may in the end have more far-reaching consequences than is suggested by their rather modest dimensions and the absence of ruffles and flourishes surrounding their introduction.

At least this is how it appears, viewed from the perspective of New York City, where one-third of all the medical care and half the cost of institutional care received by city residents has long been paid for out of public funds and where the new administration has recorded its intention of developing a systematic network of health services that would, at a cost the community can afford, better serve the unmet needs of the city's poor, help to contain the rising costs of health insurance premiums and of health care in general for middle as well as low income families, and deal with the desperate lack of arrangements for the elderly infirm and the mentally ill of all ages and all classes.

196

Basically, the professional community agrees that what is required in New York, in broad outline, is regionalization that will permit economical grouping of expensive and rarely used resources at the apex of a planned system on the one hand, and that will on the other hand provide broad-based, adequately staffed neighborhood medical services for common conditions and for ongoing health maintenance.

To accomplish this it will be necessary for the city to weld together four presently separate city departments providing health care for New York City residents; to mold into one system 22 municipal hospitals and nearly a hundred voluntary institutions, in which more than a million people are hospitalized each year. Even prior to Medicare and Medicaid, on an average day nearly half of the 33,000 New Yorkers in general care hospitals were ward patients: some of them may have had health insurance; all of them, whether in voluntary or municipal hospitals, were already receiving some degree of subsidized care, whether it was the contributed services of physicians, the contribution that high-charge private patients perhaps unknowingly make to the ward deficit, or the directly subsidized care provided each year for 300,000 patients in municipal hospitals or purchased by the city for another 140,000 patients in the wards of voluntary hospitals.

The number one issue on the health care planning agenda of the city is the development, out of these separate medical care pieces, of a coordinated network of facilities so organized and so integrated as to meet the varying needs of all residents in all the boroughs of the city without waste and duplication, on the one hand, and without such glaring gaps as occur when ambulances must make half a dozen stops before finding a hospital to which the patient can be admitted. The facilities must be capable of maintaining high standards of medical excellence to attract qualified staff and afford security and dignity to the patient.

Coupled with the necessity for systematizing these in-hospital resources is the requirement of a greatly expanded pool of extended care facilities for those who no longer require the high cost services of an acute-medicine type of hospital and, at the other end of the spectrum, the expansion, particularly for the low income population—largely without access to family doctors in private practice—of adequate, accessible ambulatory care centers to provide comprehensive health services at the local community level.

The detailed inventory of problems and of proposals to deal with them is contained in a recently issued Report of the Mayor's Advisory Task Force on Medical Economics.

197

Many consider that New York City is a nation unto itself, and that its problems, and reports that discuss them, are somehow quite different from and not relevant to those of the rest of the country.

Nonetheless, in vast sections of the country public hospitals comprise an important segment of the existing resources for health care; in these areas, as in New York City, the problems of moving forward toward a rationalized system that permits the systematic use of all resources will not be too different from the problems confronting New York City.

Moreover, as the national society moves in the direction that New York long has taken, of commitment to the use of the public authority to accomplish social change, New York—once considered atypical of the nation—now becomes, particularly in the health field, one of the country's chief laboratories for implementing this commitment.

As the country becomes more fully aware of the implications of the newly enacted Titles XVIII and XIX, it will also become more concerned about the unleashing of great new waves of consumer demand for medical services; concern that it will swamp existing resources and available manpower, that beneficiaries will be disappointed and providers overwhelmed. In the short run, cause for concern is justified; but enough evidence is available to show that the promise of effective demand is beginning to break a number of log jams on the supply side, to stimulate response in areas where need has long been known to exist, but action despaired of. The construction of extended care facilities, plans to hire and provide on-the-job training for large numbers of people who fall into no conventional category of health manpower, the attention beginning to be paid by hospitals to coping with the expected increase in utilization, the concern of medical schools with the total complex of institutions in their communities—all give promise that traditional American ingenuity will be rapidly engaged in meeting these crises. The net result will be that many innovations which have long been needed will quite suddenly begin to occur as the medical care establishment, given now the assurance that money will be available to pick up the chit, prepares to cope with the inundation.

SUMMARY

The rationalization of medical care arrangements can be expected to evolve in a variety of patterns in different localities, as a result of a kind of pincer operation, with federal action—funds and guidelines—

comprising one set of forces, and local initiative, within and outside the medical establishment the other. Together they will gradually shape into more rational systems the fragmented resources and unsatisfactory arrangements that now characterize medical care.

Provider components may be expected to continue to operate under a variety of ownerships and managements, but to become increasingly coordinated and to develop entirely new formats of service, in response to deliberate planning, both self-generated and externally imposed, and as a result of funding which will carry with it specifications as to quality, performance, specialization and responsiveness to need.

On the demand side, further federal action can be expected along the lines indicated, increasing the spread of fiscal access to the least affluent and the most vulnerable by systematic funding rather than ad hoc grants, at one end of the spectrum, and at the other end, underwriting the most expensive elements of care and thus increasingly leveling off the burdens now carried by the voluntary insurance system.

As Congress levies and appropriates larger sums for these purposes, it can be expected to become increasingly concerned with and expert in regard to the husbanding of these funds, to search for and devise and require procedures to improve the management and the yield of resources.

Within the boundaries established by the federal government these trends will undoubtedly occur at different paces and take different forms in different localities. As the scenario unrolls, new alternatives, new issues of public policy, will be revealed. In coping with these, as a by-product of new fiscal reporting systems alone, much more sophisticated analytical tools will be developed. As the area of technological competence increases, the ideological gap in dealing with these problems can be expected to narrow.

Fundamental resource allocation conflicts will continue, as between health and other social services such as education and housing, and, within the health area, as between the young and the aged, the needs of the mentally ill and the need for dental care, as between treatments for common diseases which commonly occur and treatments for rare diseases that rarely occur. In the area of choices too, the capability for measuring costs and benefits, including social costs and broadly viewed human benefits, is bound to improve as factors that are presently hidden and inscrutable become increasingly visible and measurable.

The issues will not be easy, but having at long last determined to close the book on the nineteenth century social climate, the country is now in a position to exploit twentieth century capabilities in arriving at balanced choices and in developing the management techniques and delivery systems to implement them.

ON REASONABLE COSTS OF HOSPITAL SERVICES

JOHN D. THOMPSON

Since its inclusion in the Medicare Bill, the term "reasonable cost" of hospital service has become a word-fact. If an idea is named it is often automatically considered to exist, particularly if enough people repeat the name often enough for it to assume the illusion of reality. Many are bothered with the "reasonable" part of the term, but surprisingly few are concerned about what the word "cost" really means when applied as a measurement of hospital expenses incurred in rendering patient service.

Any consideration of the implications of classifying hospital costs, whatever the descriptors may be, must start with a review of the hospital cost picture over a period of time. Table 1 presents hospital expenses per patient day over the past 21 years. Limiting the discussion to costs in non-federal, short-term general and other special hospitals, it can be seen from Table 1 that the overall increase of almost 413 per cent per patient day over the period studied represents a considerable increase in the cost of a basic commodity. Some of the burden of increased per diem expenses was offset by the fact that patients stayed in the hospital for shorter lengths of time. Though expenses per patient day increased 95.5 per cent from 1946 to 1952, expenses per patient stay for this same period increased but 72.9 per cent. From 1953 to the present, however, these two measures increased at about the same rate, 141 per cent as compared with 140 per cent, due to stabilization of length of stay, so every increase in per diem costs in the most recent period of time is a real increase of the cost of hospitalization to the patient or third party.

	Per Patient Day	Per Patient Stay
1946	$ 9.39	$ 85.57
1947	11.09	90.15
1948	13.09	114.35
1949	14.33	119.39
1950	15.62	127.26
1951	16.77	138.73
1952	18.35	148.00
1953	19.95	158.47
1954	21.76	169.67
1955	23.12	179.77
1956	24.15	186.11
1957	26.02	198.13
1958	28.27	214.67
1959	30.19	235.66
1960	32.23	244.53
1961	34.98	267.37
1962	36.83	279.91
1963	38.91	299.61
1964	41.58	320.17
1965	44.48	346.94
1966	48.15	380.39

Source: Hospitals, Guide Issues.

THE DEVELOPMENT AND CHARACTERISTICS
OF HOSPITAL COSTS

To place these numbers in their proper perspective, a consideration of the general subject of hospital costs must be undertaken, including the basic definitions, derivations and limitation of hospital costs, cost trends and the use of cost data. Hospital costs are different from hospital expenses even if both are often divided by the same denominator and expressed as cost or expense per patient day. Expenses are just what the term means—all the money paid out to operate the institution. Costs are expenses 1. specifically classified by a standard chart of accounts, 2. allocated directly or distributed to service units according to a uniform method of apportionment and 3. transformed into unit costs by dividing them by consistently defined and generally accepted units of service.

Hospital costs have been and are notoriously gross measurements of actual expenses occurred in rendering services. Costs per patient day, the average cost of a day's care in a hospital for a period, must still be viewed with skepticism particularly when comparing the costs of one hospital with those of another, until it is determined how the above three standards are met. First and probably most important, just what categories of cost does the average patient-day cost include? Is allowance made for depreciation and interest expense? Does the per diem cost include nursing education expenses and medical education expenses? Does it include expenses incurred in the operation of an emergency room or outpatient department?

The second limitation of hospital cost analyses is that apportioned cost, that is, cost not directly pinned to the patient's bed or his unit of service, is a very substantial proportion of total costs. Although standard methods of apportioning these costs have been recommended, these distributions are on a much broader basis than is usually found in manufacturing or other nonservice industries. Strict adherence to uniform apportionment is therefore critical.

Even though the service unit "patient day" has been standardized, when one leaves this measurement and attempts to find uniformly accepted definitions of an "outpatient visit" or a "laboratory examination" or "surgical operation" to determine unit costs based on these services, consistent agreement among hospitals soon fades.

One fundamental limitation in interpreting hospital costs is the difficulty of using an average cost at all. Within the hospital one finds "very expensive patients" and some "fairly inexpensive patients." Since costs are not kept on an individual patient basis, but are allocated from departmental expense, substantial effects on the average cost figures could result from completely different mixes of patients.[1]

To further confound or complicate an already murky measurement, the problem arises of variation in services offered by hospitals. This is the factor that has been confusing the hospital size-cost relationship, which has attempted to determine "the economically sized hospital" based on cost figures. Are large hospitals just "different" from small hospitals, offering a different pattern of services and probably catering to a different mix of patients, or is the mere size of the hospital an important determinant of hospital costs?

In reviewing the development of uniform cost accounting in hospitals, one is struck by two characteristics in its evolution, the comparatively recent interest in cost analysis and the variety of uses to which such analyses have been put.

The first known attempt at sophisticated unit cost finding is dated

1908, and appears in *The Forms of Hospital Financial Reports and Statistics*.[2] This little volume is interesting reading, not so much because it evokes a feeling of nostalgia for the days when patient-day costs were $2.425 for private patients and 16 cents an outpatient visit, but to illustrate that even then attempts were being made to separate inpatient costs from ambulatory service costs.

Although references in the literature indicate that the first American Hospital Association publication on recommended accounting procedures appeared in 1922, it was not until 1935 that the Association published its first manual on a standard chart of accounts.[3] That manual contained the basic charts of accounts recommended for hospitals, along with some basic statistical definitions of hospital service units, and did consider allocation of costs so classified between inpatient and outpatient departments. The manual was revised in 1940,[4] 1950[5] and 1961.[6] Not until 1957, however, were these recommended statistics and accounts classified into a complete cost-accounting system through uniform apportionment to cost and service centers.[7]

Outside the official national association, local associations and even branches of the federal government promoted the notion of uniform cost accounting for hospitals and presented methods to accomplish this end. The United Hospital Fund of New York evidenced early interest in cost comparisons, and its manual,[8] published in 1946, was the most complete available at that time. Probably the most important stimulant to uniform cost accounting was the E.M.I.C. reimbursement form developed by the Children's Bureau to pay hospitals for maternity services during World War II. A further explanation of this program will be attempted in a later section of this paper.

Attempts at refining cost data are under way at the present time, stimulated by a concern for improved management techniques and by the cost reimbursement policy of Medicare. At least one such refinement is specifically directed to the uniform derivation of critical cost and functional "indicators" by the Hospital Administrative Services (HAS) of the American Hospital Association. These indicators, both in terms of costs and labor hours, are directed at measuring departmental performance as well as the cost of units of service.

The degree of desired sophistication and standardization in a costing system depends upon how the derived information is to be used. A review of the available literature seems to indicate that cost analyses were undertaken 1. for internal control, 2. as a basis for setting rates, 3. for cost comparisons between hospitals and 4. in mounting special studies of the costs of specific critical departments. No references are found in the early literature that use costs as direct reimbursement rates, nor, in any literature, about using costs as the criteria for the evaluation of specific hospital programs.

Obviously, if the primary use of cost information is internal, whether analyzing trends of or setting rates for one institution, the primary requirement for that information is simply that it be consistent over time. On the other hand, comparisons with other hospitals, if they are to be at all useful as indicators of relative operating efficiency, require that each hospital classify, allocate and apportion expenses the same way. The same uniformity is necessary if many hospitals are to be reimbursed by a single third party on the basis of costs.

A few excerpts from Davis and Rorum illustrate the prevailing attitude toward the use of cost data before World War II. "A carefully planned system of cost analysis would be of immense benefit to a superintendent not only in the control of hospital expenditures, but also in the enlistment of public support. . . . If the total costs of each hospital service were determined separately, unit costs could be calculated for board and room, x-ray service, etc. and these costs compared with existing fees.[9]

"Cost per patient day could be regarded as an accurate measure of hospital efficiency, if all hospitals were to calculate this quantity according to the same formula. Unfortunately no uniformity is followed in hospital accounting.[10]

"The public's interest in hospital care requires that some fees be established at levels presumed to cover only portions of their respective costs. The very low daily rates in most hospital 'wards' are evidence of this public policy, for these rates are presumed to be lower than the costs of services to which they apply."[11]

Of particular importance is the last excerpt because it represented the feeling of many in the hospital field before the days of "cost reimbursement." Hospitals feared that if they were paid full cost for services they would lose their charitable immunity, their nonprofit status.

The first important service benefits, cost-based reimbursement program was the Emergency Maternity and Infant Care (E.M.I.C.) Program of the Children's Bureau, from April, 1943, through December, 1946. It is impossible to overemphasize the influence of this war-time, temporary, emergency program on the subject of this paper and on subsequent federal legislation. Fortunately, an accurate, objective rec-

205

ord of the total experience of this program is presented in a monograph by Sinai and Anderson.[12] Rereading this report now, when the implementation of Medicare is at the top of everyone's priority list, gives one an almost frightening feeling of *deja vu*.

The program was characterized by the provision of a direct comprehensive service benefit (covering physicians and hospital services), without a means test, under quality controls, where reimbursement was paid directly to the providers by a varying fee schedule for physicians and through a cost reimbursement formula for hospitals.

Without negating the importance of the first four characteristics, indeed it is recommended that all reread this monograph, an overview of the cost reimbursement principle and its derivation, its application, its acceptance and the problems associated with its administration is central to any consideration of reasonable costs.

The then radical principle of payment to hospitals based on the costs of service emerged from the previous experience of the Children's Bureau in administering certain sections of Title V of the Social Security Act. As stated by Sinai and Anderson, "Out of the experience with maternal and child care and especially with the program for crippled children, certain policies had emerged with respect to hospitals. Thus the Bureau was in position to initiate hospital payments with certain background of 'know how'."[13]

In fact, the principle of cost reimbursement was established in May, 1942, when the Bureau was operating under its "B Fund" of Title V of the Social Security Act (the first Emergency Maternity and Infant Care appropriation was not passed until March, 1943). A memorandum to state health agencies, under a section dealing with rates of payment for hospital services, states that such service will be based on "the actual per diem cost of operating the hospital, to embrace all costs of care while mother and newborn infant are in the hospital, including delivery room, laboratory service, drugs, and so forth, except the medical services of the attending physician. Hospital care for sick children should also be paid on a per diem cost basis."[14] The specific definition of per diem cost was clarified three months later; a definition that was refined in a series of memoranda to the various state health departments, who were functioning as overseers of the quality criteria and as the "fiscal intermediary" between the hospitals and the Bureau.

The reimbursable cost report, which reflected the final refinements of the Bureau's cost reimbursement approach, became effective July 1,

1944. A review of the derivation of the per diem cost is illustrative of the way total costs are classified into reimbursable and nonreimbursable costs. The exclusions begin with research expense and medical education expense. Unfortunately, the Sinai-Anderson monograph does not review examples of completed statements; it would be interesting to determine how many hospitals deducted anything on this line and how much was deducted by those hospitals that did enter a value.

On the other hand, salaries and maintenance expense of house staff and "other" physicians were included. However, the pattern was set. The authors, in commenting on the exclusions, pointed out, "Certain features of this basis of hospital payment are prominent. . . . Excluded are the costs of research and education. . . . Since the principle of reimbursable cost appears to be spreading, its application on the above basis should serve to direct public attention to the need of a more stable support of hospital research and education . . ."[15]

Other deductions are also worth noting. The deduction of depreciation was not a true deduction; it served to clear the books for a later overall allowance of ten per cent of the per diem cost. It is probable that this allowance was also presumed to cover bad debts as well as miscellaneous deductions.

It was the deduction of the estimated value of donated or voluntary services that caused the real problems. This meant that those hospitals where a portion of the services were being provided by the religious could not charge equivalent salaries for donated services, which in other kinds of hospitals would have to be purchased. Only maintenance expense of religious orders was allowed. When the Children's Bureau, the Veterans Administration and the Office for Vocational Rehabilitation jointly agreed to pay for hospital services on a revised reimbursement formula in 1947, a limit of $75 a month, to be paid to the mother house for each sister on duty in the hospital, was included in the reimbursement formula.

In spite of these restrictions and deductions, and even though the Bureau never could, for example, enforce its requirement for an independent audit of the hospital's expense statements, this revolutionary idea of payment of cost was well accepted by hospitals. In 1944, the Board of Trustees of the American Hospital Association approved the Bureau's reimbursement system[16] and a 1947 editorial in *Hospital Management* stated, "This rule was so reasonable, and yet so entirely unusual, that it struck hospital people everywhere as one of those wonderful things which somebody should have thought of much earlier; and it naturally resulted in a general demand everywhere that all governments do the same thing."[17]

It is a bit surprising, therefore, that the Commission on Hospital Care in its report of 1947, did not directly endorse or recommend the principle of cost reimbursement. Though it was stated that "hospital care for indigent patients should be provided in both voluntary and governmental hospitals. Basic services should be purchased at rates *related* to cost and adequate to maintain a high quality of hospital care, etc."[18] Later in the report, when considering patterns of Blue Cross payments to member hospitals, the following appears: "Cost of service is a third method of payment. This method is not in general use because of the unwillingness or inability of hospitals to make available actual costs of furnishing hospital service. Also because of the lack of uniformity in the accounting methods used by member hospitals, costs are not comparable."[19]

Though the cost reimbursement idea has steadily expanded since this early example, through its acceptance by many state and local governmental units and by many Blue Cross Programs, it is interesting to note that today with "reasonable cost" written into the Medicare Bill, many in the hospital field consider everyone's hospital costs except their own open to question.

The real paradox in the history of hospital costs is that as interest rose in cost reimbursement, little, if any, comparative cost information was developed as an administrative or research tool. It can still be said that "the researcher into hospital cost must be prepared to face at least two difficulties. . . . The second difficulty is more common to research in general: data series are not always consistent across hospitals or consistent within a single hospital over time. Furthermore, many of the series necessary for research have not been collected."[20]

The medicare reimbursement formula negotiated by the Social Security Administration and the hospitals was an equitable one within the framework of reasonable costs for services received. One could state that the ratio of costs to charges, rather than average cost, presumes a broader knowledge than is now available of the actual costs to care for a patient over 65 years of age in a hospital. Although the density of ancillary services per patient day is probably less on the average for the elderly patient, it may well be that each of these services "costs" more[21] or that routine services, including nursing services,[22] cost more for a patient over 65 than for a patient under that age,

208

This very problem came up in the congressional hearings on the E.M.I.C. Program when Representative Hare noted that he had received some complaints that it was unfair for hospitals to receive the average per diem for E.M.I.C. patients because the costs for these patients, being almost all maternity patients, were probably higher than for the average patient. Miss Lenroot in answering this question states that she would be glad to consider a per diem cost for maternity patients only if hospitals could give data and isolate the costs of maternity care patients from those of general care patients. It was obviously impossible to do so then, and not too many hospitals in the United States could do it in 1966.

CONNECTICUT'S COST EXPERIENCE

A detailed review of the pattern of increasing hospital costs in one state where cost data are both available and consistent will illustrate the severity of this problem. Connecticut was the first state to apply the cost reimbursement idea as the basis of reimbursement for inpatient services rendered to state and town welfare clients. As a consequence, beginning in the late 1940's, a uniform chart of accounts and separation of inpatient costs from outpatient costs were adopted by the 35 general, short-term hospitals in the state. As confidence in, and acceptance of, the validity of the data increased, inpatient costs were divided into routine (room and board costs) and special service costs. Later these were subdivided into non-maternity, maternity and newborn costs. A review of these costs is presented below.

As seen in Table 2, overall costs per patient day have increased 78 per cent over the last ten years, from $28.80 in 1957 to $51.25 in 1966. Routine bed and board costs increased by 66.6 per cent and special service costs increased by 94.8 per cent.

When the special service costs are examined further, the increased cost in that area becomes even more evident. Special service costs are further subdivided into direct and indirect costs. The direct costs reflect those expenses clearly assignable to the ancillary services; the indirect costs are those general operating and administrative expenses allocated to special services such as heat, light, power, housekeeping and general administrative expense. Table 3 reveals that direct special service costs increased by 107.7 per cent over the ten-year period. The indirect costs, on the other hand, increased at about the same rate (66.5 per cent) as routine room and board expenses (66.6 per cent).

TABLE 2. ACTUAL AND RELATIVE INCREASE OF COSTS—ROUTINE, SPECIAL SERVICES AND TOTAL COSTS PER PATIENT DAY, 35 CONNECTICUT HOSPITALS

	Cost of Routine Services Per Patient Day	Relative Increase	Cost of Special Services Per Patient Day	Relative Increase	Total Cost Per Patient Day	Relative Increase
1957	$17.13	100%	$11.66	100%	$28.80	100%
1958	18.67	109	12.99	111	31.66	110
1959	19.29	116	13.82	118	33.10	115
1960	20.04	117	14.62	125	34.67	120
1961	20.48	120	15.71	135	36.19	126
1962	21.95	128	16.86	145	38.81	135
1963	23.00	134	17.95	154	40.95	142
1964	24.49	143	19.14	164	43.63	152
1965	26.29	154	20.57	176	46.86	163
1966	28.54	167	22.72	195	51.25	178

Source: Connecticut Hospital Association

TABLE 3. COST PER PATIENT DAY SPECIAL SERVICES, DIRECT AND INDIRECT COSTS, 35 CONNECTICUT HOSPITALS

	Cost of Special Services (Indirect Cost) Per Patient Day	Relative Increase	Cost of Special Services (Direct Cost) Per Patient Day	Relative Increase
1957	$3.47	100%	$ 8.20	100%
1958	3.56	103	9.43	115
1959	3.73	108	10.08	123
1960	3.55	103	11.07	135
1961	4.22	122	11.49	140
1962	4.51	130	12.35	151
1963	4.77	138	13.18	161
1964	4.96	143	14.17	173
1965	5.20	150	15.37	188
1966	5.78	167	16.94	207

	Cost Per Non-Maternity Patient Day	Relative Increase	Cost Per Maternity Patient Day	Relative Increase	Cost Per Newborn Patient Day	Relative Increase
1960	$34.43*	100%	$36.51**	100%	$12.60**	100%
1961	35.99	105	37.76	103	13.33	106
1962	38.40	112	42.43	116	14.99	119
1963	40.45	118	45.45	125	16.16	128
1964	43.13	125	48.44	133	17.21	137
1965	46.33	135	52.30	143	18.61	148
1966	50.66	147	57.84***	158	21.28***	169

* 35 Hospitals.
** 34 Hospitals.
*** 33 Hospitals.
Source: Connecticut Hospital Association.

The proportion of the total costs accounted for by the *direct* special service costs rose from 28 per cent in 1957 to 33 per cent in 1966.

In 1960, the Connecticut hospitals began to order their costs by non-maternity patient day costs and maternity patient day costs, costs per newborn day having been considered separately since 1957. To reset these cost figures, as opposed to those above, which considered costs over ten years, the general baseline figure of an increase in total costs per patient day was 47.9 per cent over the seven-year period. Table 4 reveals that though the non-maternity day costs had increased by 47.1 per cent over the seven-year period, cost per maternity day increased by 58.3 per cent and cost per newborn day by a factor of 68.8 per cent. Though approximately 47 per cent of the increase in the latter two categories would reflect general salary increases, the additional 11.2 per cent and 20.7 per cent increase in relative costs cannot be explained by advances in medicine, since the practice of delivering babies and caring for them have not changed that much over the seven-year period. Maternity admissions fell from 58,626 to 55,190 during the same seven years, and one hospital closed its maternity service.

The Connecticut cost data are presented for two reasons: first, to illustrate the increasing size of the problem the federal government faces with the Medicare reimbursement based on reasonable cost, and second, to examine the cost data to determine the course of action with a significant payoff to reduce this federal commitment.

211

The data support findings by others,[23] that increases in hospital costs, averaging more than six per cent annually for the past ten years, reflect an increase in general operating expenses—primarily personnel expenses, increases in wages and increases in the number of personnel per bed. In addition, a five per cent yearly increase for the 30 per cent of hospital costs reflects use of new, and the increasing use of old, ancillary services. All of this has occurred without an increase in productivity, as measured by standard econometric model.

Implications derived from the maternity-newborn data point out special factors operating in the costs of this clinical service.[24]

With the passage of Medicare, increasing hospital costs became a national concern rather than one of an occasional state insurance commission or Blue Cross Plan, as was the former rule. Many of these confrontations on the state level—in Michigan, New Jersey and New York, for example—did produce programs designed to attack the problem of escalating hospital costs.

Though many of the recommendations of these various studies were included in the Medicare law, the first year of experience with Medicare has been characterized by a preference to deal with the mechanics of paying reasonable costs rather than a concern toward controlling them. It is hoped that after the "year of the accountant" has passed, several years will be devoted to the examination of basic reimbursement policies. The following three-point program is offered to assist in these considerations: it is felt that provisions should be made to monitor, partition and study hospital costs; to make maximum use of the medicare utilization review process, and to coordinate federal and state planning efforts toward developing an integrated medical care delivery system.

MONITORING HOSPITAL COSTS

At this time, little valid, carefully controlled, comparative cost data are available as a basis for policy formation, research or administrative decision. The nearest approximation of such data is that gathered by the Hospital Administration Services of the American Hospital Association. The data are limited, however, particularly in consideration of outpatient expense, and it is not possible to determine cost indicator information by clinical services, such as obstetrical service as separate from the general medical and surgical service. The Connecticut data reveal that newborn and maternity patient day costs behave differently than do general medical and surgical costs.

212

Basic operational data are lacking on hospital costs detailed enough to monitor the system, refined enough to derive performance standards, or of sufficient accuracy to permit sophisticated multivariate analysis. It is hoped that the National Center for Health Services Research and Development will address itself to this question.

PARTITIONING HOSPITAL COSTS

Even before Sinai began to divide consumer costs from costs to which at least public attention should be drawn, Davis and Rorum were considering what costs the public should be responsible for, as opposed to the hospital. They stated, "The data for analysis of hospital costs would enable the hospital superintendent to show clearly which of the various services were not self-supporting from patients' fees . . . the need for public funds may be traceable directly to the cost of education for student nurses."[25] These authors were a little more specific in other references. "It is the public's responsibility to remove from the superintendent that portion of the economic burden resulting from the community's demand for hospital care and from the unwise investment of that community in plant and equipment."[26]

Another cost study specifically points out, "The Committee believes that a hospital is ethically justified in maintaining a nursing school only if it is desirous and capable of providing an effective program of nursing education and if it can secure for this purpose adequate financial means. The Committee further believes the hospital is justified in expending hospital funds for its schools up to a point where the cost of the school is no greater than the value of the nursing service rendered by the school."[27]

Later consideration of the separation of patient care expenses from non-patient care expenses were not so definitely expressed. In 1962, McNerney, et al., stated, "Although education costs are incurred for the benefit of the entire community, these may be properly included in the cost of care in view of the significant amount of services rendered by the trainees."[28]

This study went on to recommend that almost all the points at issue in the E.M.I.C. formula, i.e., depreciation, dollar value of services by members of religious orders, research expense (with some controls), education costs, both nursing and medical, should be included in reimbursement formulas as reasonable costs.

Regardless of inclusion or exclusion in reimbursement formulas, hos-

213

pital costs must be partitioned into what Pollack[29] has classified as Hospital Community Services and Patient-Centered Services, since as this report points out, "Certain hospital services benefit the community as a whole, rather than the individuals who use the hospital." The committee then goes on to recommend payment by the community as a whole of various costs of services to the community. This recommendation is taken up in chapter six of the report, which points out serious obstacles to implementing this recommendation and recommends that only certain carefully selected costs be shifted; those that promise that the shift can, in fact, be accomplished. Specifically, one of the committee's recommendations is for payment from state revenue to voluntary hospitals for the support of nursing schools in voluntary hospitals.

Before going into the consideration of this recommendation, it might be well to review how the hospital got into the "education business" in the first place. Hospitals have historically regarded themselves as institutions with a triple mission—patient care, education and research. It was considered correct to spend income from patient care to achieve the other two goals because of the presumed direct relationship between the quality of patient care and the quality of the educational and research programs. In other words, if a hospital had any ongoing programs in medical education and was the seat of medical research, it was therefore a better hospital and the patients should be expected to pay a "premium" for this quality.

As noted above, the E.M.I.C Program deleted costs of research from its reimbursement formula. The recent availability of research funds, primarily from the National Institutes of Health, has resulted in a situation, where little of the patient income dollar is now being spent on research It may be possible under the Heart, Stroke and Cancer Program to pick up some of the medical education expense in certain of the hospitals. Both these programs were reflections of public concern that medical research and education were not receiving sufficient emphasis or funds under past arrangements—whatever the sources of funds happened to be. A byproduct of these programs is that perhaps less underwriting of these activities will take place with the fees paid by the consumers of hospital services.

Viewing the problem of nursing education expense in this frame of reference, one might question whether the concern of public policy might better be directed toward the overall problem of nursing education, and specifically to the question of whether nursing education should continue to be seated in the hospital at all. The arena of hospital

214

costs is not a proper place to determine the future of nursing education. Nursing education today should be undergoing as radical a revision as are the educational programs in engineering and other professions considered critical by the public. As long as most of the nurses are being trained in hospitals outside the mainstream of professional education, this reevaluation will not occur, nor will the needs of the nation for nurses (particularly for different kinds of nurses) be met.

The nursing profession and the hospitals have been playing with this question for years. As yet the public is confused between the claims of the nurses that any "true" professional education must take place in an academic locus,[30] and the claims of the hospitals that if they depended entirely upon university education programs for nurses, they soon would not have enough trained manpower to care for their patients. Would not the isolation of these costs from within the more general patient day costs focus public attention on the problem and eventually free the consumer of hospital care from being the sole contributor to this expense?

This is not the place to discuss the future role of the professional nurse, the proper seating of nursing education programs or the curriculum content of these programs. Public concern in this area is beginning to be reflected in lesiglation. The Nurse Training Act of 1964 provides grants-in-aid for construction, grants toward the operating expenses of schools planning to improve the quality of their nursing education programs, and grants for traineeships. The federal government is now paying nursing education costs in its Medicare reimbursement formula, thus underwriting about 30 per cent of the net costs of many hospital nursing schools. Nursing schools seated in colleges or universities are not eligible for these funds. Separation of these expenses from the reimbursement formula would permit general tax funds to be used in a directive way to influence the total system of nursing education.

STUDYING HOSPITAL COSTS

Little in this area remains to be added to the recent review of hospital costs studies by Lave.[31] The Connecticut cost data referred to earlier was studied in an attempt to relate variations among hospitals in cost per available bed day to a set of independent variables representing selected characteristics of these same hospitals. The characteristics selected were: 1. size of the hospitals as measured by admissions, beds in service and average daily census; 2. utilization as measured by per cent occupancy; 3. patient turnover as measured by discharges per bed and average length of stay; 4. quality as measured by a facilities and education index and a local price index as measured by average annual wage per employee.

Comparing such analyses of maternity and non-maternity costs, the effect of utilization as measured by per cent of occupancy in both of these services was clearly indicated. In fact, using this factor alone explained some 53 per cent of variation in cost per non-maternity available bed day in the 35 hospitals in Connecticut. The same factor explains up to 57 per cent of the variability in cost per available bed day in the maternity service.

This finding, though it agrees with some theoretical hypotheses of Klarman,[32] is contrary to the findings in the McNerney study[33] which states, "no consistent relationship was demonstrated between occupancy and cost."

Such lack of agreement is not unusual in this field and points up the absolute necessity for further studies if the implications of payment based only on reasonable costs are to be understood.

UTILIZATION REVIEW PROCESS AND AREA WIDE PLANNING

One wonders if too much concern is being directed toward the essentially limited area of hospital costs, expressed as cost per patient day, whether that cost be reasonable or unreasonable. The acute general hospital bed is rapidly becoming the most precious of community resources. At an investment cost of around $35,000 a bed and an annual operating cost of 12 to 15 thousand dollars a bed, it is obvious that the use of this expensive commodity must be considered a critical resource allocation problem.

The problem must be attacked in at least two ways. The first is to control the proper use of this resource: the fact that the right patient is in the right bed at the right time for the right period of time, and furthermore that he is receiving the correct kind of care while he occupies that bed. These, in essence, are the goals of the Utilization Review Process which now has the force of law, having been included in Medicare under Title XVIII A.

Various attempts have been made in the past to achieve these goals, in the AID program of New Jersey, for instance, and in various Blue Cross utilization review programs. It is evident, however, from the study of some of these plans that in spite of fairly sophisticated centralized information gathering processes, without strong reinforcement and commitment at the local level the desired utilization pattern will not be achieved.[34] This places the burden of proof—that the right patient is in the right bed at the right period of time and is receiving the care—on the shoulders of the medical staff of each institution.

Evidence[35] indicates that though hospitals have responded to the utilization review requirement of Medicare, much remains to be done in this area. A stepped-up review of what happens to a patient once he is in a hospital would be much more effective if it were coupled with a pattern of medical practice that has demonstrated that fewer patients needed to be admitted in the first place.[36]

The second approach in allocating this precious resource is through total medical delivery system planning to be certain that new resources will flow into the system at a rate and kind needed to achieve maximum utilization of old and new facilities.

These two approaches are somewhat divergent, because, on the one hand, if the right patient must be in the right bed, and, on the other hand, these beds must be utilized to their full capacity, the number of beds available must, in the future, be balanced with the demand.

These two attacks, therefore, consider hospital costs not as the price of a unit of a service, but as the cost of decreased units of service per unit of population served. This may be the only way to assure the delivery of hospital services at a reasonable cost.

REFERENCES

[1] Feldstein, Martin, S., Hospital Cost Variation and Case Mix Differences, *Medical Care,* 3, 95–103, April-June, 1965.

[2] No author listed, *The Forms of Hospital Financial Reports and Statistics,* Boston, Thompson-Brown Company, 1908, Appendix i.

[3] *Hospital Accounting and Statistics, A Manual for American Hospitals,* Chicago, American Hospital Association, May, 1953.

[4] *Hospital Accounting and Statistics, A Manual for American Hospitals with Specific References to Smaller Hospitals,* Chicago, American Hospital Association, 1940.

[5] *Handbook on Accounting, Statistics and Business Office Procedures for Hospitals: Section One, Uniform Hospital Statistics and Classifications of Accounts,* Chicago, American Hospital Association, 1950.

[6] *Uniform Chart of Accounts and Definitions for Hospitals,* Chicago, American Hospital Association, 1961.

217

[7] *Cost Finding for Hospitals*, Chicago, American Hospital Association, 1957.

[8] Rosewell, Charles G., ACCOUNTING, STATISTICS AND BUSINESS OFFICE PROCEDURES FOR HOSPITAL, New York, United Hospital Fund, 1946.

[9] Davis, Michael M. and Rorum, C. Rufus, THE CRISIS IN HOSPITAL FINANCE, Chicago, The University of Chicago Press, 1932, p. 109.

[10] *Ibid.*, p. 115.

[11] *Ibid.*, p. 110.

[12] Sinai, Nathan and Anderson, Odin W., E.M.I.C.: A STUDY OF ADMINISTRATIVE EXPERIENCE, Ann Arbor, Bureau of Health Economics, University of Michigan, 1948.

[13] *Ibid.*, p. 140.

[14] *Ibid.*, p. 57.

[15] *Ibid.*, pp. 142–143.

[16] *Ibid.*, p. 39.

[17] *Ibid.*, p. 147.

[18] Commission on Hospital Care, HOSPITAL CARE IN THE UNITED STATES New York, The Commonwealth Fund, 1947, p. 174.

[19] *Ibid.*, p. 577.

[20] Lave, Judith L., Review of Methods Used to Study Hospital Costs, *Inquiry*, 2, 80, May, 1966.

[21] Ingram, James C. and Colman, J. Douglas, Implications of a Study of the Age Differential in Hospital Costs, Associated Hospital Service of New York, March 1, 1967, mimeographed.

[22] Patients over 65 Receive More Nursing Care. Preliminary Report: Hospitals, *Journal of American Hospital Association*, February 16, 1967, pp. 23a and 23b.

[23] Klarman, Herbert E., THE ECONOMICS OF HEALTH, New York, Columbia University Press, 1965, pp. 108–110.

[24] Thompson, John D. and Fetter, Robert B., The Economics of the Maternity Service, *Yale Journal of Biology and Medicine*, 36, 91–103, August, 1963.

[25] Davis and Rorum, *op. cit.*, p. 110.

[26] *Ibid.*, p. 109.

[27] Pfefferkorn, Blanche and Rovetta, Charles A., ADMINISTRATIVE COST ANALYSIS FOR NURSING SERVICE AND EDUCATION, Chicago, American Hospital Association and the National League of Nursing Education, 1940.

[28] McNerney, Walter J., *et al.*, HOSPITAL AND MEDICAL ECONOMICS, Chicago, Hospital Research and Educational Trust, 1962, p. 955.

[29] Report of the Governor's Committee on Hospital Costs, New York, December 15, 1965, p. 63.

[30] A.N.A.'s First Position on Education for Nursing, *American Journal of Nursing*, 65, 106–111, December, 1965.

[31] Lave, *op. cit.*

[32] Klarman, *op. cit.*

[33] McNerney, *op. cit.*, p. 799.

[34] Bailey, David R., An Exploratory Analysis of Length of Stay Statistics of the Hospital Service Plan of New Jersey's Approval by Individual Diagnoses Program (AID), essay submitted for Master of Public Health degree, Yale University School of Medicine, June, 1967.

[35] Greaney, Francis, Morisse, Robert and Wilson, James, A Study of Utilization Review Mechanisms Employed in Connecticut Hospitals, Hospital Administration Program, Department of Epidemiology and Public Health, Yale University School of Medicine, May 30, 1967, mimeographed.

[36] Densen, Paul M., Balamuth, Eva and Shapiro, Sam, PREPAID MEDICAL CARE AND HOSPITAL UTILIZATION, Hospital Monograph Series No. 3, Chicago, American Hospital Association, 1958.

Manpower:

Some Illustrative Economic Issues

RESEARCH INTO MANPOWER FOR HEALTH SERVICE

DALE L. HIESTAND

Manpower has often been said to be the key problem in the expansion of the health services, despite the fact that health manpower resources have expanded extremely rapidly (about four per cent per year in the 1950's, and 2.5 per cent per year so far in the 1960's). Yet, as in all services, manpower remains the crucial resource in health services. How rapidly and how well manpower is developed essentially determines how rapidly health services rise.

This paper provides an appraisal of the recent research into manpower for the health services, both to indicate its accomplishments and to suggest the main lines which should be pursued in the future.

The key question has always been: How can research on manpower contribute to the expansion and improvement of health services to the nation? Since the number of those who are engaged in health manpower research is quite limited, this paper has been written particularly with the potential, but inexperienced, researcher in this field in mind. The intent has been to make the key issues explicit, to indicate what has been emphasized to date and to point out open research areas where specific efforts are likely to yield significant contributions. At this stage, more rapid progress will be gained from solidly constructed, finely focused efforts rather than from grand designs.

THE CONTENT OF MANPOWER STUDIES

Research into manpower for the health services represents the juncture of many areas of interest. Both health and manpower economics have grown rapidly in the last decade, and have begun to take definite shape. Health economics, long the preoccupation of health professionals, is becoming a recognized field in economics itself. Manpower or human-resources economics is also relatively new.

Manpower studies are concerned with both the supply of and the demand for workers, including the various forces and institutions which affect the development of potential and actual workers in a field. These forces include the education, training, selection, hiring and assignment of workers. The manpower concept also includes the utilization of workers, i.e., the particular functions which workers in different occupations perform, and the way these functions change as a result of other changes in the economy, technology and society.

Manpower research deals with the economics of supply, demand and utilization, but also with nonmonetary factors, motives and institutional forces. Thus, manpower research borders on the fields of management, administration, education, training, psychology and sociology.

Research into health manpower is still in its infancy. The literature is already voluminous, but one is impressed more with what has not been learned than with what has. This paper is concerned with empirical research, rather than theoretical and *ad hoc* discussions of health manpower. The impact of the total educational system on the number and quality of workers in the health services is also not within the scope of this paper. Neither is the research bearing on the structure, functioning and financing of hospitals, governments and professional schools being examined, even though the amount and quality of manpower available for health services depends directly on the economics of the public and nonprofit sectors.[1]

The present paper is organized along six separate axes:

1. The availability of basic data on health manpower.
2. Shortages and future demands for workers in particular fields.
3. The inflow of workers into particular fields, including the development and training of personnel; the incentives, disincentives and opportunities to enter various fields; etc.
4. Losses from the health fields through retirement, leaving the labor force, transfer to other occupations, etc.
5. Current manpower utilization patterns and their changes over time.
6. The qualitative dimensions of manpower in the health services.

224

This rather structured approach is used because the field is so new that most manpower research has been of an *ad hoc* nature. Persons from different disciplines have investigated one or another problem relevant to their own work and, as a result, manpower problems in health services have usually been studied from relatively narrow points of view. By looking at topics rather than occupations one can appraise relative progress in different fields and indicate methods to deal with related problems of the different occupational groups.

TENDENCIES IN EXISTING RESEARCH

The most striking aspect of research into manpower for health services to date has been its concentration on a few groups and problems and its spotty nature otherwise. In 1960, as Table 1 shows, some 2.6 million persons were employed in the health services industry, and 291,000 were in selected health occupations in other industries. The central concern in health manpower research has been with physicians, who number only 230,000 (234,000 including osteopaths) or only eight per cent of the total. Indeed, most attention has been paid to physicians in private practice, who comprise perhaps six per cent of all health services manpower. Secondarily, attention has been centered on registered nurses, who comprise one-fifth of the total, and particularly on hospital nurses, who comprise less than one-seventh of the total. The other manpower groups employed in health services have received only sporadic attention. Of course, more up-to-date estimates may be found for some of these manpower groups, as is shown in Table 2. Although these data are not quite comparable, the central point remains.

The overriding attention given to physicians is clear in the literature and data on manpower discussed by Klarman[2] and Harris.[3] Of course, attention has centered on physicians and nurses for many reasons. These two occupations are the key manpower groups with specialized skills which are essential to the maintenance and improvement of health. Indeed, in a way unparalleled in any other industry, the physician controls and influences his field and all who venture near it. For many functions, no direct substitute for the physician exists. This has a great impact on the manpower problems of the health services industry.

However, other personnel groups may substitute directly and indirectly for physicians and nurses. Because nonprofessional nursing

TABLE I. OCCUPATIONAL DISTRIBUTION OF PERSONS EMPLOYED IN HEALTH OCCUPATIONS

	Hospital, Medical and other Health Services Industry	Health Occupations Outside Health Service Industry	Total in Health Occupations
Professional and technical	1,167,218		
Physicians and surgeons	218,301	11,370	229,671
Osteopaths	3,861	220	4,081
Nurses, professional	528,771	52,518	581,771
Nurses, student professional	57,746		57,746
Technicians, medical and dental	127,947	10,866	138,813
Dentists	85,263	1,624	86,887
Dietitians and nutritionists	18,190	8,280	26,470
Chiropractors	13,630	223	13,853
Optometrists	13,073	3,132	16,205
Pharmacists	6,504	85,729*	92,233
Veterinarians	382	14,823	15,205
Therapists and healers, n.e.c.	25,272	11,296	36,568
Other	68,278		
Service workers, except private household	799,887		
Attendants, hospital and other institutions	365,690	25,446	391,136
Midwives	896		896
Practical nurses	144,045	63,921	207,966
Other service workers	289,256		
Clerical	399,703		
Attendants, physician's and dentist's office	70,607	1,564	72,171
Other clerical	329,096		
Craftsmen, foremen	67,742		
Operatives and kindred workers	62,441		
Managers, officials and proprietors, except farm	50,092		
Laborers, except farm and mine	12,172		
Sales workers	1,838		
Occupation not reported	28,160		
Total	2,589,253		

* In addition, are 25,456 managers and proprietors of drug stores, an unknown number of whom work primarily as pharmacists.

Source: United States Census of Population, 1960, Occupation by Industries, pp. 132–136.

personnel and paramedical personnel in other than nursing service have received far too little attention, this paper calls attention wherever possible to them. Practically no research has been reported in connection with personnel who are necessary to the provision of health services, but who are not substantially identified with health fields per se. This would include cooks, clerical workers, housekeepers, mechanics and the like. As the health services industry grows, health specialties in such fields are being developed. Ward clerks, medical secretaries, hospital masons and so on are becoming a part of the health manpower complex. As they become a more integral part, the need for research on these groups is becoming pressing.

Basic Data

Whatever the reasons for inadequacies in health manpower studies, they cannot include lack of basic data with which to work. The decennial censuses of 1940, 1950 and 1960 contain a great deal of data about the occupational, educational, income, locational, demographic

TABLE 2. HEALTH SERVICE WORKERS, BY LEVEL OF TRAINING

Level of Training and Occupation:	Number of Persons
Total	2,417,000
Doctoral level	
Physicians (including osteopaths)*	288,000
Dentists*	93,000
Other	44,000
Total	425,000
Allied health professions	
Dental hygienists†	15,000
Medical record librarians**	10,000
Medical technologists††	32,000
Occupational therapists	8,000
Physical therapists	12,000
Professional nurses (BS)	70,000
Speech pathologists and audiologists	13,000
X-ray technologists***	70,000
Other	160,000
Total	390,000
Diploma nursing	522,000
Other 1–3 year post-high school	
Certified laboratory assist.	1,100
Cytotechnologists	3,000
Dental assistants	95,000
Dental laboratory technicians	27,000
Inhalation therapists	4,000
Practical nurses	265,000
Other	159,900
Total	555,000
Short training	525,000

* Active.
† Licensed (some baccalaureate, primarily 2-year programs).
** Employed in hospitals.
†† Registered (both baccalaureate and less than baccalaureate).
*** Both baccalaureate and less than baccalaureate.
Estimates by Public Health Service on basis of available data from professional organizations.

Source: United States House of Representatives. *Report of the Committee on Interstate and Foreign Commerce on H.R. 13196* (Allied Health Professions Personnel Training Act of 1966). House Report No. 1628, 89th Congress, Second Session, 1966, p. 9.

and other characteristics of persons in the health service industry and health occupations. The various professional associations collect similar data from their members. A wealth of data on the personnel and operating characteristics of hospitals are collected and reported each year, and some data will be available on a monthly basis in the future. Indeed, annual occupational data are reported separately for practically every hospital in the country. The various educational and training institutions regularly report on their student bodies and their operations individually and through their associations. The relevant licensing agencies in the various states are also sources of valuable and detailed data, much of which is collected, classified and published by government or the various professional associations. Governmental agencies which employ, train, assist or in other ways deal with health manpower publish great quantities of relevant data. In addition, special surveys have been made from time to time by various governmental agencies and professional groups as a part of their continuing studies of one or another subject of interest.

In few other sectors of the economy are so much manpower data reported in comparable detail on a regular basis. In many cases, moreover, these data have been further processed to make them more useful to the researcher. The United States Public Health Service has published some 19 Health Manpower Source Books since 1952, providing data which have been partially processed but not analyzed to any significant degree.[4] Indeed, since the medical service industry is largely carried on under governmental and nonprofit auspices, new data are relatively easy to obtain. The only significant exceptions are independent practitioners, health workers employed in industry and the employees of privately owned hospitals. Even in these cases, responses to surveys have been good.

The development of research in health manpower has not been particularly impeded by a lack of data. Rather, vast amounts of information have not been well exploited. Some may question the quality of the data, but it is better than most manpower information in other sectors of the economy. New and better data can be relatively easily obtained if that appears advisable. But manpower researchers are exceedingly scarce, and priority ought to be given to analysis, rather than data collecting. That is particularly true for those newly entering health manpower research. As new concepts and relevant distinctions are developed, they can be fed into existing data collecting systems with relative ease.

228

Shortages

The preoccupation of manpower analysts in the health fields has been the estimation of shortages and the establishment of manpower goals for the future. One way in which shortages are measured is through the gap between minimum quantitative and qualitative standards and what exists in fact. For instance, in 1956, the American Psychiatric Association issued guide-lines on personnel-to-patient ratios for a variety of occupations and types of services in public mental hospitals. The number actually employed consistently fell short of the estimates of need based on these standards: by 55 per cent in the case of physicians, by 35 per cent in the case of psychologists, and so on.[5]

Another example of an estimate of shortage is the report of the Surgeon General's Consultant Group on Nursing. The Group based its estimate of a need for 850,000 nurses in 1970 largely on the finding of one study that in general hospitals "highest patient satisfaction was achieved when professional nurses gave at least 50 per cent of the direct care." This was in contrast to the existing proportion of 30 per cent. Realistically, considering the potential supply of students and the potential capacity of schools of nursing, the Group concluded that this total need could not be met by 1970. It then set a total of 680,000 professional nurses as a feasible goal for 1970.[6] Just prior to the time of the report, a total of only 582,000 nurses were employed in the United States.[7]

Another approach is the accumulation of data on budgeted vacancies. Hospitals, health departments and other units regularly provide data comparing actual employment with budgeted positions for various occupations and types of services. The vacancy rates thus computed vary greatly from one occupation to another and are lower for the higher administrative and other specialized nursing personnel than for general duty staff nurses.

Surprisingly, such estimates of shortages are received with little enthusiasm by many manpower analysts. The term shortage tends to be used in one way by non-economists and in a distinctly different way by economists. Non-economists use the term to describe a discrepancy between the situation which they view as necessary or desirable, and the situation which does in fact exist. That is, "shortage" often has meaning primarily in relation to the norms and value systems of those in the leadership of particular professions. Such professional leaders use a variety of terms: minimum standards, necessary levels of care, desirable staffing practices or optimum standards.

Whatever standard is employed, the usual judgment is that more services and resources are needed than can in fact be provided by the amount of funds which the community is spending either as individuals or through its public and private institutions. Economists point out that in a market economy the community indicates its own judgment as to what is necessary and desirable within the limits of the total resources available to it. It often decides to allocate its funds in ways which various groups in health, education and even business do not think wise or desirable.

From the economist's point of view, the difference between what some persons think the community should spend in a particular area and what it does spend is essentially irrelevant. For example, in 1957, the Joint Information Service of the American Psychiatric Association and the National Association for Mental Health stated that in staffing public mental hospitals, "no state even approaches the minimum standards."[8]

The public clearly differs with health leaders as to what is adequate or what is minimum. This point is difficult for the leaders of any field to accept. Complaints about deficiencies and inequities merely mask the fact that different standards of value exist in the community. Only as health proponents persuade the public at large to spend more for health services and manpower does the purported shortage become economically relevant. This is essentially a problem of value shaping and politics, not manpower research.

From the economist's point of view, a shortage indicates some discrepancy between the actual level of manpower supply and that which is possible, given the existing structure and level of demand for services and manpower in health and in all other fields. Any difference between what is possible and what actually exists can occur in two ways.

The first has to do with discrepancies which occur with a change in the conditions of supply or demand which have not had sufficient time for the essential resources to be re-allocated through the market place by way of the attraction and retention of personnel, the readjustment of demand and the like. This kind of shortage normally solves itself with time. A second kind of shortage is due to deficiencies or imperfections in the market system, such as artificial or institutional limitations to the flow of manpower because of monopoloid tendencies or ignorance.

Thus, every discussion of shortages is shot through with different opinions and confusion as to what is desirable and what is the result of supply and demand factors. The point can be made clearer by suggesting that if by some magic the supply of most kinds of health professionals were large enough to meet the stated minimum adequate needs, consumers would not increase their spending by nearly as much, many professionals would find themselves fully or partially unemployed and income levels would fall. Most governments and nonprofit institutions would not have the necessary funds to fill their reported vacancies and would reduce both the number of budgeted positions and salary levels. Many health professionals would flee to other occupations and enrollments in training programs would drop sharply.

But if the governmental and nonprofit agencies could somehow find the funds to absorb the minimum number considered to be adequate, one could be reasonably sure that the professional groups would soon announce new and higher minimum adequate standards. Such standards will almost always advance in front of what can exist in fact. In a progressive, increasingly affluent society, this is perfectly normal.

Estimates of manpower shortages based on conceptions of need rather than demand do have their uses. But most studies purporting to estimate present or prospective shortages of manpower are woefully inadequate. The primary problem is the lack of any way to evaluate such shortages or to appreciate their significance. Most estimates of shortages are based on some apparently arbitrary relations between the population and the various manpower groups. But the connection between the total population, its health needs and the precise needs for any particular manpower group are indeed tenuous. A complex of factors affects the health needs of a population. Among them are its age distribution, the natural, economic and technological environment within which it lives, and so forth. Public health practices change, and with them the frequency of various conditions. The skill and means for diagnosis and treatment change. Health treatment may become more institutionalized, as it has in the past, or a reverse trend may set in. The relative availability of different classes of personnel and the particular functions assigned to them also change. To be meaningful, estimates of needs will have to pin down the probable course and effect of each of these factors. Generalities do not suffice.

In addition to estimates of need, estimates of the demands for health manpower, that is, estimates of what will in fact occur, are necessary. Demands are subject, of course, to all the changes enumerated above. But, in addition, estimates would be needed of changes in incomes, insurance and public funds, as well as how much would be spent for various types of health care and personnel. Surprisingly, arbitrary ratios of health professionals to population have shown remarkably stable trends over the past several decades. Since 1938, every 100,000 persons in the population have been served by between 131 and 135 physicians. On the same population basis, the ratio has been eight or nine osteopaths since 1931, and 56 or 57 dentists since 1947. The number of active professional nurses per 100,000 population increased from 175 in 1930 to 280 in 1960, but the increase has been at a remarkably stable pace—a little more than 30 per 100,000 during each decade.

These stabilities are remarkable in view of the great changes which have occurred over these periods in the factors affecting the supply of and demand for health services and health manpower. Some of these changes have tended to increase and others to decrease the supply of and demand for professional health manpower, sometimes in conflicting ways. The steadiness of the trends has been, of course, the net result of these conflicting influences. Canadian experience shows the danger of assuming that conflicting forces will counterbalance in any regular way. There the ratio of physicians per 100,000 moved irregularly upward from 97 in 1931 to 117 in 1961; and that for dentists irregularly downward from 38 in 1931 to 30 in 1962. Both ratios are lower than in the United States. In contrast, the ratio for nurses increased from 181 in 1941 to 338 in 1961, more rapidly in the latter decade. It is now much higher than in the United States.[9]

Almost every writer on the needs and demands for health manpower denigrates the use of simple population ratios—and then proceeds to use them with little real qualification. If ratios are inadequate—and they are—considerably more research is needed to assess the relative effect of the diverse trends which have occurred in the past so that more useful methods can be found to estimate the impact of diverse future developments. The Bureau of Labor Statistics has a study underway on future employment in the health occupations, but a great deal of basic work will continue to be necessary.

Most discussions of demand have centered on physicians.

At the very least, alternative estimates ought to be made of the expected demand in the various secondary and tertiary occupations, given various estimates as to what will obtain in the key manpower groups. This involves an estimate of the consequences of shortages in terms of the availability and quality of health services as well as in terms of utilization practices. The various health manpower fields both complement and substitute for each other. A shortage of physicians could have two possible effects. If physicians are uniquely necessary, any shortage of them will be accompanied by a lack of demand for nurses and other paramedical personnel, while an increase in the number of physicians will be accompanied by a nearly equivalent increase in the employment of various auxiliary personnel. On the other hand, to the extent that nurses and other paramedical personnel are substitutes for physicians, a shortage of physicians will add to the demand for paramedical personnel, while an increased supply of physicians reduces the demand for paramedical personnel. Similar relationships exist between registered nurses and other nursing and non-nursing personnel, and wherever diverse groups of workers are combined directly or indirectly to provide a service. Some clues as to the nature of diverse relationships appear in the literature, but no research has been directed specifically at the degree to which complementarity and substitutability exist. This topic will be raised again in the discussion of utilization practices.

Besides national estimates of health manpower demands, an equally interesting question concerns the level of demand in the various states and communities. Every inventory of health manpower reveals the wide differences which exist among the states in terms of health manpower per capita. A number of analyses have shown a correlation between income levels or urbanization and the number of physicians and dentists.[10] The urbanized states tend to have higher per capita incomes, educational levels and hospital admission rates; they also have higher per capita expenditures for mental hospitals and more employees per patient in hospitals.[11] Health manpower also tends to be scarce where the population is widely dispersed.[12] Urbanization, income levels, population density and education are all highly correlated, and cause and effect cannot be traced. They are, however, far from a full explanation of the variations in the level of demand for health service personnel. The subject deserves considerably more investigation.

The few demand estimates which have been attempted suggest that both national and state studies of manpower demands can be more fruitfully undertaken if they are deaggregated as much as possible. That is, studies should be limited to specific areas of demand or particular types of institutions. A good example of this approach is that of Albee.[5] By concentrating on the problem of manpower demands for mental health, he was forced to keep in the forefront the very crucial questions of competition between that and other fields for manpower, as well as the functional relationships among the various professional and nonprofessional groups.

The various studies of dental health manpower also illustrate the value of constricting the scope of demand studies. These studies have made substantial progress in estimating trends in demand in the states, regions and nation. The earlier studies commented on expected changes in some of the factors affecting the demand for dentists, but finally resorted to manipulating conventional ratios of population per dentist. The later studies, however, include rather complex estimates of the increased demand for dental services based on trends in population, per capita expenditures for dental services and income levels, as well as an estimate of expected decreases in the incidence of caries through fluoridation. The resulting estimates of the demand for services were compared to estimates of the likely increase in the number of dentists, as well as to changes in their productivity through improved equipment, better office management, and the increased and improved use of auxiliary personnel.[13]

The dental manpower studies were perhaps fortunate in that a few key implicit assumptions about the methods of practice, the degree of specialization, the rate of increase in improved equipment and so forth could be made with some confidence. By restricting the scope of other studies, the usefulness and validity of other similar assumptions can be progressively explored. Other studies might be made of the demands for health manpower for, say, public health, general hospitals, rehabilitation service, services to the aged and research and development. Clearly, such studies would overlap and cause problems in reconciling them. But if the focus is kept on demand rather than hopes and goals, such studies can be of immense value.

Types of Shortages and Research Policy

As a summary judgment, the nature and extent of shortages in the health occupations vary greatly among different fields. In the case of physicians, the evidence overwhelmingly indicates a shortage in the senses mentioned earlier. The demand for physicians' services is increasing rapidly. Nearly all those trained as physicians work as physicians. The number of qualified applicants to medical schools substantially exceeds the number of openings available.

Very few medical students withdraw prior to graduation. Nearly 20 per cent of all new physicians' licenses issued each year go to graduates of medical schools outside the United States and Canada. Some are American citizens who were qualified, but were not accepted to enter domestic schools, and went abroad for training. Finally, the income levels of physicians have consistently exceeded those in other professional fields, even after considering the time and cost of education. On any grounds whatever, the shortage of physicians and, more importantly, of opportunities to enter medical school is evident.

On the other hand, in an economic sense, little or no evidence indicates a shortage of registered nurses. In the first place, nearly half of those who have been trained as nurses and a third of those who are currently registered as nurses are not employed. Since nearly all nurses are women and many have family responsibilities, the significance of these unemployed trained and licensed nurses is not unequivocal. But many are not working simply because the incentives are not great enough, or because hospitals and other employers are not willing to make the necessary adjustment in hours, part-time work, etc. In contrast, female physicians and dentists usually work at least part-time during all but a few months prior to and after delivery.[14]

Secondly, rather than having a surplus of qualified applicants, hospital schools of nursing typically operate at only 90 to 92 per cent of capacity.[15] Thirdly, as noted later, utilization practices with respect to registered nurses continue to be inconsistent with the purported fact that they are a scarce manpower resource. Finally, no evidence shows that salaries in nursing are unusually high or have advanced rapidly as normally occurs in a shortage. Rather the incomes of nurses are equal to or lower than women of similar educational level, whether or not one takes into account other factors which might affect income, such as race or regularity of employment. Yett reports that professional nurses' salaries increased by only about 50 per cent during the 1950's, compared to 70 per cent for teachers or all female professional and related workers.[16] From the point of view of the "need" for registered nurses in some abstract sense, shortages may well exist. But these needs are unsupported by private or public expenditures for them.

The situation in the nonprofessional nursing and other paramedical professions is somewhat less clear. In part that is because these fields are relatively new and rapidly growing. Evidence, one way or the other, is almost nonexistent either in terms of the number and quality of applicants, the experience of training programs, or employment patterns and income. The single most relevant fact is that the supply of personnel in nearly all nonprofessional nursing and paramedical fields is increasing rapidly and new occupations are appearing. This warrants the hypothesis that what shortages exist in these fields are primarily the result of imbalances of a rapidly increasing demand continuing to outdistance the supply. If so, achieving a better balance between supply and demand is more or less a matter of the market working out training programs, incentives, etc., making opportunities available and attractive, and attracting the necessary manpower into the fields.

The nature of the shortages in the different fields has significance for research into health manpower. Priority in research depends on an evaluation of what the important problems are and what the significant policy decisions are likely to be. With the excess of qualified applicants for positions in medical schools and as long as practically all persons trained as physicians continue to work as physicians, research into the characteristics and motives of those who enter medical school may prove interesting, but will make little contribution to policy, for it will not show how to increase the number of medical school opportunities. Rather, the significant research will lie in the area of predicting the demand for physicians' services to justify more medical schools, in studying such alternative sources of physicians as those trained abroad, and in learning how to improve the utilization of physicians for maximum benefit from these scarce resources. In the case of nurses, the principal questions would center on why purported shortages and poor utilization practices have not been rectified, and particularly on the incentives of nurses and their employers in these matters. In the case of paranursing and paramedical personnel, research into every aspect of manpower would be relevant: the determinants of demand, the recruitment and retention of personnel, the effects of different training mechanisms, their allocation among different types of health activities and their utilization on the job. The

236

goal would be both to help supply become more responsive to demand and to insure that wasteful efforts are not undertaken.

CHARACTERISTICS AND MOTIVES OF THOSE ENTERING HEALTH SERVICE

Who enters the various health fields? Considerable research has been done on the social, economic and intellectual characteristics and goals of medical, osteopathic and dental students. In part, this reflects the considerable concern during the last dozen years with the quality of medical school applicants.

In the early 1950's, the proportion of newly admitted medical students who had had an "A" average in their undergraduate education declined, with a corresponding increase among "B" students. During those same years, the number of applicants to medical schools decreased by over 40 per cent, and the proportion admitted increased from less than one-third to over one-half. This apparently was a temporary situation, perhaps related to the changes in the supply of students in connection with World War II, the Korean War and the low birth rates some two decades earlier. Since 1954, the quality of medical school students has been stabilized and quite high. Although some schools accept students who do not rate particularly high, this is more likely to occur at some state-owned schools which seem to accept local applicants rather than more highly qualified out-of-state applicants.[17] This point could be verified, but it has not.

Actually, a ratio of admissions to applicants of about one-half held throughout the 1930's, the early 1940's and since 1952. This ratio probably has no particular significance. Students and their advisors are aware of the standards of admission, and those not likely to be accepted do not apply. The standards of admission are generally considered somewhat less demanding in dental than in medical schools, but in both a ratio of one-half has held in recent years. This was true even when dental schools were willing to accept more students, but did not think those being rejected were qualified. In dentistry, no decline in quality of students occurred during the 1950's.[18]

The evidence of a decline in quality is not convincing on more basic grounds. Quite consistently, studies have found little relationship between undergraduate grades, aptitude test scores, or other criteria used in admitting students and subsequent performance in medical school. Even more important, almost no evidence relates quality as

237

conventionally gauged in student applicants and ultimate quality in medical practice.[19] The question of further research in this area will be examined later.

What are the motives for entering the health professions? The popular discussion and the analyses of economists suggest that income factors are of overriding importance. Medicine is the highest paying profession of all.

Primarily because of the long training period, the investment in actual expenditures and foregone income of the student and his family are also quite high. Friedman and Kuznets found that, considering both of these factors, the rate of return on this investment to both physicians and dentists was above that in other occupations.[20] In more recent analyses, Hansen concluded that the relative incentives to enter dentistry were adverse in 1939, quite attractive in 1949, but about balanced in 1956. In the case of physicians, he concluded that the relative incentives were about balanced in 1939, strongly in favor of medicine in 1949, and somewhat less strongly in favor of medicine in 1956. Hansen suggests that these shifts may be partially responsible for the reported decline in the quality of medical school applicants in the 1950's.[21] Serious difficulties cast doubt on the accuracy of income data, and whether Hansen's income data were increasingly influenced downward by the influx of foreign trained physicians during the 1950's is not clear. More importantly, one may question whether the manpower market in the medical or any other field operates so neatly and quickly. Complaints as to the quality of medical school applicants began to appear in 1951, just two years after the differential in favor of medicine was at its widest. No record exists of complaints on the quality of students in the late 1930's, when the incentives to enter medicine were apparently balanced.

Composite estimates of costs and returns are only a starting point. The length of the training period, the level of tuitions, the availability of loans and scholarships, the level and rate of growth in income during internship, residency and different forms of practice may each have somewhat different effects which may be relevant to manpower policy. Altenderfer and West made an exceptionally complete study of medical and osteopathic students and the types and levels of their money receipts and expenditures classified by the source of the funds and their marital status, number of children, living arrangements, geographical location, year in medical school and public versus private school,[22] but did not face the effect of these financial factors.

238

In varying forms, salary increases, changes in the amount and rate of increase in salaries over a career, lower tuition costs and greater availability of grants and loans have all been used in the several health fields and new proposals appear regularly. The effects of these alternative mechanisms in different occupations ought to be carefully appraised. More follow-up studies of the recipients of federal and other scholarship or traineeship grants are needed over longer periods of time. Particularly in the case of women, the results of investments in occupational training may not be clear for 20 years or so.

A careful appraisal of the various steps in the education and training process with a view to finding the extent to which it can be shortened might produce significant results. Various proposals have been made, for instance, to reduce the time in premedical and medical school, as well as to reduce or even eliminate internship. A shorter training period would add to the incentives to enter a program. It would also permit training more manpower with the same training resources of faculty and facilities. This all presupposes no essential qualitative changes in the training process due to a shorter period.

The non-monetary incentives to enter the health occupations have been speculated upon but have not received enough attention. The health professions have been characterized as fundamentally appealing to deep motives of service, the application rather than the development of science, and involving quite unique responsibilities in many cases along with a unique measure of independence.

More's survey of dental students is exceptional for a study of a health occupation in the extent to which he sought to compare them with other groups in ways which were relevant.[23] Davis has also distinguished medicine from nine other (generally broader) career interest fields in his large-scale study of college seniors and their occupational choices. In this way he was able to compare the aspiring medical student to others in socioeconomic terms, academic performance and expressed values.[24] In the health fields, as in many ubiquitous fields, one would expect to find a high proportion who are committed to a particular occupation very early. One would also expect many to be deeply interested in the health field, but with the final occupational choice slow to emerge, perhaps depending on circumstance. He will also find many who are seriously interested in a health occupation, but also in other fields. At some margin, occupations and fields compete for students,

239

and the students compete for entry. The key points in these two processes should always be the central focus. This requires the knowledge of the fields with which health service competes at each level (doctoral, bachelor, diploma, associate, technician or even lower) and the factors which affect these decisions. So much work is going on with respect to the career patterns of highly qualified persons that better insights should appear regularly; the lesser level occupations have been neglected.

Alternative Career Paths

The professional associations are beginning to make rather extensive longitudinal studies of the career patterns of those entering their fields. The American Association of Medical Schools, for instance, is making a longitudinal study of the class of students which entered in 1957. The American Dental Association has data on the class which started in 1958, and may follow them up. The National League for Nursing Education is following up the class which entered and graduated from the various types of nursing programs in 1962. Longitudinal studies covering the entire occupational spectrum are also under way under several auspices. Such longitudinal studies cannot fail to be interesting, but they will be slow to produce data. They ought to be supplemented by studies following up the students of earlier years as well as surveys of the educational and work histories of those now in various types of practice and responsibility. The rapid growth of continuing education suggests that it be periodically examined for its effect on skills, mobility, utilization patterns and the like.

One of the major sources of medical manpower which has not received the attention it deserves consists of persons trained in other countries. Between 1950 and 1959, the proportion of all new medical licenses issued to persons trained outside the United States increased from 5.1 to 19.7 per cent, and it has remained at or near the latter level since. Foreign-trained physicians include both the citizens of other countries and Americans who studied abroad, usually after being rejected by a medical school in the United States. The increased number of alien physicians is directly related to the increase in the number of physicians who are members of hospital house staffs, i.e., interns and residents. Between 1951 and 1963, the total number in approved programs at hospitals increased by nearly 60 per cent. Aliens accounted for about half of this increase and they comprised about one-fourth of both residents and interns in the latter year.[25]

240

The role of middle-aged women as source of manpower for the health professions has been noted but perhaps not explored as adequately as it might. Yett estimated that the return of women past age 35 accounted for at least one-third of the increased employment of registered nurses between 1948 and 1962.[26] Just how important they have been among practical nurses, nurses' aides and the like ought to be ascertained. Several other questions might be raised in each of these fields having to do with just where middle-aged women have gone to work, why they went to work and the extent to which they obtained training of one sort or another after or in preparation for their return.

Very little has been done to portray with any accuracy the various routes by which technical assistants and other paramedical personnel enter their occupations. Most of the literature in the field describes the few programs which are in operation and the formal systems of certification which are developing. Many changes are occurring here, particularly as junior college programs are expanding and special programs have been instituted under the Manpower Development and Training Act and through the Poverty Program. Research into the education and training, the actual functions performed and the deficiencies of those now employed as technicians and in other paramedical jobs might point up possible approaches to improve their quality through various training mechanisms.

Upgrading: An Unexplored Area

A crucial area which needs research is the opportunities and problems in connection with the transfer of persons from one level of practice to another. In most non-medical fields, recruitment from the next lower level on the basis of experience, with such additional education and formal training as is warranted in the individual case, is often as important as the prescribed formal route of entry into the field. Semiskilled workers are the major source of craftsmen,[27] persons without college degrees are a major source of engineers,[28] and so on.

Alternative routes into the various health fields have often been foreclosed by tight control of training requirements for licensure, or have been obscured or denigrated by leaders of various occupational groups. One-third of the degree candidates in nursing already have an R. N., but the leaders of the nursing profession assert that this is an unusual situation which will disappear with time.[29] Special degree programs for registered nurses are being closed out in favor of basic nursing programs. However, this tends to increase the length of time in school, with the predictable results that the number entering and graduating after an R. N. has declined and the total number of graduations at the bachelor's level has failed to grow significantly for several years.

Research, including experimental programs, should investigate ways to encourage upgrading and transfers among the health occupations. The need for such mobility is likely to increase as a greater degree of differentiation occurs in nursing and other health occupations. Research would probably disclose that advancement by stages is a sensible course for those with limited means and uncertain ambitions and opportunities; that is, that it reflects some very normal exigencies of life. Research also ought to further illuminate the effects current practices in upgrading of health personnel are having on recruitment and retention of personnel.

More specifically, research needs to be done on the qualities of nursing, technical and paramedical personnel at each level to see whether new sources of manpower for the next higher level might be found. Can ways be found to elevate experienced nurse's aides to the practical nurse level, short of having them take the entire practical nurse program? Can experienced practical nurses be similarly upgraded to the associate or diploma nurse level? How can associate and diploma school graduates be most effectively upgraded to the bachelor nurse level? How can laboratory helpers be upgraded to technicians, and technicians to technologists? Research might indicate ways in which new occupations in patient care and diagnosis might develop between the physician and the bachelor-level nurses and technologists.

Crucial policy questions are involved here. The practice is so common in other fields, however, that upgrading might become a major source of manpower in each of the various levels of nursing, technical and paramedical service. In a similar vein, Kissick points to the need to explore the opportunities for lateral transfer among the various paramedical occupations. He also suggests the need for experiments in core courses in the various health occupations, not only to conserve educational resources, but also to encourage both vertical and lateral mobility.

Losses of Health Manpower

A number of earlier comments about the effectiveness of various training devices in terms of the extent to which trained personnel

242

remain in their fields is only part of the larger problem of the retention of personnel. A number of illuminating hospital turnover studies have been made in recent years. A major shortcoming of these studies is that they usually fail to distinguish between losses of people who immediately go to work elsewhere in health services and losses which reduce the total health manpower supply through retirement, leaving the labor force or entering some other occupation.

The evidence is that physicians rarely leave medical functions short of retiring, and that dentists are almost as persistent. On the other hand, about five per cent of all nurses are said to leave the field each year, primarily due to marriage or pregnancy.[30] This is somewhat lower than the annual loss rate of seven to eight per cent among school teachers, which contrasts sharply with the finding that job turnover rates for nursing personnel are about three times as great as among public school teachers.[31] Of course, high losses among young women are to some extent counterbalanced by their return at a later date when their family responsibilities have been reduced. Data on loss rates among other health service occupations do not seem to have been published.

Physicians in independent practice face no problem of compulsory retirement. One observer notes that physicians tend to be retired as their practices shrivel, in part due to competition from younger physicians.[32] Dentists start to reduce the number of weeks they work per year in their forties, and the number of hours per week in their fifties.[33] Salaried employees may face the prospect of compulsory retirement, although pension plans may not be so prevalent in nonprofit institutions. The process of retirement in the various health fields, however it occurs, deserves investigation to determine its effect on the manpower supply.

The spate of hospital turnover rate studies in recent years has undoubtedly given hospital administrators valuable tools to improve personnel practices, lower turnover and thus lower their costs. In the process, too, they have probably reduced losses from the health manpower field. About 20 to 25 per cent of the losses in one study, and about 75 per cent in another were considered avoidable.[34]

Levine has studied turnover of nursing employees in general hospitals in the midwest and northeast relating it to length of employment, size and ownership of hospitals, particular nursing occupations and whether or not the hospital had a school. Turnover of nursing personnel in these hospitals was higher than for female factory workers; among aides, orderlies and attendants it was twice as high.[35]

243

Turnover can be quite costly. One study in a Minneapolis hospital found that direct costs amounted to three per cent of the payroll. The study noted but did not measure the costs that would have to be incurred to reduce this turnover or would result from lower turnover. The simple reduction in turnover drives up salary costs because of the longer tenure of employees. Again, higher salaries might discourage turnover, but would lead to higher salaries to other employees, not just those who would otherwise leave. Other costs might be incurred to improve other personnel functions to reduce turnover.[36] Of course, some efforts might lead to reduced costs in other directions. For instance, expenditures to improve on-the-job training, supervision, the definition of responsibilities or communications might lead to reduced turnover while improving the effectiveness of the enterprise as a whole. These tradeoffs between costs and benefits have not been carefully studied, however.

THE UTILIZATION OF HEALTH SERVICE MANPOWER

As has become evident, utilization of manpower in the health fields is an extremely complex and crucial issue. Changes in utilization practices can make key professional workers, and thus the health enterprise, more efficient. Changes in utilization practices may partially convert the demand for manpower from occupations which are in short supply to those in which manpower can be more easily obtained. Utilization practices are crucially determined by the character of training that health workers have received. On the other hand, utilization practices are highly relevant to the character of the training health workers ought to receive. Utilization practices directly affect the incentives to enter and stay in different fields. Moreover, to the extent that improved utilization practices affect the efficiency of an organization and the economy, the quantity and quality of services may be raised, and expenditures to help increase and improve staffs may be made.

Most of the knowledge about actual utilization practices is really confined to assertions, rather than being determined by research. The assertion has been made that, because of shortages, physicians have become less accessible, less communicative and busier; that they keep longer hours, have reduced night and home calls, rely more on telephone consultations and schedule office visits more closely; and that they have reduced their role as family counselors.[37] Presumably, therefore, variations in the extent of these practices in different communities

244

at the present time would be related to the size of local complements of physicians versus the local population, income levels, etc. This has not been investigated.

National surveys of utilization practices appear to have only limited value. Utilization practices must be judged against the costs and returns of alternative possibilities, and these can only be judged in the specific instance. By looking at the amount of time various kinds of workers spend at various tasks, one may identify time which is wasted and tasks which could be more economically performed by others. Tasks which can be more efficiently performed by more highly skilled persons should be shifted to them, provided such personnel are available at a lesser cost for the same amount and quality of work. If not, the task should remain with the workers performing it, but they may require additional training to improve their skill. Tasks which can be more efficiently performed by less skilled, lower paid workers should be shifted downward. Such workers can usually be more easily obtained, but the requirement of reducing costs while maintaining the amount and quality of service always holds.

The question of the relative availability, cost and productivity of different personnel groups can only be answered in the context of a local situation. What can large-scale research contribute to this process? This is certainly not just an academic question. Research showing utilization patterns, that is, the tasks performed by various personnel groups and the costs involved, can serve as norms to guide individuals and administrators. Gathering the data for comparative utilization studies can be directly useful to administrators, for they immediately indicate some situations which can be altered for the better on the spot. Utilization studies can call attention to persistent and generic problems, leading to concerted efforts to better understand and rectify them. Moreover, studying changes in utilization patterns over time can illuminate the conditions under which practices are likely to change, the types of changes which occur and the problems which are likely to accompany them. But studies showing the amount of time nurses or any other group spend on one task or another are not, per se, evidence of good or bad utilization.

Almost no aspect of health services can be overlooked in its effect on utilization patterns. Careful examination of the interaction between each of the several professional and nonprofessional groups may reveal ways to more effective utilization of the available manpower resources. The assertion that registered nurses have been delegated many functions

245

once performed only by physicians has never been investigated. Are the functions of nurses different in different geographical areas? To what extent are differences in utilization practices among communities a reflection of different availabilities of manpower? How is this related to relative wage and income levels for nurses and other types of personnel?

Levine and others have been analyzing utilization and staffing patterns of hospitals according to their size and other characteristics. Great variation has been found from hospital to hospital in terms of the hours of nursing service available per patient. To some extent, this is related to the size of the hospital, in that the smaller the hospital, the more hours of nursing service available per patient.[38] This may be interpreted to mean either that in small hospitals patients receive better care or that nursing personnel are being utilized inefficiently. No clues are given as to exactly what tasks were being performed by registered or practical nurses and aides.

Although the number of nursing hours per patient is steadily increasing in each smaller size class of hospital, the pattern is more complex for both registered nurses and nurses' aides. These data provide some clues on the extent to which aides are substitutes for nurses. In general, however, one is impressed with the great unexplained variations in nursing staff patterns among hospitals of the same type and in the same general location. Other variables could easily be introduced into these and similar analyses which would provide insight into the question of whether nursing and other salaries, local supplies of nurses and relatively unskilled women, local income levels and similar variables have anything to do with these variations in staffing patterns.

Also, hospital design, including the layout and size of each unit, clearly affects the extent to which scarce nursing personnel must be relied upon and the extent to which auxiliary nursing and clerical personnel may be used.[39] The larger the unit, the more options that become available, although the maximum could probably be reached, depending on the precise situation, types of patients, etc. This topic deserves research in connection with hospital architecture.

In recent years, a rapid increase in the number of detailed management analyses of work performance in nursing service and in the other departments of hospitals has revealed innumerable half-concealed and inadequately understood problems. Such management research at the working level is ultimately the responsibility of local administrators. From a larger point of view, some better insight into the utilization

246

problem might be gained by examination of the administrative process itself. What explains the great variations in utilization practices from hospital to hospital? Which hospitals are making internal surveys, which are not, and why do they not? To what extent have surveys led to the introduction of new practices? What difficulties arose in making changes? What apparently poor utilization practices turned out to be not so inefficient after all? Studies which would illuminate this aspect of the management process might be of considerably greater value than the examination of global ratios and percentages.[40]

One reads the material on the utilization of nursing personnel with the feeling that the major problem is inadequate organization and supervision. Another apparently pervasive problem is the mismatch between training and function. Registered nurses seem to be trained for patient care, but are primarily engaged in supervisory and administrative tasks, including paper work, while the nurse's aides and orderlies, who actually spend most of their time in patient care, are essentially untrained. Most people involved seem to be unhappy with this situation. This is especially true for nurses, in part because they were motivated to enter their fields by ideals of patient service, which motives may be accentuated by the training program itself. If nursing function studies were more concerned with what actually is occurring or is likely to occur on the job, rather than with what ought to occur, they might provide a better guide to what ought to occur in training programs. Moreover, studies are needed on the question of whether training programs which are closely aligned to the actual functions workers subsequently perform on the job are related to better work performance, improved recruitment and improved retention.

Innumerable examples could be cited of specific cases where utilization practices were changed and new health occupations developed, leading to lower total costs for salaries and training, the tapping of new labor supplies and improvement in the quality of service. The health services industry is ubiquitous, and essentially the same conditions are faced by a great many institutions across the country. Because of the fragmented nature of the American health service system, individual administrators under pressure can relatively easily resort to unconventional tactics in the assignment of function and in the types of personnel utilized. Some of these tactics turn out to be feasible, and the result is new occupations, new utilization patterns and so forth.

Sometimes, however, fragmentation and lack of funds inhibit creative experimentation with new utilization patterns or new occupations.

Legal limitations which surround the performance of many functions in the health field also inhibit change. Special institutes or other type of institution may be needed which could establish experimental units for carrying on research in different personnel patterns. In addition, considerable research should be carried out on utilization practices in the armed services and in foreign countries to see what could be translated into American civilian practice.

One problem which ought to be studied is how utilization practices have changed over time in local areas in relation to other variables. Much data on employment in the various health occupations generally and in hospitals and health departments are available over time and for geographical areas at the regional, state and even county level. These data ought to be more fully explored to see how a geographical health complex grows, or even declines. How are changes in the number of physicians, nurses and other health personnel related? How has change in the health fields in new and rapidly growing areas differed from that in depressed or slowly growing areas? What is happening in the city and in the suburbs? Do areas where active campaigns have been carried out to solve health manpower problems have any greatly different experience from other areas?

The increasing degree of specialization of health manpower, either within a health occupation or in the form of new health occupations, is the direct result of improvements in utilization practices. In the literature on physicians, however, specialization often is looked upon with some disfavor. This theme was popular a generation ago, as it is now, despite the fact that specialization has steadily increased for over a century.[41]

Specialization is often said to flow from increased scientific knowledge, forcing a practitioner to limit himself to a smaller and smaller part of the whole. From economics, however, one learns that specialization is a function of the scale of the enterprise or market. As the population became more concentrated, as transportation improved for both patient and physician, and as patients were concentrated in hospitals, increasing numbers of physicians could occupy themselves fully while restricting their types of patients. With a limited practice, they gained increased skill and productivity through deeper explorations into particular disease entities and medical techniques. Specialization is the source of increased knowledge, not the result. More importantly, it leads to higher quality and an increased supply of services, since the specialist can usually handle a given problem

248

better and in less time than a less skilled practitioner. The relative size of the medical and dental professions may, therefore, be the major reason why less than half of all physicians, but practically all dentists, are in general practice.

Considerable difficulty has been encountered with the integration of specialists' services under a system of independent private practice. Not enough is known about just how referrals are handled at the present time. A particular effort ought to be made to ascertain both the incentives and the inadequacies of the existing system, as seen by specialists, general practitioners and patients.

Many physicians utilize specialists less than they might, either because they want to avoid extra expenses to their patients, because they fear a loss of face or because they really do not know how to use the skills and services of the various specialities. Many physicians seem to be reluctant to call in paramedical people, such as social workers, visiting nurses or occupational therapists. Some even seem to be ignorant of the resources available to them, or how to call them into action.[42] Studies might well be made of the extent to which different physicians utilize the services of the wide range of personnel. That could yield some clues as to how to utilize them more efficiently. Although some might object that these are matters for the professional person to determine for himself, these decisions could hardly be compromised if the individual physician had some useful information as to what is being done by others.

Quality

Leaders in the health occupations have been increasingly concerned with the low quality of many entering or in their fields. In some cases, the leaders may have despaired of obtaining significantly greater numbers into particular fields and have turned to quality and skill as the only way to obtain an effective increase in the quantity and quality of health services. At a number of earlier points, research questions bearing on the quality of health manpower resources have been noted.

Certain difficulties arise in dealing with the concept of quality, however. Quality and quantity often go together, and the ability to attract a better quality of applicants is usually equivalent to the ability to obtain larger numbers of applicants in general. An increase in number of applicants means that educators, administrators and others can be more selective, raising the quality of the personnel

249

actually entering training or employment in a field. Research to find ways to increase the flow of applicants to any field is thus directly relevant.

In the second place, a key route toward expanding the quantity and quality of health services has been the addition of lower quality manpower, for the employment of paramedical and paranursing workers has expanded much faster than that of physicians and nurses. Bringing in more persons of lesser skills to perform less demanding functions has released the time of the more highly qualified professional, making him more productive. The result has been the growth of various technical specialties and paramedical groups. Wherever research can illuminate ways to use persons of lesser quality, it makes a great contribution because high quality is always in short supply.

For reasons which are not entirely clear, those who make decisions in the health service industry often seem to choose quantity over quality. The rapid growth in auxiliary nursing personnel in recent years suggests that hospital and nursing administrators have systematically been saying in effect that they can get more nursing service from three nurses' aides than from two registered nurses. Otherwise, they would have competed in the market for registered nurses, bidding up salary levels, and ultimately attracting more students into nursing and inducing more nurses to re-enter employment. A really careful research effort is needed into the productivity of the different kinds of nursing personnel and the incentives to which administrators are responding in their staffing policies.

Quality has often been equated with training and skill, and rightfully so. But improved quality has often been equated with longer training programs. Since the length of a training program is a crucial incentive, attempts to improve quality through longer training programs tend to be self-defeating, adding to the difficulty in recruiting more and better applicants.

Research which indicates ways in which training in the various fields can be improved with no increase in training time, or even with a decrease in training time, might be most productive in terms of raising both the quality and quantity of manpower in the several fields. Research into the qualities, functions and backgrounds of workers in the various paramedical occupations, with a view to devising appropriate upgrading opportunities, on-the-job training programs and supervisory structures which encourage training, also appears to be a promising route to follow.

250

In a broader sense, research bearing on quality in health manpower may not proceed fruitfully until the concept, criteria and measurement of quality are more fully explored. That is true whether one is concerned with the quality of persons entering a field, the quality of their education and training, the quality of their school performance, or utlimately the quality of their service. These aspects of quality are arousing great interest, not only in manpower, but also in education, economics and many other disciplines. With the service sector of the economy growing in importance, quantitative measures of output no longer suffice as they have with goods, and economists are faced with the question of how to measure intangibles. Conceptually, this is akin to the measurement of such intangibles as intelligence, aptitude and performance. The inadequacies of aptitude tests or school grades as predictors of later performance suggest how difficult is the problem of measuring quality. The point is that the assessment of quality is a major problem, and research on it will have to be of a quite fundamental nature.

CONCLUSION

This paper has been concerned to clarify priorities in research into health manpower. That is quite diffierent from priorities in manpower policy. As noted earlier, manpower is the crucial resource for health services. Manpower research can help indicate how the attraction, retention and utilization of manpower might be improved. But manpower research cannot solve manpower problems. Only manpower policy can do that.

The most striking things to one who has been preoccupied with manpower studies in many fields, and not health manpower studies alone, are: 1. the rapid growth in employment and training in most occupations in health service; 2. the continued complaints about shortages of health manpower; and 3. the continuation of essentially the same problems with respect to utilization, high losses, turnover and the like over a long period of time. Given these conditions, the collection of more data of essentially the same nature as in the past does not seem to be particularly promising. The question must finally be raised as to why, when so much has been changing, the issues seem to remain the same.

An easy answer is that policies have been wrong. But this begs

251

the question as to what the public and private policies have really been designed to accomplish. For this reason, the difference must be clarified between the goals of leaders in the health fields and the goals of those who make public and private policy as indicated by their spending and employment policies. The determinants of demand for health manpower must be clarified if realistic planning is to be accomplished. Apology for, but continued reliance on, simple population ratios must be called into question.

A considerable redirection of the occupational orientation of research seems particularly necessary. For researchers to continue their preoccupation with physicians and nurses is anomalous while the paramedical and paranursing occupations proliferate and expand so much more rapidly. The social, economic and technological reasons for these developments need to be explored in depth and the functional relationships between the various groups clarified. Whether this is a temporary response to shortages or a more fundamental change in the technology of producing medical services, akin to the shift from handicraft to mass methods of manufacture of goods, deserves exploration. The problems of management, work organization, selection, training and placement take on entirely new meanings as the work force becomes increasingly differentiated in function and skill level.

Studies of career choice and motivation are improving, but more is needed in the way of comparisons which are relevant to the choices people make. In particular, studies are needed which explore the effectiveness of various financial and other incentives as means to increase the manpower in particular fields. Greater attention needs to be given to the irregular sources of manpower, particularly the import of manpower and the entry of nonprofessionals into health service. The highest priority should be given to research and experiments on upgrading personnel from one level of health service to the next through experience and training. New routes for the development of skilled manpower could be a powerful recruitment device.

Finally, one must ask why utilization patterns which distress health leaders continue to prevail. Global surveys have shown great differences in utilization patterns from one situation to the next, and these data could be used to determine whether utilization patterns are related to the relative availability of health manpower, pay rates or to other factors. Even more important are surveys of utilization patterns which seek to identify the role played by cost factors and the desires of the people concerned. Research is needed into the process of effecting

252

change in utilization patterns to find out why and how greater rationalization occurs in some situations than others.

The emphasis on what exists rather than what might be may appear to be retrogressive. However, a careful examination of why goals have not been achieved—or when they have been achieved, how and why—ought to illuminate the goals themselves. Impossible goals can stultify progress which could be made; attaining realistic goals can be a stimulus to further progress.

Even so, the growth of employment in most of the health occupations has been quite extraordinary by the standards of other industries. If the demand for health services continues to grow rapidly, as it may for the foreseeable future, one must ask the question of whether employment in the industry should also grow as rapidly. The health services are now becoming major consumers of the nation's manpower. In the past, rapidly growing industries, faced with mounting manpower problems in numbers and costs, have often turned to technology as a way out. At some point, capital equipment and relatively smaller numbers of highly trained manpower become cheaper and produce a better product than the utilization of gross aggregates of people. This shift has occurred throughout the goods producing sector, and it has occurred or is occurring in many parts of the service sector: in communications, in entertainment and in information processing. Indications are that in various aspects of laboratory analysis, medical information systems and so forth, the substitution of capital for manpower may be imminent. It is also occurring in many of the non-medical and non-nursing functions of hospitals, as in housekeeping, food services, inventory control, etc. The expanding manpower costs of health care provide increasing incentives to search out places for economizing on manpower. Where this will occur is difficult to see, but the possibility must always be kept in mind. As it does, entirely new perspectives on manpower for the health services will surely emerge.

REFERENCES

[1] For one attempt to clarify this subject, *see* Ginzberg, Eli, Hiestand, Dale L. and Reubens, Beatrice, THE PLURALISTIC ECONOMY, New York, McGraw-Hill Book Company, 1965.

[2] Klarman, Herbert E., THE ECONOMICS OF HEALTH, New York, Columbia University Press, 1965, Chapter 4.

[3] Harris, Seymour E., THE ECONOMICS OF AMERICAN MEDICINE, New York, The Macmillan Company, 1964, Chapters 5–9, 23.

[4] United States Department of Health, Education and Welfare, Public Health Service, HEALTH MANPOWER SOURCE BOOK, Sections 1–19, Washington, 1952–1965.

[5] Albee, George W., MENTAL HEALTH MANPOWER TRENDS, New York, Basic Books, Inc., Publishers, 1959, Tables 17–22.

[6] Surgeon General's Consultant Group on Nursing, TOWARD QUALITY IN NURSING: NEEDS AND GOALS, Washington, United States Department of Health, Education and Welfare, 1963, pp. 15, 20.

[7] American Nurses' Association, FACTS ABOUT NURSING, 1965 Edition, New York, pp. 10, 13.

[8] Albee, *op. cit.*, p. 41.

[9] Based on data in Royal Commission on Health Services, REPORT, Volume I, Ottawa, Roger Duhamel, 1964, pp. 238, 258, 266.

[10] Friedman, Milton and Kuznets, Simon, INCOME FROM INDEPENDENT PROFESSIONAL PRACTICE, New York, National Bureau of Economic Research, 1945, pp. 161–199; Judek, Stanislaw, MEDICAL MANPOWER IN CANADA, Ottawa, Roger Duhamel, 1964, p. 139.

[11] Albee, *op. cit.*, p. 60–61.

[12] National Manpower Council, GOVERNMENT AND MANPOWER, New York, Columbia University Press, 1964, pp. 123, 126–136.

[13] American Council on Education, THE SURVEY OF DENTISTRY, Washington, 1961, Chapter I and Appendix A; New England Board of Higher Education, DENTAL MANPOWER NEEDS IN NEW ENGLAND, Winchester, Massachusetts, 1958, Chapters II, III; United States Department of Health, Education and Welfare, Public Health Service, Division of Dental Resources, A STUDY OF DENTAL MANPOWER REQUIREMENTS IN THE WEST, Boulder, Colorado, Western Interstate Commission for Higher Education, 1956, Chapter IV; ———, A STUDY OF OKLAHOMA'S DENTAL MANPOWER NEEDS, Washington, 1954.

[14] American Council on Education, *op. cit.*, pp. 544–545.

[15] Yett, Donald, The Supply of Nurses: An Economist's View, *Hospital Progress*, 96, February, 1965.

[16] *Ibid.*, p. 97.

[17] National Manpower Council, A POLICY FOR SCIENTIFIC AND PROFESSIONAL MANPOWER, New York, Columbia University Press, 1953, p. 239.

[18] American Council on Education, *op. cit.*, p. 282.

254

[19] Gough, Harrison G., Hall, Wallace B. and Harris, Robert E., Admissions Procedures as Forecasters of Performance in Medical Training, *The Journal of Medical Education*, 38, 983–998, December, 1963.

[20] Friedman and Kuznets, *op. cit.,* pp. 291–295.

[21] Hansen, W. Lee, "Shortages" and Investment in Health Manpower, *in* University of Michigan, Bureau of Public Health Economics and Department of Economics, THE ECONOMICS OF HEALTH AND MEDICAL CARE, Ann Arbor, Michigan, 1964, pp. 75–90.

[22] Altenderfer, Marion E. and West, Margaret C., How MEDICAL STUDENTS FINANCE THEIR EDUCATION, Washington, United States Department of Health, Education and Welfare, 1965.

[23] More, Douglas M., The Dental Student, *Journal of the American College of Dentists,* 41, March, 1961.

[24] Davis, James A., UNDERGRADUATE CAREER DECISIONS, Chicago, Aldine Publishing Co., 1965, pp. 165–180.

[25] Datagrams, *The Journal of Medical Education,* 39, 1056–1057, November, 1964.

[26] Yett, *loc cit.,* p. 95.

[27] National Manpower Council, A POLICY FOR SKILLED MANPOWER, New York, Columbia University Press, 1954, p. 212.

[28] Blank, David M. and Stigler, George J., THE DEMAND AND SUPPLY OF SCIENTIFIC PERSONNEL, New York, National Bureau of Economic Research, Inc., 1957, pp. 86–92.

[29] Council of Member Agencies, Department of Baccalaureate and Higher Degree Programs, National League for Nursing, Statement of Beliefs and Recommendations Regarding Baccalaureate Nursing Programs Admitting Registered Nurse Students, *Nursing Outlook,* 57–58, June, 1964.

[30] Albee, *op. cit.,* p. xvii.

[31] Surgeon General's Consultant Group on Nursing, *op. cit.,* p. 47.

[32] Hall, Oswald, The Stages of a Medical Career, *American Journal of Sociology,* 53, 332, March, 1948.

[33] American Council on Education, *op. cit.,* pp. 492–493.

[34] United States Department of Health, Education and Welfare, Division of Hospital and Medical Facilities, HOSPITAL PERSONNEL, Public Health Service Publication No. 930-C-9, October, 1964, pp. 3–12; Christopher, W. I., Jr., Personnel Management, Planned and Controlled, *Hospital Progress,* 77, September, 1963.

[35] Levine, Eugene, Turnover Among Nursing Personnel in General Hospitals, *Hospitals,* 31, 51–53, 138, 140, September 1, 1957.

[36] A Study of Turnover and Its Costs, *Hospitals,* 29, 59–62, May, 1955.

[37] Means, James Howard, Homo Medicus Americanus, *Daedalus,* 712–713, Fall, 1963.

[38] Levine, Eugene, Some Answers to the "Nurse Shortage," *Nursing Outlook,* 30–34, March, 1964.

255

[39] For some discussion of this point *see* the comments by Tonkin, Thomas E., Planning the Nursing Unit, *Hospitals,* 39, 95–98, February 1, 1965.

[40] For an example of one management analysis, *see* HOSPITAL PERSONNEL, *op. cit.*

[41] Klarman, *op. cit.,* p. 82–88.

[42] Means, *op. cit.,* p. 716–717.

ACKNOWLEDGMENTS

My thanks go to William L. Kissick, M.D., Deputy Chief, Division of Public Health Methods, Office of the Surgeon General, United States Public Health Service; Stanislaw Judek, Ph.D., Professor of Economics, University of Ottawa, and other members of the Health Services Research Conference.

HEALTH MANPOWER IN TRANSITION

WILLIAM L. KISSICK

Doctor Michael M. Davis, one of the pioneers in the study of medical care and health policy in the United States, identified the basic elements of medical services as 1. people, 2. professionals, 3. facilities, 4. organization and 5. finances.[1] In his opinion, finances represented the foundation that supported professionals, facilities and organizations, which functioned as a ". . . complex aggregate of human beings and material facilities . . ." to deliver health services to people.

The frame of reference for this discussion of health manpower differs slightly. Manpower will be considered as one of three *basic* health and medical resources—1. health manpower (professional, technical and supportive); 2. facilities, including equipment and supplies; and 3. biomedical knowledge, or "state of the art." In this context, organization and financing are the intangible resources or mechanisms that serve to translate the three basic resources into health services for the consumer. An adequate analysis of health manpower at a minimum requires its consideration in this, or an alternative context that attempts to relate these variables, which together make up a highly complex, interdependent system.

In general, health manpower has not received the attention accorded to the other two basic resources. Although not impressive when contrasted with expenditures for defense or space exploration, society's investments in the resources of biomedical knowledge and facilities over the last two decades are substantial. Expenditures for medical and health related research have totaled almost $14 billion since the end of

World War II. More than two-thirds of the two billion dollars spent in the pursuit of new biomedical knowledge during 1966 was derived from public sources, and expenditures for this type of research will be even higher in 1967. For the construction of hospitals, nursing homes, health departments and other facilities for the delivery of health services, the Hill-Burton Program has been appropriated more than $2.7 billion since 1948, and these funds have been matched through the appropriation of public monies at the state and local level, through private philanthropy, loans and other means of financing, to achieve a total investment of $8.5 billion.

Until 1963, on the other hand, investments in the development of health manpower were relatively neglected, especially as a responsibility of the federal government. Although a substantial portion of the educational costs of health manpower have been publicly financed, largely from appropriations by state legislatures,[2] federal support of manpower development has been limited to grants for research training, except for some specialized efforts on a small scale; e.g., support of graduate preparation of nurses for careers as teachers, supervisors and administrators; support of preparation at the graduate level of public health personnel; and a relatively few fellowships and training grants in maternal and child health, rehabilitation and related disciplines. One major exception to the rule has been the program of the National Institute of Mental Health, which from 1948 through 1965 supported 35,000 trainees in psychiatry, psychology, social work, psychiatric nursing and related fields; the trainees were in service, as distinct from research positions.

A federal concern for the preparation of adequate numbers of health manpower was established, however, with the passage of the Health Professions Educational Assistance Act of 1963. Passage of this act represented the culmination of a legislative effort lasting 15 years. In 1965, the legislation was amended to add formula and project grant support of basic educational costs and scholarships to the original program of construction grants and student loans, in an effort directed toward increasing the nation's supply of physicians, dentists, pharmacists, optometrists and podiatrists. The Nurse Training Act, enacted in 1964, has comparable provisions, and the Vocational Education Act of 1963 emphasizes the support of programs geared to those areas in the nation's economy which have ". . . actual or anticipated opportunities for gainful employment." These Congressional actions signify the beginning of what will undoubtedly become sustained and increasing support by the federal government of the education and training of health manpower.

258

But at this juncture, thorough review and analysis of the forces influencing both the preparation and the utilization of health manpower deserves the highest priority. Careful assessment of the relevant issues is needed as a prerequisite to the formulation of a rational manpower policy to guide the investment of vast sums of public monies during the years ahead. Lacking such a policy, billions of dollars could be expended without significantly increasing the availability and accesibility of health services to meet the population's rising expectations.

CURRENT STATUS OF HEALTH MANPOWER

Definitions

An even more basic prerequisite to policy formulation is definition of terms. In its usual connotation, the term *health manpower* does not extend beyond the categories of physician, dentist and nurse. Such a definition is both restrictive and deceptive, as well as unrealistic in view of the diversity and array of personnel necessary to sustain a complex social enterprise that now represents expenditures in excess of $45 billion annually. Health manpower should rather be considered as comprising individuals ranging from the highly sophisticated, extensively educated biomedical scientist, who requires many years of postgraduate education and training, to the aide or attendant working in a hospital after only limited on-the-job training.

Two major classifications of health manpower are currently in use, frequently cited in the literature, sometimes interchangeably. The first of these classifications is used by the Bureau of the Census, which divides the civilian labor force into 71 separate industries. The "health services industry" at the time of the 1960 census ranked third among these industries, employing 2,578,214 persons. Between the 1950 and 1960 census, the "health services industry" gained almost a million workers, for a growth rate of 54 per cent. Only seven of the 71 industries experienced a higher growth rate.[3]

Approximately one-third of the individuals employed in the "health services industry," however, are clerical workers, craftsmen, laborers and others who assist the provision of health services by functioning in a supportive role, but whose skills and work are not unique to health services. The importance of the approximately one million clerical, technical and kindred workers in health services is not to be ignored, but their recruitment, education and utilization constitute problems that are generic to most enterprises in an industrialized, specialized society.[4]

259

The second classification of health manpower—"health occupations" —is more appropriate to this discussion since it focuses on those individuals possessing knowledge and skill unique to the health establishment. Also, this classification includes health manpower counted in industries other than "health services" by the Bureau of the Census; e.g., only three per cent of veterinarians and seven per cent of pharmacists are counted in the "health services industry." The "health occupations" are the categories of manpower that come to mind when one hears the often repeated statements of "shortage," "gaps" and "limited supply."

The National Center for Health Statistics has been collecting manpower data for these health occupations categorized into 35 fields, and it has been estimated that the health manpower in these fields totaled nearly three million in 1965 (Table 1). When these categories are subdivided into more discrete units, the range and diversity of health careers can be more readily appreciated. The *Health Careers Guidebook*,[5] published recently by the United States Department of Labor, identifies approximately 200 health career opportunities, subdividing each of the 35 general categories—"health careers briefings" as they are called in the book, several of which cover more than ten individual careers—into the distinct and separate careers each comprises. Thus each medical specialty is presented as a separate career.

Trends

The changes in the types and characteristics of health manpower are perhaps the most striking to be found in the health establishment—an area where striking changes are the order of the day. It is estimated that the health professions requiring college education or professional preparation accounted for approximately 200,000 persons in 1900. In 1920, the number of individuals in these categories increased to 409,000; in 1940 to 692,000; and in 1960 to 1,140,000.[6] Whereas, at the turn of the century, three out of five health professionals were physicians, by 1960, rapid growth in other disciplines reduced the proportion of physicians to one out of five professional health workers; a continued decline is to be anticipated as other disciplines experience more rapid rates of growth and new categories of personnel emerge. Also at the turn of the century, individuals in the health occupations accounted for 1.2 per cent of the experienced civilian labor force. This proportion increased to 2.1 per cent by 1940; 2.4 per cent by 1950; and 3.0 per cent by 1960.[7] A projection of this trend forecasts a total of between four and five per cent of the civilian labor force employed in health occupations by 1975.

260

TABLE I. HEALTH MANPOWER—1965

Health Field	Estimated Persons Employed[1]
All fields	2,778,900 to 2,893,700
Administration of health services[2]	31,500 to 37,000
Anthropology and sociology	600 to 800
Automatic data processing	300[3]
Basic sciences in the health field	44,200
Biomedical engineering	7,500
Chiropractic and naturopathy	25,000
Clinical laboratory services	85,000 to 95,000
Dentistry and allied services	230,900[4]
Dietetic and nutritional services	30,000[5]
Economic research in the health field	500
Environmental health	32,500 to 35,000[6]
Food and drug protective services	16,500
Health and vital statistics	1,400 to 2,400[7]
Health education	16,700
Health information and communication	5,000
Library services in the health field	8,000[8]
Medical records	37,000
Medicine and osteopathy	305,100[4]
Midwifery	5,000
Nursing and related services	1,409,000[9]
Occupational therapy	6,000[6]
Orthopedic and prosthetic appliance making	3,300
Pharmacy	118,000[6]
Physical therapy	12,000[6]
Podiatry	7,600
Psychology	9,000
Radiologic technology	70,000
Secretarial and office services	150,000 to 230,000
Social work	17,500[6]
Specialized rehabilitation services	5,300 to 5,900
Speech pathology and audiology	14,000
Veterinary medicine	23,700[4]
Visual services and eye care	40,400
Vocational rehabilitation counseling	4,200
Miscellaneous hospital services	6,200.[10]

[1] Each occupation is counted only once. For example, all physicians are counted in "Medicine and osteopathy" even though certain specialists perform in other health fields.

[2] Excludes business, clerical and maintenance workers.

[3] Estimates not available for programmers, operators and electronic technicians.

[4] Includes total personnel (active and inactive) for dentists, physicians and veterinarians.

[5] Estimates not available for food service supervisors, clerical workers and other workers.

[6] Estimates not available for aides and technicians.

[7] Estimates not available for statistical clerks.

[8] Includes technical and clerical workers in medical libraries. Estimates not available for patients' librarians.

[9] Estimate not available for ward clerks.

[10] Estimates not available for electrocardiograph technicians and hospital aides—obstetrical, pediatric, surgical and so forth.

Source: Health Resources Statistics: Health Manpower, 1965. United States Department of Health, Education and Welfare, Public Health Service Publication No. 1509, Washington, D.C., 1966. p. 177.

During the decade ending 1960 alone, the number of workers in health occupations increased at a rate twice that of population growth —from 1,531,000 in 1950, to 2,176,700 by 1960, an increase of 42 per cent in contrast to a population growth of 19 per cent. The rate of increase among occupational categories differed, being greatest among those with the shortest periods of training (e.g., practical nurses, x-ray technicians and hospital attendants) and among the occupational categories that have arrived relatively recently (e.g., medical technology, medical record librarians, physical therapy, occupational therapy and speech and hearing therapy).

The trend toward new careers is yet to be fully appreciated. Among the 200 plus careers listed by title in the *Health Careers Guidebook,* the majority represented but a small segment of total health manpower prior to World War II. Many careers, including inhalation therapist, nuclear medical technologist, radiologic health technician, cytotechnologist and medical engineering technician, did not exist. Admittedly, the three basic careers—medicine, dentistry and nursing—still constitute approximately 40 per cent (1.0 of 2.7 million) of persons in health occupations; however, specialization within these fields and the emergence of new disciplines are major factors to analyze in any discussion of health manpower. Although the data are limited, it can be anticipated that specialization and diversification will continue as the two foremost characteristics of health manpower in future decades.

The institutionalization of health services, and the effects of this institutionalization on health manpower, is an issue yet to be faced. The anachronistic features of the "one doctor-to-one patient mythology," the changing technology, and the emergence of new skills and professions are well illustrated by a recent account of the diagnosis and treatment of a 28-month-old girl with phenylketonuria (PKU). The patient's physician was backed up by a team of 14, including medical specialists, microchemists, psychologists, speech pathologists and social workers, not to mention nurses, aides and other hospital personnel. In situations such as these, organization is essential. Health services has moved from the era of the "cottage industry" to that of space exploration, and as more and more medical care is provided within an institutional structure—118,000,000 visits were made to the hospital outpatient departments, emergency rooms and specialty clinics in 1963[8]— mechanisms for effective utilization must be sought. The goal is one of maximum efficiency in delivery of services without compromising the quality of those services.

262

The growth of institutionalization and specialization is an effort to cope effectively with the requirements for depth and thoroughness in a wide range of tasks. These are essential to adequate provision of many new services. The exponential growth of scientific knowledge has contributed to both this inexorable trend and to a vast potential for improved health care. A physician could provide a wide range of services in the early part of this century, but now these services are provided more effectively, with greater skill and competence and in greater depth by several individuals with professional and technical skills, no one of whom represents the diversity of service that was once found in a single practitioner.

Specialization in medical practice, a post-World War II occurrence, and concentration of health manpower in hospitals, or institutionalization, have reached major proportions. As recently as 1940, 80 per cent of physicians had not specialized. In 1941, a total of 5,256 residency positions were offered and 78 per cent of them were filled. At the present time, the situation is rapidly approaching in which almost nine out of every ten graduates of the nation's medical schools enter specialty training. In 1964, 1,317 hospitals had sponsored 5,440 approved residency programs offering a total of 38,373 residencies; 80 per cent of these were filled. For the young physician seeking specialty training in July, 1966, more than 40,000 positions were offered.[9] This represents almost a ten-fold increase during the past 25 years and a doubling of the residencies offered since 1951. It is estimated that now seven of every ten physicians in private practice are full-time specialists.[10]

In 1941, hospitals had approximately one professional nurse for every 15 beds and one practical nurse, aide, attendant or auxiliary person for every ten beds. Personnel increased over the next ten years so that by 1952 the figures were one to seven and one to five. By 1962 the continued proportionate increase of nursing personnel resulted in one professional nurse for every five beds and a practical nurse or auxiliary person for every three beds.[11] This increasing concentration of nursing personnel per hospital bed may come as a surprise to many who are familiar with the complaints of lack of personal service and attention being voiced by many of the millions of Americans hospitalized in a general hospital during a single year. These comments beg the question, "What are the services provided and tasks performed by these categories of manpower?" This of course bears on the whole question of utilization of health manpower. In addition to nursing personnel, hospitals are increasing the numbers of personnel in other occupational categories, e.g., occupational and physical therapists, dieticians, medical record librarians, medical technologists, x-ray technicians, pharmacists and social workers, at a rate that exceeds both the expansion in hospital beds and the climb in the total annual admissions to short-term general hospitals.

In summary, one finds divergence in the types of health manpower and a convergence of the settings in which services are delivered. Organization becomes the ranking imperative, but it is hardly the full solution to the problem.

REQUIREMENTS AND RESOURCES

This, then, is health manpower. The next step is to establish what the boundaries of *needs* are to be, for any statement of need for health manpower, as for health services, is to a certain degree arbitrary. Few would disagree that a person suffering from acute appendicitis is in need of specific health services—particularly those of a surgeon. Likewise, a patient with diabetic acidosis is in need of an array of health services to save his life. But in many areas need is determined by a highly judgmental process. How many times does a patient with well-controlled diabetes need to see a physician? How many times does a patient with hypertension need to see a physician? How many times ought an infant to see a pediatrician during his first year of life? If one definitive answer could be cited to each of these questions, a definite need would exist for a specific amount of health manpower.

However, economists and manpower specialists agree that manpower forecasts based even on a finite need for future health services are unrealistic. Instead they suggest approaching manpower forecasting in terms of demand for health services in the classic economic sense of supply and demand. For the most part, demand is the economic expression of need, but some suggest demand may go beyond actual need. Illustrative of this point of view is the affluent hypochondriac who may be expressing a demand for health services that is in excess of actual need. Others feel that anxiety expressed by a patient for a physician's services is a valid need and not an inappropriate demand.

Both need and demand for health services are greatly affected by biomedical advances. Using Phenylketonuria as an illustration shows dramatic needs and demands for health services, neither of which existed prior to the discovery of the technique for detecting, diagnosing and treating inborn errors of metabolism and congenital malformations. It might be argued that preventing mental retardation and correcting

264

heart lesions achieves a net saving in the utilization of health services. In the absence of data to support such a contention, these advances have increased rather than decreased the requirements for health services. The same applies to the developments in renal dialysis, exfoliative cytology, rehabilitation and the like, not to mention an advance such as the discovery of insulin, which has transformed a once-fatal disease to an abnormal varient of the metabolic process with late sequelae that require extensive and, frequently, intensive health services.

In any case, demand for health services has and will continue to increase. Anne Somers identified the "significant long-run social and economic trends over the past century that have already greatly enlarged the demand for medical services and altered the character of that demand." The trends listed were: 1. overall increase in population, 2. the increase in the over-65 population, 3. the rising proportion of nonwhites in the population, accompanied by their improved socioeconomic status, 4. increasing portion of women in the population, 5. steady increase in urbanization and industrialization, 6. steady increase in educational levels, 7. steady rise in income levels, and 8. rise in national income.[12]

The purchasing power of the aged for health services has increased with the establishment of the Medicare program, which, it is estimated, will cost well over three billion dollars in 1967. How much of this sum represents displacement of funds that were expended for health services and how much represents added expenditures is not known. Many take the position that this increased purchasing power, whatever the amount, will allow the aged to translate needs into demand, while others state that this will allow the aged to generate demand for health services in excess of actual need.

Instead, this issue will be set aside and health manpower requirements will be considered, recognizing that the term *requirements* blurs the difference between need and demand. It may mean primarily need or mainly demand; or it may mean a mix of need and demand. As one reviews the literature of projection of manpower requirements, the distinction between need and demand is frequently unclear.

In many respects the requirement for health services can be virtually insatiable, depending on a society's level of expectation and the resources it wishes to allocate. This was suggested by participants in the first seminar when they alluded to "a visit to the dentist every six months," "a complete medical check-up each year" and Nelson's aspiration, "an analyst for every adult." At any rate, it would appear that any characterization of the dimensions, quantitative and qualitative, of requirements for health services is arbitrarily defined, at least within the limits of the present scientific ignorance.

Determination of Manpower Requirements

Whatever the definitions employed, predicting or forecasting the requirements for health manpower is a hazardous enterprise. As Hechinger commented in the *New York Times*,[13]

> Why, then, make projections? The answer appears to be that modern society's dependence on highly skilled talent has made obsolete the theory that if everybody just pursues his interests, everything will come out all right.

Forecasting has become essential.

To date efforts to forecast health manpower requirements have used various methods, each with its own deficiencies, each risky:

1. *Population Ratios:* The application of existing health-manpower-to-population ratios to the projected population base is the most frequently used and accepted method for predicting future manpower requirements, but this technique is seldom used without qualification and recognition of its limitations. Admittedly, it is a crude indicator that ignores changes in patterns of utilization and increases in productivity. Furthermore, it does not take into account anticipated changes in economic conditions, awareness of health problems, sophistication in seeking health services, general level of educational attainment and availability of resources, each of which can result in an increased demand for health manpower.

This method was used by the Surgeon General's Consultant Group on Medical Education (the Bane Committee)[14] in 1959, to project physician requirements by 1975. The maintenance of the ratio of 141 physicians per 100,000 population existing in 1959 was accepted as a minimum goal for 1975. The committee recognized and discussed the implications of the various factors that would probably serve to increase the need and demand for medical services (chronic disease, aging population, specialization, regional disparities and changing patterns of practice) and concluded that the existing physician to population ratio was a "minimum essential to protect the health of the people of the United States."

2. *Economic Projections:* A second method employed in attempts to forecast manpower requirements uses a formula in which projected

expenditures are the numerator and expenditures per worker are the denominator. This is an effort to translate effective demand into manpower requirements.

Using this formula and assuming a national biomedical expenditure of three billion dollars and a cost of $39,000 per professional research worker in 1970, the National Institutes of Health has forecast a medical research manpower requirement of 77,000. Allowing for attrition from among the 39,700 research workers in 1960, a net additional requirement (1961–1970) of 45,000 was calculated.[15]

The Center for Priority Analysis of the National Planning Association has been using this technique to estimate the manpower requirements in health for 1975. Two premises have been used for the calculations: 1. continued expansion of total expenditures for health and medical care at the existing rate—a maintenance of effort level—and 2. expansion of effort to pursue realistically the health goal of narrowing ". . . the gap between the potentialities of the modern health technologies and the availability of medical care for most Americans," recommended in 1960 by the Presidential Commission on National Goals. The Center estimates that the attainment of this goal would result in an increase in ". . . public and private spending for health and medical care rising . . . to 8.7 percent of GNP in 1975"[16] or between $85 and $90 billion. Using these alternative premises, the projected manpower requirements for 1975 are: physicians (M.D.) 310,000 to 400,000; dentists, 118,000 to 140,000; registered nurses 840,000 to 1,091,000; licensed practical nurses 442,000 to 575,000; hospital attendants 930,000 to 1,229,000; and medical and dental technicians 279,000 to 352,000.[17]

3. *Professional Judgment:* The Lee-Jones' study, completed in 1930, for the Committee on Costs of Medical Care, remains the major effort to calculate manpower requirements on the basis of professional judgment, or expert opinions as to medical needs. Roger I. Lee and Lewis W. Jones examined the nation's morbidity experience and computed the manpower required for preventive, diagnostic and curative health services. The authors estimated the requirements at 135 physicians per 100,000 population, 220 nurses per 100,000 populations, and between 99 (with use of dental hygienists and assistants) and 179 (if dentists do all the work themselves) dentists per 100,000 population. Although all of these requirements fell below existing ratios, the authors doubted that the country during the Depression had the economic capacity to respond to this need.

The Surgeon General's Consultant Group on Nursing[19] based its calculations of nurse requirements, totaling 850,000 by 1970, on the opinion that adequate services were provided when 50 per cent of the inpatient nursing care was provided by registered nurses, 30 per cent by licensed practical nurses and 20 per cent by aides or attendants. Qualitative judgments were also made as to the requirements for public health, occupational health, nursing education and so forth. The need was considered unobtainable, fully 25 per cent in excess of a feasible goal of 680,000 professional nurses by 1970, 920,000 in 1975.

More recently, professional judgment was used to estimate the requirements of some ten million disabled Americans for rehabilitation services, including the services of certain allied health specialists. Assuming a 2,000-hour work-year for professional personnel, the author concluded that present service requirements called for seven times the existing number of physical therapists, eight times the number of occupational therapists and five times the number of medical social workers.[20]

The State of Health Manpower—1966

In 1966, using both the tools of economics and professional judgment, the American Hospital Association, in cooperation with the Public Health Service, undertook a survey of hospital staff and staffing requirements. The study was made to determine the number of personnel employed, current vacancies and estimates of personnel needs, and thus to provide a more adequate picture of the present health manpower situation. Data from the first 4,600 hospitals that reported, have been used to estimate totals for all 7,100 hospitals in the United States registered by the American Hospital Association. These reports indicate that the total number of professional, technical and auxiliary personnel employed in hospitals is about 1.4 million. About 275,000 additional professional and technical personnel would be needed to provide optimum patient care, an increase of about 20 per cent over present staffing. Over 80,000 more professional nurses and more than 40,000 practical nurses are needed. Some 50,000 aides are needed in general hospitals; another 30,000 in psychiatric institutions. Over 9,000 more medical technologists, almost 7,000 social workers, and about 4,000 more physical therapists, 4,000 x-ray technologists and 4,000 surgical technicians are required.

Resources

The main pool of manpower resources from which the health occupations can draw to fill these requirements is that of the nation's youth.

268

Viewing the situation in terms of numbers, the nation has a virtually unlimited pool of manpower from which to draw, each year bringing a bumper crop of 18-year-olds—more than 3.5 million in 1966—all of them seeking careers and making choices, many of them potential recruits to the health occupations. This figure will increase gradually over the next 15 years to reach 4.2 million in 1980.

Two other dimensions of this manpower resource warrant consideration. During the 1963–1964 academic year, three-fourths of those 17 years old graduated from high school, and during recent years the percentage of young people completing high school has steadily increased. Further increase in this percentage is projected, reaching almost 85 per cent by 1975. Furthermore, approximately one-half of all high school graduates in 1962 went to college (44 per cent of 18- to 21-year-olds were enrolled in institutions of higher education during 1964). Five hundred thousand bachelor degrees were awarded in 1965, and this number will increase to almost 750,000, a 50 per cent increase, by 1975.[21] The size of this manpower resource is impressive.

The growing proportion of women in the labor force will also be of benefit since, by and large, the health occupations are a woman's field. The proportion of women in the labor force has been increasing steadily during the past several decades, from 24 per cent in 1940, to 27 per cent in 1950, to 32 per cent in 1960. Also, the working wife or working mother is an increasing phenomenon in society. In 1940, one-third of the women who worked were married; in contrast, by 1965, almost two-thirds of women who worked were married.[22] In 1960, 70 per cent of workers in the health services industry and 75 per cent of individuals working in hospitals were females.[23] Within the health occupations, of course, the proportion of women varies—ranging from 90 per cent in fields such as nursing and dietetics to less than ten per cent in dentistry, medicine, optometry and pharmacy.

If other nations can be taken as a guide, more women will choose the health professions in the future. Dentistry, for example, is a woman's field in other societies. More than 50 per cent of all medical students in the Soviet Union are women, as are about 25 percent of those in the United Kingdom. In the United States, women have never accounted for more than 12 per cent of all M.D. degrees awarded in any year. In 1965, only 7.3 per cent of these degrees went to women.

Looking at the resources for health manpower in the context of the total economy, the signs are encouraging. The decline in agriculture as as a source of employment—a 38 per cent decrease in manpower between the 1950 and 1960 census—automation in industry and the development of a productive capacity that exceeds consumption of goods, would suggest a greater availability of manpower for the service aspects of the economy. As has been noted earlier, health and educational services represent the two most rapidly growing segments of the service economy. As the society pursues the policy of full employment, health services will be viewed increasingly as a source of employment.

Attempting to develop health manpower from these basic resources is when problems arise. In the fall of 1960, one first-year medical student was admitted for every 45 baccalaureate degrees awarded the previous June. One first-year dental student was admitted for every 100 baccalaureate degrees. Projecting these ratios ahead ten years, one can anticipate for the fall of 1975 a potential for 16,500 first-year medical students and 7,400 first-year dental students. Can the medical and dental schools accommodate them? Not on the basis of current estimates; these figures exceed the probable school capacity in 1975 by at least 50 per cent.

Federal Manpower Programs to Develop Resources

Action has already been taken by the federal government to avert the full effects of health manpower shortages by promoting efforts to increase the nation's training capacity in the health field, as well as by encouraging health personnel and institutions to accompany this expansion by the most productive use of existing health resources.

Within the past few years, several significant legislative measures have been enacted whose impact upon the nation's supply of health personnel can already be measured. Under the Health Professions Educational Assistance Act of 1963, the federal government has provided grants to certain professional schools—medical, dental and others—to expand and modernize their teaching facilities and to support student loan programs. In 1965, the Act was amended to continue these programs and to add two new categories of assistance: grants to support basic educational costs and student scholarships. Awards made in the first 18 months for which funds were available are adding 2,442 first year places in schools of medicine, dentistry, public health, nursing, pharmacy and optometry. Eight new schools of medicine, one new school of dentistry, and one new school of public health are being established under health professions assistance.

The Nurse Training Act of 1964 has comparable provisions. These include: grants to enable collegiate, associate degree and diploma schools of nursing to strengthen and expand their teaching programs; a

270

loan program for students of all types of professional nursing schools; and grants for the construction of new schools and the expansion or modernization of existing teaching facilities.

Significant progress has been made also in training allied health personnel. The Vocational Educational Act of 1963 emphasizes support of programs geared to those areas in the nation's economy which have "actual or anticipated opportunities for gainful employment." This Act, which authorized greatly increased federal aid for vocational and technical education at less-than-baccalaureate level, is already stimulating the growth of educational opportunities in high schools, technical schools and community and junior colleges for existing and new categories of technical and supportive health manpower. The Vocational Rehabilitation Amendments of 1965 authorized increased project grants for traineeships, and fellowships to assist with the training of physical therapists, occupational therapists, rehabilitation counselors and other categories of rehabilitation personnel.

The most recent legislation in this area, and perhaps the most responsive to many of the problems produced by current changes within the health occupations, is the Allied Health Professions Personnel Training Act of 1966, passed by Congress on November 3, 1966. The goal of this Act is to fill a critical health manpower gap: meeting a growing need for supervisors of subprofessional workers, for teachers in the allied health professions, for highly skilled technical specialists and for new types of allied health professionals.

The qualitative aspects of this program are important in view of the limited number of people to be trained in relation to the total demand. The legislation encourages the creation of broad, multidisciplinary training programs and the expansion of many high-quality existing programs. Improvement grants will be awarded to selected schools with three or more interrelated allied health professions curricula. Some universities with medical centers have developed comprehensive groupings of health curricula, including medical technology, physical therapy, occupational therapy, x-ray technology. In such coordinated programs, individuals who will later work together in providing health care are trained together.

Traineeships will help prepare teachers, administrators, supervisors and specialists in the various allied health professions. They will permit people with basic preparation or work experience in their field to return to school for limited periods to obtain the further training needed to fit them for teaching or supervisory duties.

271

Finally, project grants for developing, demonstrating or evaluating new curricula to train new types of health technologists yet unknown will allow educators flexibility and room for experimentation. This is perhaps the most important aspect of the program since the organization and technology of health care will continue to change. New kinds of technologists will both use and develop radically new diagnostic and therapeutic equipment, which in turn will require changes in allied health professions personnel training.

FACTORS INFLUENCING FULL REALIZATION OF MANPOWER POTENTIALS

The improvement in the capacity for training, which the above legislative measures are designed to insure, is a first and vital step, but the full realization of manpower potentials for health services requires consideration of the effectiveness of both the preparation and utilization of professional, technical and supportive health workers. It also requires consideration of the obstacles that will be encountered in improving effectiveness and fully realizing potentials.

Income and Salaries

One of the foremost obstacles encountered is presented by the economics of health manpower. As the opportunity to fulfill humanistic drives has been diffused throughout a variety of social institutions, health services can no longer rely principally on this value for attracting manpower. Consequently, the multiplicity of elements that together constitute working conditions must be considered. For physicians, the opportunity still exists for the satisfaction of both altruistic drives and economic needs. A recent study by the United States Department of Labor reported that physicians enjoyed the highest median annual earnings ($14,561) of male workers in 321 selected occupations,[24] and a survey conducted by *Medical Economics*[25] found that the average physician in private practice netted in excess of $28,400 during 1964, up from $25,000 in 1963, and ranging from $26,000 in the East to $31,000 in the Midwest. Admittedly, the work week is closer to 60 hours than 40; however, this intensity of work is probably not greater than that undertaken by most professionals. For physicians at least, participation in the healing of the sick does not require significant financial sacrifices.

The same cannot be said for the profession of nursing. A survey of the annual salaries received by school teachers, not a particularly high-paid

272

occupational group, reveals that on the average women with comparable educational experiences can earn $1,000 per year more in teaching as contrasted to nursing. A 1962 study of 810 selected agencies revealed the median salary of a staff public health nurse to be $4,442 in a voluntary agency, $4,902 in an official health agency and $6,090 with the board of education.[26] This disparity has led to a particularly acute situation in which nurses have left nursing practice to take positions with boards of education or school systems, where their knowledge and skills are not fully utilized.

As noted recently,[27] this is not the only unfavorable comparison—"In New York City, a nurse starts at an annual salary some $400 lower than that of a beginner in the Sanitation Department." A 1963 survey of short-term general hospitals revealed average weekly earnings of $86.50 for general duty nurses, $98.50 for head nurses and $110.50 for nurse supervisors.[28] The recent demands for higher wages by nurses suggest that the issue of wages and working conditions must be faced realistically in the near future.

Other health occupations do not fare much better. Average weekly earnings in mid-1963 were: dietitian, $103.50; medical record librarian, $106.50; medical social worker, $116.50; medical technologist, $94.00; physical therapist, $106.50; and x-ray technician, $82.50.[29] Even though these salaries reflect the disparity in incomes of men and women in society, the figures are substantially below the earnings of individuals with comparable education and training in other fields.

The low earning potentials in health occupations take on added significance if one hopes to increase the attractiveness of the health occupations for men. It has been suggested that a definite association exists between the increasing portion of teachers who are men and the rising salary scales in elementary and secondary education; the $6,164 estimated average annual salary for a nine-month contract exceeds all of the salaries for the health occupations listed above.

Educational Inflexibility

Restricted opportunities for job enlargement through continuing expansion of the individual's horizons and opportunities present another obstacle. For the most part, a recruit to the health endeavor is expected to select his or her ultimate goal and then enter a highly structured—"locked step"—curriculum that presents first general and then specific information. Once graduated, the individual is supposedly prepared to perform certain functions for the ensuing decades. In general, any

273

attempt to move from the discipline or profession originally selected—from practical nursing to professional nursing, pharmacy to medicine, social work to clinical psychology, or physical therapy to physiatrics—requires individuals to return to the beginning of the educational sequence. This is less true among the most extensively prepared members of the health professions; for example, it is not unusual to see interchange in career lines among M.D.s and Ph.D.s in the biological sciences. But since both the individual and the society gain when each citizen achieves the fullest potential within the limits of his innate capacity, this would seem to be ample stimulus to establish a more flexible educational framework.

At the same time a point of entry to the educational continuum commensurate with the individual's general capacity should be considered. At present, is it not ludicrous that a recent college graduate and a middle-age matron who has successfully raised a family of three through adolescence during the 20 years since she graduated from college, require, or for that matter necessarily benefit the most from the same two-year graduate experience? Such is the case in social work, and innumerable similar cases may be found in the health field.

Consumer Expectation

In attempting to modify or change the existing patterns and mechanisms for the preparation and utilization of health manpower or for the delivery of health services, the factors exerting influence on patient acceptance must be identified for consumer expectation will be one of the more formidable obstacles to many contemplated improvements. As noted by George Silver,[30] a patient may desire to consult with a physician and only a physician even when the difficulty could better be handled by another professional who has more suitable training—in this instance, a social worker for problems of social and psychological adjustment. Reluctance on the part of patients to settle for a dental hygienist as the most appropriate practitioner to administer dental prophylaxis is another illustration, and use of private-duty nurses by the affluent patient who wishes every whim catered to is characteristic of the inappropriate utilization of scarce manpower.

The prevailing philosophy of allocation and provision of services according to one's ability to pay is another obstacle to rationalization of the utilization of health services. Income and not medical need appears to determine whether one is treated by a psychiatrist or a social worker, an ophthalmologist or an optometrist, an orthopedist or a podiatrist.

274

The disparity between need and utilization of professional manpower in the case of maternity services was discussed in a recent lay publication.[31] The authors, in discussing infant mortality in the United States in contrast with other countries, note:

> No country on earth has enough obstetricians and pediatricians to supply . . . [the full scientific resources of medicine] to all mothers and all newborn babies. But it is relatively easy to supply top-quality care to the 25 to 35 percent of pregnant women who really need it and to their babies. It is in this selection of high-risk women for high-quality care that the United States lags far behind countries like Sweden and the Netherlands.

The authors inform the reader that Fellows of the American College of Obstetricians and Gynecologists or an obstetrician who is board-certified are qualified to handle "high risk" pregnancies. The logic of the presentation notwithstanding, it is doubtful that the middle-class reader of the magazine will settle for less than "top-quality care" no matter how normal her pregnancies. Thus do many obstetricians become the highest paid midwives in the world.

Professional Conservatism and Isolationism

Health professionals are likewise unwilling to accept modifications of traditional patterns. Most established professions are conservative in orientation—a desirable trait when viewed as an effort to safeguard standards and enhance quality. But professional conservatism produces a natural reluctance on the part of a profession to share functions or responsibilities previously recognized as its sole prerogative. This attitude frequently can create conflicts between the older and newer professions as each seeks the same end—patient well-being—by different means. The resultant "jurisdictional disputes" are comparable to those prevalent in other sectors of the economy. The defenses on the grounds of quality are frequently noteworthy for their lack of supporting evidence. Moreover, these conflicts can be socially devastating when the fight over prerogatives occurs in the midst of a need and demand for health services that surpass the present capacity of health manpower.

Some of the problems inherent in this subject are related to those posed by the educational framework. Frequently, the pressures for annexation of new responsibilities and expansion of the scope of interests results from individuals who have selected a discipline or profession that ultimately fails to place the greatest demand on their intellectual resources. These individuals are prevented from moving up into more prestigious and privileged groups that have greater responsibilities.

In anticipation of encroachment, some professions; e.g., physical therapy, have resisted the inauguration of training programs for assistants. Interdisciplinary relationships within health services are of critical importance. Herein both existing and emerging health disciplines must be considered. As new specialties take form in an effort to cope successfully with the potential offered by scientific and technological breakthroughs, one can anticipate additional careers. Since few, if any, new disciplines confine their activities to new techniques or problems, areas of overlap can be expected.

Resistance to the pressure for change can be even more difficult to overcome when the *status quo* is firmly imbedded in a multiplicity of statutes, accreditation procedures and criteria for certification. Even these can be minor obstacles, however, when compared to the economic vested interests that are supposedly a hallmark of guilds rather than professions. In such situations the forces of logic and rationality may be no match for tradition and vested interest.

The irrationality of many standards that become fixed in state statutes is evidenced by the differing privileges accorded dental hygienists in various states. Almost one-half of the states prohibit a dental hygienist from providing dental prophylaxis that requires scaling beneath the margin of the gum. "Why should a dental hygienist who can successfully scale and polish teeth below the margin of the gingivae in Michigan be forbidden to do so in New York?" asked the New York State Committee on Medical Education.[32]

The problems raised in accreditation have been forthrightly reviewed by William K. Selden, former Executive Director of the National Commission on Accreditating and an interested student of the problems associated with the accreditation of professional programs of study. Increasing the supply of health manpower, through both the expansion of existing programs and the creation of new curricula, often faces the dilemmas of quality versus quantity in the arena of accreditation. As noted by Selden:[33]

> Professional accrediting, most of which is supported indirectly by licensure laws in the various states is intimately related to the desires of individuals to attain a high vocational status. When individuals in a particular group discover that they are using a common body of knowledge . . . inevitably they band together . . . [and] develop an impelling motive to raise individual status by restricting admission to the profession—sometimes with more emphasis on the interests of the practitioners than on public welfare. The issue of control over admission is extremely important to

any profession. This is especially true in the formative stages of a profession as it fights for recognition and struggles against the superior attitude of the established professions.

These comments can also apply to a host of "semiprofessional," "subprofessional" and technical areas in which the individuals in an occupational category share an identifiable common body of knowledge that is transmitted through educational programs.

The issues vary from the "delicate balance between the institutional and the public interest" that are of a general nature and ever present, to the more discrete conflicts in which each of the protagonists claims to represent the public interest, as in the present struggle between the National League for Nursing, advocating accreditation of professional programs, and the American Association of Junior Colleges, arguing for institutional accreditation. Some observers have suggested that inclusion of more generic concerns within the accreditation procedures of individual fields is required.

Since "quality" as a criterion for accreditation has been discussed up to now, a pause is in order to recognize that although the expression "quality of health services" is widely used, discussed and argued, it is imprecise and lacks an accepted definition. The expression usually connotes a value judgment as to whether or not the professional is performing his tasks to the best of his ability and in accordance with some generally accepted standards. Actually, as suggested by the Surgeon General, standards promulgated by a profession are but one part of a notion of quality of health care. The other basic dimensions to any determination of the quality of health services are the criteria established by the consumer and the society. Admittedly some overlapping occurs; nevertheless, each set of criteria has distinct features.

The criteria established by the professional are those of peer judgment and are concerned with diagnostic excellence, the scientific validity of one's decisions and the technical skill manifested in one's provision of service. These are some of the factors with which record audits and comparable approaches to measuring and evaluating standards are concerned. This is also the dimension that is most severely challenged by the growth in scientific knowledge that has resulted in shortening the performance half-life of the practitioner and created an awareness of the need for well-developed and utilized continuing education.

The second dimension of quality of health services is that advanced by the consumer. Although he recognizes the importance of the "science of medicine," he is also concerned with the "art of medicine." His assessment of quality of health services is subjective and emphasizes the patient's emotional needs. For the consumer, accessibility and compassion are very important elements in determining the quality of health services. That is not to suggest that he is willing to sacrifice scientific quality to have accessibility and compassion; but neither is he particularly desirous of sacrificing them to receive care of the highest caliber.

The third dimension of the quality of health services is that developed by society. In some respects this dimension is concerned with achieving a balance between the previous two. For a society, efficiency, reasonable costs and unit productivity are all extremely important variables. A fair statement would be that the societal dimension seeks the most effective utilization, the lowest cost and the greatest unit productivity without sacrificing the expectations of the professional or the consumer. It is here that conflicts are found as those concerned with the formulation of social policy take cognizance of individual and group expectations and seek to achieve satisfactory resolution of incompatibilities. This emphasizes the importance of seeking an arena in which the interests of both the provider and consumer of health services can bargain over the requirements for preparation and utilization of health manpower.

Organization and Utilization

On the more positive and slightly less problematic side, with the growth in the size and complexity of the institution of health, an increasing organization has been noted in an effort to achieve more effective utilization of skilled manpower. The institution of health has been slower than many of the other institutions in society to adopt the principles of organization and many of its benefits are therefore only now beginning to be reaped.

Also, slow but continuous changes have occurred in the utilization of manpower. Attempting to analyze these changes from 1940 to 1960, Weiss[34] grouped health occupations into three levels of job content—high, medium and low—using as measures, in the absence of more concrete data, relative earnings and estimates of educational and training requirements. Comparing employment at each level over this period, he found the largest percentage increases in the occupations with low job content and the smallest increases in the occupations with high job content. This inverse relationship was valid also when the data were analyzed by region and sex. Furthermore, his analysis showed that "if the 1950 job coefficients [earnings and educational requirements] for

278

health manpower had been maintained [in 1960], an additional 100,000 health jobs with a high level of job content and 113,000 health jobs with a middle level of job content, would have been required to produce the 1960 output of health services. Instead, 117,000 with a low level of job content were substituted for these 113,000 jobs." In addition, analysis of specific groups of jobs indicated improved utilization of health manpower. For example, productivity of dentists has increased from 1950 to 1963, and the evidence suggests that this increase is partially due to additional dental auxiliary personnel. Similarly, the field of nursing has seen an increase in the productivity of nursing care and the proportion of low-level content jobs.

Therefore, although not actively pursued as a policy, in effect improvement has taken place in some fields in utilization and organization of health manpower. But this is only a beginning.

Problems of Under-Utilization

Traditionally qualified manpower has been under-utilized by "capital-poor institutions," such as universities and hospitals, in the service section of the economy. As Ginzberg has stated: [35]

> Partly because we have so many non-profit institutions which tend to be capital poor, productivity tends to be low. . . . The kinds of supporting personnel that even a broken-down business organization would have on the payroll to economize the use of the more expensive personnel are scarce in non-profit institutions. Being capital poor, these institutions squeeze their dollars and try to make them go as far as they can. From a productivity point of view, I think you have a substantial under-investment in capital, with corresponding under-utilization of personnel which on balance gives you a bad result.

Everyone can cite examples of the waste of talent and training in hospitals and other institutions as well as in private medical and dental offices. Hospitals, the major employers of health manpower, generally are unable to afford supportive clerical and administrative personnel in the numbers needed to free their professional and technical staffs from the routine and the repetitious. The result, as they recognize and as Ginzberg points out, is a less-than-desirable method of operation that requires specialized personnel—who must be employed—to function for a good portion of their time at less than their highest levels of capability.

A recent time-motion study of practicing pediatricians by Bergman, Dassel and Wedgwood[36] raises many questions concerning the appropriateness of training and utilization of pediatricians. Although the

279

study included only four pediatricians, the data revealed that 48 per cent of the pediatrician's day was spent with patients, 12.5 per cent on the phone, and nine per cent on paper work. Fifty per cent of the time with patients was spent with well children and 22 per cent with children who had minor respiratory illness. Less than two per cent of the total work week of the pediatricians studied was spent on the types of illnesses that constituted the vast majority of pediatric residency training, namely on the inpatient care of nephrosis, meningitis, inborn errors of metabolism, leukemia, cardiac disease and severe infectious disease. As a result, the authors concluded, "intellectual understimulation seems to arise from spending the majority of time with children who did not require their special talents." One consequence has been a trend to subspecialization in a search for intellectual challenge. With rising demands for child health care and an increasing population, the pediatrician manpower gap will become larger and larger. If current manpower trends continue, it has been estimated that by 1980, 59,000 additional physicians would have to be trained to maintain the current physician-child ratio.[37] Obviously, that is not going to be possible. Different patterns of child health care will be necessary.

Ross, commenting on this study, has made some suggestions for new patterns:[38]

> Can we not set up teams comprising trained individuals to interpret normal growth and development, give advice on nutrition, and carry out planned immunization procedures, and reserve to the pediatrician a supervisory role, the performance of physical examination, and the care of illness? As the head of the team the individual pediatrician should be able to provide good care to a much larger number of children and satisfaction not only to his patients and their parents but also to his professional teammates themselves.

The issue—an issue relevant to every discipline—is how long even a wealthy society can rationalize the investment of years of education and training beyond high school in individuals who will subsequently devote significant portions of their time to routine duties that might be provided very effectively by people trained in half the number of years.

ESSENTIALS OF A MANPOWER POLICY

The number and variety of health occupations considered in juxtaposition to society's pool of manpower resources is a challenge to formulate a rational policy for health manpower. A continuum must be

280

developed in which the preparation and utilization of different types of professional and technical workers are related in an optimum fashion. This will require consideration of health manpower at all levels of knowledge and skill.

The range of skill, aptitude and general interest required of health manpower is as great as that found in virtually any societal endeavor. Careers exist in the health disciplines for individuals with highly disparate backgrounds, diverse levels and duration of preparation and significantly divergent interests and capacities. Moreover, critical shortages exist of highly trained and specialized manpower. Efforts to create jobs that comprise only circumscribed tasks and a limited number of skills can contribute ancillary and supportive activities that aid highly competent manpower to achieve a greater output of health services. Individuals with innate capacities that will enable them ultimately to pursue higher levels of education need to be considered. So do individuals with lesser talents who can be expected to perform work that requires the mastery of only limited skills.

Education Programs

To clarify the various levels of preparation in health occupations is difficult since every group considers itself professional and use of the terms technician and technologist and vocational and technical is interchangeable. The confusion in nomenclature notwithstanding, education and training for the health occupations occurs essentially in six levels or clusters, namely:

1. *Advanced professional:* programs that admit students holding a baccalaureate degree to study at the graduate level; four years for an M.D., D.D.S. or Ph.D. in the behavioral or biological sciences and two-year curricula leading to masters degrees in social work, hospital administration, etc.

2. *Intermediate professional:* programs that require two years of college prior to a four-year curriculum leading to a Doctor of Optometry, Doctor of Pharmacy, Doctor of Podiatry or Doctor of Veterinary Medicine.

3. *Basic professional:* programs based in colleges or universities and leading to a baccalaureate degree. Included are physical therapy, occupational therapy, speech therapy, medical laboratory technology, medical record librarianship, dietetics and nursing. In some instances as much as a full year of clinical or practical work in a supervised

281

setting is required for professional certification; in the four-year program, the practical or clinical work is frequently accomplished during summers and vacations. Programs for the preparation of cytotechnologists and dental hygienists represent a variation on this level of preparation since six months and one year of practical training respectively follow two years of general education in a college or junior college.

4. *Technical:* programs offered by community colleges, vocational institutions or hospitals, are usually of two-year duration, although less when little, if any, general education is included in the curriculum. Illustrations include programs for associate degree nurses, diploma nurses, x-ray technicians and dental laboratory technicians.

5. *Vocational:* training offered primarily by vocational high schools or hospitals, usually six to 12 months in duration and almost completely practical in orientation. Training programs for licensed practical nurses, inhalation therapists and certified laboratory assistants are illustrations.

6. *On-the-job training:* programs that have virtually no educational prerequisites and are limited to short orientation courses or in-service instruction in limited procedures.

The differences between the technical and vocational clusters are the least distinct. The terminology used is arbitrary and attempts to distinguish between training programs of one year's duration or less and those requiring two years of study beyond high school.

The relations between the two principal types of programs for the preparation of health manpower—educational institutions (universities, colleges, community colleges, vocational schools or departments of education) and service institutions (mainly hospitals)—needs resolution. The recent trend is toward increasing the portion of training sponsored by primarily educational institutions with hospital affiliations for the clinical or practical component of the program. Expansion of this trend will require a major shift of administrative responsibility for technical and vocational training service to educational institutions. This trend is being stimulated by the tremendous growth of two-year community colleges in the United States and a redirection of public, vocational education from industrial trades to those of service careers.

Two benefits of a merger of educational and service institutions with respect to the preparation of health manpower are to be anticipated. A majority of the programs for training health technicians have less than ten students. Many have as few as two. The question is being raised as to whether or not a program of this size has the necessary "critical mass" to justify the energies of a faculty, no matter how small its numbers or the portion of time devoted to that effort. The character of the training approximates apprenticeship far more than an organized curriculum. Another salutary effect of this merger would be the expanding influence of educational accreditation. Currently, regional accreditation, the main mechanism through which society assesses and acknowledges the adequacy of its programs of formal instruction, is not used for the technical areas.

In any event, an adequate health manpower program should be aimed at obtaining the most effective yield possible from the nation's educational resources, represented by almost 600 junior colleges, universities and other institutions offering four or more years of higher education, augmented for purposes of supervised practical experiences by the approximately 1,000 short-term general hospitals with 200 or more beds.

Theory-Skill Spectrum

Developing new educational programs and changing existing ones will constitute one of the most important avenues to the improvement of utilization. Kinsinger, who has been concerned with developing increasing numbers and kinds of health technicians, has proposed a "theory-skill spectrum in the health field."[39] Such an idea with the added dimension of "capacity for independent action," as proposed by Mase,[40] offers a context in which to deduce the interrelationships among specific disciplines with respect to both their preparation and utilization. Approaching health manpower as an interrelated whole rather than merely an agglomeration of disparate categories of personnel is essential.

The "theory-skill spectrum" suggests a hierarchical continuum in which generalizable academic and experience equivalents are common to several levels of functioning. The technical or professional health worker is faced with the necessity of mastering varying portions, in both range and depth, of biomedical knowledge and specific skills. Flexibility in both the development and use of health manpower requires that educational and experience equivalents must be identified and measured wherever they might exist. This, together with the development of adequate measures of capacity for independent action, is a prerequisite to accomplishing a downward transfer of functions from the higher-trained to the lesser-trained individuals (see below), as well as to de-developing "job enlargement," i.e., assuming increasing responsibility commensurate with one's skills.

283

It is suggested that the curricula found in the various clusters of health manpower described above (advanced professional, intermediate professional, basic professional, technical and vocational) could be examined both for the common elements within each cluster and the relationships among the hierarchy of clusters. A determination of the portion of each curriculum devoted to generalizable knowledge and to technical skill could assist and enable an individual completing a program in one cluster to receive advanced standing in a curriculum in another cluster located above it in the hierarchy. In addition to facilitating and encouraging each individual to obtain the fullest margin of his capacity, the existence of such a continuum could open positions in the clusters of "basic" through "advanced" health professions to students making a lateral or diagonal transfer.

For example, the nation's medical and dental schools lose approximately ten per cent of their students between enrollment and the start of the third year. It would seem that the possibility of filling these 800 plus vacancies in the third year medical class and the 300 vacancies in the third year of dental school with "transfers" from other programs in the health professions through the vehicle of related curricula is worth exploration. The increasing portion of the medical curricula given over to electives (two of the four years in the new curriculum at the Duke Medical School) increases the options for developing overlaps with curricula in other professional schools. Advanced placement is now a widespread phenomenon in the movement of the student from high school to college. Honors study offered to students of nursing, pharmacy, optometry, physical therapy and so forth to qualify them for advanced placement in a medical curriculum should not be impossible to devise.

At the present time, high school graduates spending three years in a diploma school of nursing in a hospital receive no credit toward a college degree; the assumption is, therefore, that the program has zero academic equivalents. On the other hand, a girl spending two years in a community college qualifies for licensure as a registered nurse at the same time that she receives academic credit, suggesting that the program has fewer technical equivalents. The Bachelor of Science in Pharmacy degree, however, that required five years beyond high school, represented four years of academic equivalents for enrollment toward a Ph.D. in most universities.

284

Core Curricula

New curricula may well have to be devised and planning and inauguration of core curricula at various levels of health manpower must be pursued. With an increasing number of health professions, relationships among the various members of the health team who will be sharing responsibilities will become critical, and interaction among these health workers must be encouraged. At the same time, consideration must be given to making maximum use of limited educational resources through such mechanisms as the sharing of faculty, which the development of core curricula would facilitate.

Indications are that community colleges will attempt to develop core curricula as they consider initiating programs for a whole range of health technicians.[41] The similarity of the curricula for many of these programs with respect to the biological sciences supports the logic of such an approach. One program in Minneapolis, Minnesota,[42] using core curricula, currently offers preparation in seven health occupations: 1. medical laboratory assistant, 2. medical record technician, 3. medical secretary, 4. nurse technician, 5. occupational therapy assistant, 6. radiologic technologist and 7. food service supervisor.

In addition, the use of core curricula is found in graduate schools and universities where the basic science faculty provides instruction for students in the biomedical sciences, medicine and dentistry. Some faculty also teach in several clusters by varying the scope and intensity of the subject matter covered—for example, in teaching clinical pathology and medical technology. Efforts to develop core curricula at the basic professional and intermediate professional levels, as well as increasing the effort at the other levels, would appear to warrant careful study and implementation.

Education as a Continuous Process

But the education of health manpower cannot be considered solely a preparatory experience, as it has tended to be to date. The increasing rate at which scientific and technological advances are being achieved indicates the foolhardiness of considering any preparation as terminal. It has been suggested, and advocated, that the intimate relationship between educational and service programs discussed above would enable education to become a truly continuous process. The individual health worker could learn new techniques relative to his or her discipline, and he might also have more chance to enlarge his theoretical knowledge.

285

Opportunities for the latter—that is, increasing the level of one's mastery of theory and generalizable knowledge—are essential to upward movement on a career ladder.

Career Mobility

Any increase in opportunities for movement on a career ladder will be of paramount importance in achieving the most complete utilization of health manpower. At the present time, mobility is limited in either a lateral or vertical direction among health careers. As noted above, with the present system of education and training an individual has to select one of the many possible health careers prior to enrollment in a specific program. In effect, the student who chooses one health career bars himself from all others, unless he chooses to go back and begin at the beginning in a new course of study that may well repeat what his previous training and experience have already taught him. But, as noted by Ginzberg and his associates,[43]

> A person's occupational choice is not a one-time decision but the cumulative result of many decisions over time. These decisions re-enforce each other until the occupational path open to an individual has been narrowly delineated.

A more flexible system fostering both lateral and vertical career mobility among health disciplines could serve to offset premature restriction or closure of occupational choice.

The absence of vertical mobility among the health disciplines and the restriction of occupational decisions to only one or at most a couple of "points of entry" virtually close the majority of the health careers to the socially and culturally disadvantaged in society. The odds against motivating an impending high school dropout to complete secondary schooling, four years of college, four years of medical school and four years of post-graduate work so that he might practice medicine are beyond his comprehension, his innate intelligence and aptitude notwithstanding. Providing him with a series of short-range goals encompassing a step-by-step elevation in responsibilities—all accompanied by general educational opportunities—might provide the individual with sufficient challenge and motivation to reassess his career aspirations in the light of recent achievements and newly perceived horizons.

Can several of the health disciplines be related in an education continuum to provide multiple points of exit to jobs and reentry for further study preparatory to a higher level of functioning? It seems that combinations of some parts of existing curricula reinforced by the current thinking about education as a continuous process could produce a plausible first step to truly exciting opportunities. One of the major policy recommendations of the Conservation of Human Resources Project[44] is that of work-study programs designed to stimulate the "awareness of occupational opportunity," an approach that warrants scrutiny.

A continuum of enlarging experiences through a work-study program could enable an individual to derive motivation from an "awareness of occupational opportunities." Although it is usually argued in educational circles that the general or broad education should precede training for specific activities, this sequence is not always possible and frequently is impractical. A widely recognized example of specific or technical training occurring before rather than after general education can be found in many case histories of "self-made" men. In these situations, so frequently idealized and venerated in folklore, circumstances necessitate the individual's entrance into the labor market through the performance of menial tasks. Energy combined with innate ability and good fortune enables the individual to progress to a point where he can acquire a broadened and general education through the vehicle of life experiences.

Similarly, the opportunity to work in health services, even at a very basic or rudimentary level, could represent the beginning of a broader horizon of basic education, adult education, self-study and similar experiences. It is important to recognize that efforts aimed at adapting jobs to individuals do not preclude consideration of the educational facets of these programs. On the contrary, these efforts ultimately can contribute to the educational enhancement of the individual. Thus, he can grow to fill larger, more complex and more demanding responsibilities in the future. The experience of the armed forces in preparing hospital corpsmen, laboratory technicians and personnel for other health occupations suggests that career ladders in health are feasible, and it should be noted that one-quarter of the medical students in the Soviet Union have had prior education and experience in one of the health occupations.[45]

The widely publicized two-year, post-high-school curriculum initiated recently at Duke University Medical Center to train physician assistants could be used as part of a foundation for construction of a career ladder. This program is aimed at increasing the productivity of medical practitioners by preparing a new category of paramedical manpower to perform a large array of procedures under supervision. The information available to date does not suggest that the graduates of this program

287

will possess skills that vary significantly from those found in many nurses, but a great contribution of the program may be in establishing new opportunities in the health field for men as an alternative to nursing, characterized as predominantly a female profession. The most far-reaching impact could be achieved, however, if thought is given to devising future educational opportunities, in combination with work experiences, that would permit one of these or subsequent "physician assistants" to move up the occupational ladder to become a physician.

The subject of the "indigenous, nonprofessional" is stimulating the curiosity of many service professions. The idea of career development is included in the thinking on this subject, and the shortsightedness of concentrating on jobs, and therefore failing to look for careers, is recognized. As noted by Reiff and Riessman: [46]

> The concept of employing indigenous nonprofessionals calls for the possibility of promotion to various levels of subprofessional and professional positions. For this to occur, both public and private sector requirements will have to accept combinations of work experience plus education which can be acquired concomitantly with employment or intermittently with leaves of absence.

Downward Transfer of Functions

Complementary to establishment of career mobility as an approach to effective utilization is a downward transfer of functions. Giving each service the level of skill it needs, no more and no less, may be the principal challenge to health manpower. Meeting this challenge requires detailed study of health services and a subdivision of specific functions into the component tasks. Then individuals possessing only a limited range of skills and competencies can be drawn into the manpower pool to perform many of the tasks, freeing those more highly trained and skilled for the performance of duties requiring their more advanced level of competency.

Extensive research and analysis to determine the limits of safety is, of course, a necessary prerequisite to this approach. Then, attention must be focused on those services that can be provided by more than one discipline and on the fact that the greatest economy is realized when disciplines in shortage areas are devoting the greatest possible percentage of their time to those services that they, and they alone, are equipped to provide.

Success in programs of "downward transfer of functions" usually hinges on effective organization and supervision of the services performed, and, accordingly, the approach requires an institutional setting for effective implementation. That should not present a problem in the health enterprise, however, since health comprises a variety of institutions and agencies—hospitals, health departments, nursing homes, group practices and voluntary health agencies—located throughout the nation and extensive in both number and kind. Moreover, as was noted earlier, the trend toward institutionalization of health services, in a functional sense, suggests an increased opportunity for new approaches.

The increasing use by dentists of auxiliary personnel is one illustration of a downward transfer of functions. A recent survey of dental practice,[47] which assumed dentists' incomes reflected productivity, found that their income or productivity increased with each additional dental auxiliary that they employed. Furthermore, the addition of a second assistant increases income more than the addition of the first assistant, and the addition of a third assistant increases income more than the addition of a second. Since most dentists now employ one or two full-time assistants, the study implies the need for further improvements in utilization.

A downward transfer of functions has frequently resulted in the creation of new disciplines and some interesting innovations involving assistants to physicians now being tried may well create more. Of these, the following programs are illustrative:

1. Training of personnel as "medical emergency technicians" for emergency service, being conducted at Ohio State University.
2. Duke University's two-year program for training "physician assistants," comparable to the experienced medical corpsman of the armed forces.
3. The "pediatric public-health nurse practitioner" being trained at the University of Colorado to assume an expanded role in child health.
4. The "unit manager," developed at the University of Florida Health Center, who orders supplies, stocks, medications and linens, handles requests for and records results of laboratory and technical procedures, schedules orderly service and patient transportation and manages meal service, thus freeing nurses for patient care.

Application of Technology

Increased application of technology to provision of health services would also serve to improve utilization of health manpower. In contrast

289

to other industry, "the health service industry" has substituted technology for manpower to only a limited degree. No doubt, a variety of reasons may be cited, ranging from an inherent distrust of the appropriateness of the extensive use of automation and instrumentation in what must be a personalized, service activity, to the lack of capital for investment in developmental activities and purchase of hardware. Nonetheless, when the health endeavor is viewed as a $45 billion labor-intensive industry, with labor costs approximating three-quarters of the total, the impetus to substitute technology for manpower becomes inevitable.

Several examples of "labor-saving" developments can be cited: disposable supplies (syringes, needles, transfusion sets and gloves), pre-packaged formula and intravenous solutions, simplified laboratory tests (Clinitest for Benedict's solution) and so forth. The potential of automated laboratories, computer analysis of electrocardiograms and similar developments is suggested by the Kaiser Permanente multiphasic screening project[48] under development in Oakland, California, since 1962. Approximately 40,000 health-plan beneficiaries are screened annually with a battery of 20 automated and semi-automated tests, including a self-administered health history questionnaire. Only approximately two and one-half hours are required to complete the automated survey and it is conducted by nurses, technicians and other supportive health manpower. Conventional methods would require two days and between four and five times the $42 cost established in this program.

CONCLUSION

Careful exploration of each of these avenues to improved utilization and application of new ideas and practices encountered in this exploration can profoundly affect the capacity to insure that every individual receives the best in health care. For utilization is a critical variable. As such, it is considered in a new book by Rashi Fein of the Brookings Institution.[49] Working on the premise that manpower equirements are a function of requirements for services, now considered by some to be the only meaningful and realistic basis for forecasting, Fein asserts:

> The 'need' for medical personnel depends on the demand for medical services and on the quantity of services a given amount of personnel can and is prepared to offer. Both the demand and the supply change over time. The former is affected as the health and socio-economic characteristics of the population alter, as research in medicine advances, and as government helps transform medical needs into demand by instituting new

medical services or financing programs. The latter changes as new patterns of medical organization come into being, as new types of personnel are trained and new technology is developed, and as the productivity of personnel changes.

Not all of the variables involved are quantifiable, but estimating the effects of each to the extent possible and using existing patterns of utilization as his base, Fein projects an increase in demand of at least 22 to 26 per cent for 1975, and a 19 per cent increase in the number of physicians. For 1980, he predicts a 35 to 40 per cent increase in demand and a 29 per cent increase in physicians.

Obviously, utilization of health manpower in such a way that the benefits of modern medicine may be made available to all will require much in terms of creative energy and innovative approaches. The introduction to this paper expressed the belief that billions of dollars could be invested in the education and training of health manpower without making a significant impact on the availability of health services, and thereafter, attempted neither a thorough review nor analysis of all the relevant factors. Rather the attempt has been made to suggest issues and to provoke a discussion of health manpower policy.

Planning for the effective preparation and use of health manpower is the subject of the first two of the 23 recommendations of a task force that has spent considerable time in examining the subject of health manpower.[50] But, as always, the recommendation is easier than implementation. Nonetheless, "plan we must!" As planning proceeds, visualizing the problems and formulating solutions must precede and guide the computerization of the data.

REFERENCES

[1] Davis, M. M., MEDICAL CARE FOR TOMORROW, New York, Harper & Brothers, 1955, p. 7.

[2] The nation's 87 medical schools reported total expenditures of $695,684,904 (regular operating programs $286,157,698; sponsored programs $409,528,206) for the 1964–1965 academic year. Major sources of funds included: federal research grants and contracts, $252,284,161; federal training grants and contracts, $80,506,064; state appropriations, $75,554,188; overhead on federal grants and contracts, $40,201,471. *Source*; Medical Education in the United States, 1964–1965, *Journal of the American Medical Association*, 194, 760, November 15, 1965.

[3] *Manpower in the 1960's*, Health Manpower Source Book No. 18, Washington, United States Department of Health, Education and Welfare, Public Health Service Publication No. 263, 1964, pp. 2–3.

[4] *Ibid.*, pp. 7–10.

[5] United States Department of Labor, *Health Careers Guidebook*, 1965. The 31 "Health Career Briefings" listed in the book and the 34 fields for which the National Center for Health Statistics is collecting data differ in several instances. The *Guidebook* does not list chiropractics as a health career. The National Center combines medical and osteopathic as one category and has separate categories for "automatic data processing" and "medical secretarial" as well as "miscellaneous."

[6] *Manpower in the 1960's, op. cit.* Includes physicians, dentists, nurses, pharmacists and other persons who are college educated or professionally trained among those employed as biological scientists, biostatisticians, chiropractors, clinical psychologists, dental hygienists, dietitians, health educators, medical laboratory technologists, medical record librarians, optometrists, podiatrists, rehabilitation counselors, sanitary engineers, social workers—medical and psychiatric—veterinarians and therapists—occupational, physical, speech and hearing.

[7] Altenderfer, M. E., Trends in Health Manpower, Staff paper No. 1 for the Task Force on Health, Education and Welfare Manpower Requirements and Training Programs, November 30, 1965.

[8] Weinerman, E. R., *Dilemma of the OPD: Epilogue or Epicenter,* Hartford Foundation Conference on Ambulatory Care and Rehabilitation, October 15, 1965, publication pending.

[9] Medical Education in the United States, 1964–1965, *op. cit.*, p. 771.

[10] Health Information Foundation, Where Physicians Work, *Progress in Health Services,* 13, May–June, 1964.

[11] *Trends in Health Manpower,* Table 8.

[12] Somers, A. R., Some Basic Determinants of Medical Care and Health Policy: An Overview of Trends and Issues, in this volume.

[13] Expert Guessing, *New York Times,* July 12, 1964.

[14] United States Department of Health, Education and Welfare, PHYSICIANS FOR A GROWING AMERICA, Washington, United States Government Printing Office, 1959.

[15] *Manpower for Medical Research: Requirements and Resources, 1965–1970,* United States Public Health Service Publication No. 1001, 1963.

[16] Lecht, L. A., *The Dollar Cost of Our National Goals,* Washington, National Planning Association, May, 1965, p. 27.

[17] Estimates from study nearing completion by the Center for Priority Analysis, National Planning Association, undertaken for the United States Department of Labor.

[18] Lee, R. I. and Jones, L. W., THE FUNDAMENTALS OF GOOD MEDICAL CARE, Chicago, University of Chicago Press, 1932, Tables 7 and 11, and pp. 115 and 123.

292

[19] *Toward Quality in Nursing: Needs and Goals,* United States Department of Health, Education and Welfare, Public Health Service Publication No. 992, February, 1963.

[20] Daitz, B. D., The Challenge of Disability, *American Journal of Public Health,* 55, 528–534, April, 1965.

[21] Office of Education, unpublished data.

[22] *American Women,* Presidential Commission for the Status of Women, 1963.

[23] *Manpower in the 1960's, op. cit.*

[24] Rutzick, M. A., A Ranking of U. S. Occupations by Earnings, *Monthly Labor Review,* 88, 249–255, March, 1965.

[25] Physicians' Economic Health: Excellent, *Medical Economics,* 42, 77 and 81, December 13, 1965.

[26] Freeman, V. and Levenson, G., Salaries of Nurses in Selected Public Health Agencies: 1962, *Nursing Outlook,* 10, 815, December, 1962.

[27] Nationwide Crisis in Nursing, *Medical World News,* January 28, 1966, p. 77.

[28] Elliott, J. E., FACTS ABOUT NURSING: A STATISTICAL SUMMARY, New York, American Nurses' Association, 1965, p. 130.

[29] *Ibid.,* p. 223.

[30] Silver, G. A., FAMILY MEDICAL CARE, Cambridge, Harvard University Press, 1963.

[31] Brecher, R. and Brecher, E., The Disgraceful Facts About Infant Deaths in the U. S., *McCalls,* February, 1966, p. 82.

[32] *Education for the Health Professions,* Albany, New York State Education Department, 1963, p. 25.

[33] Selden, W. K., ACCREDITATION, New York, Harper & Brothers, Publishers, 1960, p. 56.

[34] Weiss, J. H., The Changing Job Structure of Health Manpower, Cambridge, Harvard University, unpublished doctoral dissertation, July, 1966, pp. 117–120, 156.

[35] Ginzberg, E., Manpower Aspects of the Service Sector of the Economy, Joint Economic Committee Hearings on Employment Growth and Price Levels, 86th Congress, First Session, September–October 2, 1959, Part 8, pp. 2661–2670.

[36] Bergman, A. B., Dassel, S. W. and Wedgwood, R. J., Time-Motion Study of Practicing Pediatricians, *Pediatrics,* 38, 254–263, August, 1966, Part I.

[37] *Ibid.,* p. 262.

[38] Ross, R. A., Commentary: Time, Motion and Pediatric Practice, *Pediatrics,* 38, 165–166, August, 1966, Part I.

[39] Kingsinger, R. E., *Education for Health Technicians: An Overview,* American Association of Junior Colleges, 1965.

[40] Mase, D., "The Utilization of Mindpower," paper presented to the American Public Health Association, Health Manpower Section, November 2, 1966.

[41] Kinsinger, *op. cit.*, Appendix III, lists the following 21 Community College Career Programs in Allied Medical and Auxillary Dental Occupations:

Biomedical Electronics Technician	Medical Secretary
Dental Assistant	Medical Assistant
Dental Hygienist	Medical Emergency Technician
Dental Laboratory Technician	Food Service Supervisor
Director of Hospital Volunteer Services	Inhalation Therapy Technician
Medical Laboratory Assistant	Operating Room Technician
Nursing (ADN)	Ophthalmic Dispenser
X-ray Technician	Radioisotope Technician
Occupational Therapy Assistant	Prosthetist
Medical Record Technician	Environmental Health Technician
Ward Manager	

[42] *Ibid.*, p. 17.

[43] Ginzberg, E., Anderson, J. K. and Herma, J. L., THE OPTOMISTIC TRADITION OF AMERICAN YOUTH, New York, Columbia University Press, 1964.

[44] *Ibid.*, pp. 145–158.

[45] *Medical Education in the Soviet Union,* Report of the Delegation on Medical Education, U.S.–U.S.S.R. Cultural Exchange Agreement, 1964.

[46] Reiff, R. and Riessman, F., The Indigenous Nonprofessional: A Strategy of Change in Community Action and Community Mental Health Programs, *Community Mental Health Journal,* Monograph No. 1, November, 1965.

[47] American Dental Association, Bureau of Economic Research and Statistics, The 1962 Survey of Dental Practice, *The Journal of the American Dental Association,* 66, 722, May, 1963.

[48] Collen, M. F., "Periodic Health Examinations Utilizing an Automated Multitest Laboratory," presented at a joint meeting of the Section on Preventive Medicine and the Section on General Practice, American Medical Association, June 23, 1965.

[49] Fein, R., THE DOCTOR SHORTAGE: AN ECONOMIC DIAGNOSIS, Washington, D. C., The Brookings Institution, 1967.

[50] Task Force on Health Manpower, National Commission on Community Health Service, *Health Manpower: Action to Meet Community Needs,* Bethesda, 1966.

EFFECTS OF MANPOWER UTILIZATION ON COST AND PRODUCTIVITY OF A NEIGHBORHOOD HEALTH CENTER

IRENE BUTTER
GORDON T. MOORE
ROBERT L. ROBERTSON
ELISABETH HALL

Manpower is a major cost component in today's health care system, absorbing at least one half of the average health care dollar. Growing pressures to achieve cost containment and rationalization of scarce health manpower will force health care institutions to rely increasingly on management techniques for examination of choices, for guidance of activities and for evaluation of outcomes. In recent years much effort has gone into developing analytic and quantitative techniques for application to the health field, an effort that has produced a rapidly growing literature. Some of the tools are still subjects of pilot testing and further refinement; but others, whose usefulness has been demonstrated, are available for implementation by management of health facilities.[1-4]

This paper describes a methodology for evaluating manpower utilization in ambulatory health care facilities and illustrates its uses as a management tool. Several applications of the methodology will be discussed: (a) development of staffing standards; (b) assessment of resource allocations relative to objectives; (c) allocation of departmental costs between patient care and non-patient care services; and (d) assessment of cost-effectiveness of manpower mix and manpower resource allocations. Although the methodology may be used to make comparisons within and between ambulatory health care facilities, illustrative applications are confined to a single health center.

THE SETTING

This study was carried out at the Bunker Hill Health Center, a community health service of the Massachusetts General Hospital (MGH), primarily but not exclusively for residents of the Charlestown section of Boston. The Health Center offers primary as well as specialty medical services, mental health, dental health, nursing, nutrition and social services as well as physical and speech therapy. Radiology and laboratory services are also provided. The Health Center is open five full weekdays, two evenings and several hours on Saturdays and Sundays; patients are referred to the MGH Emergency Room at other times. Thirty-three full-time equivalent salaried health professionals are employed, the majority of whom practice at the Health Center full time. Professionals are grouped into two teams for the delivery of patient care and the Health Center is organized along a departmental structure. A grant from the Children's Bureau of HEW finances care for Medicaid eligible children; other patients are charged for services. By midyear 1971, after two and one-half years of operation, the Center had a registrant file of nearly 11,000 patients.[5]

The study to be reported is one of several evaluation studies of the health center developed cooperatively by Bunker Hill Health Center and the Harvard Center for Community Health and Medical Care.

THE DATA SYSTEM

Encounter and time study forms are key components of the Health Center's data system and fundamental to the manpower evaluation study. The encounter or medical visit form is filled

296

FIGURE 1. ENCOUNTER OR MEDICAL VISIT FORM

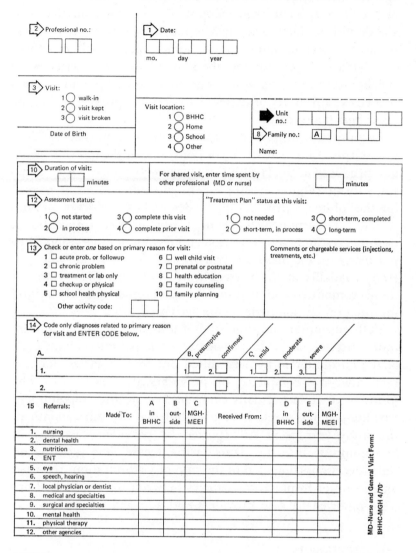

B.H.H.C.-13*

out for each face-to-face contact between patient and provider, which required more than five minutes or is a billable service. The form (Figure 1) provides information on patients, such as

297

age, sex and reason for visit; on manpower inputs, such as type of provider, specialty and amount of time spent on the visit; and on visit characteristics such as diagnosis, type of visit (check-up, acute, chronic) and location (home, school or clinic). When correlated with information about supplementary services such as laboratory tests and x-rays, encounter forms provide a comprehensive inventory of patient care services produced in clinic visits and house calls.

Encounter forms provide data on provider inputs and patient care outputs,[6] but actually record only one of the multiple products produced at the Health Center, namely patient visits. Time study forms (Figure 2) supplement encounter forms by recording the volume of provider inputs devoted to production of non-patient care outputs such as community outreach (prevention), training, research, self-education and receipt of supervision. Output measures for these non-patient care functions are not generally available at the present time, and even the volume of inputs committed and their dollar values represent fairly unique information on non-patient care activities.

Both encounter and time study forms were designed to minimize interference with providers' work patterns. Some parts of the encounter forms were filled out by secretaries, and the remainder was completed by providers after each visit. The forms were collected daily and checked against appointment schedules. Time sheets were distributed every third month of the study year, were self-reported by providers each day in fifteen-minute intervals. Direct patient care time reported on time sheets was compared to the sum of visit durations reported on encounter forms. Discrepancies between the two recordings were reported back to providers and adjusted.

THE METHODOLOGY

The data collection phase of the study covered one year, July 1970 through June 1971. Manpower utilization was examined in the departments of Pediatrics, Internal Medicine,

298

FIGURE 2. TIME STUDY SHEET

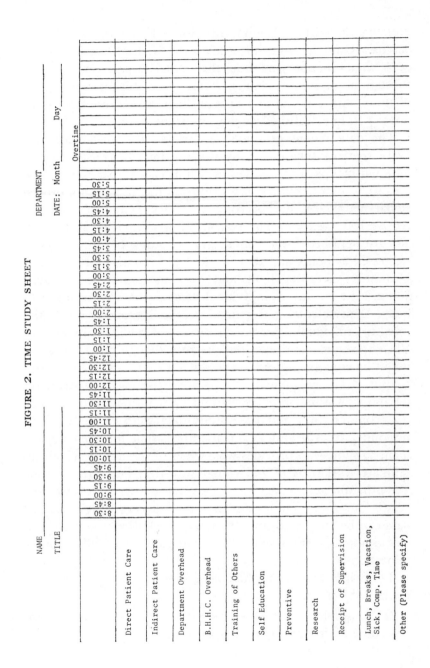

NAME _____

TITLE _____

DEPARTMENT _____

DATE: Month _____ Day _____

Overtime

	8:30	8:45	9:00	9:15	9:30	9:45	10:00	10:15	10:30	10:45	11:00	11:15	11:30	11:45	12:00	12:15	12:30	12:45	1:00	1:15	1:30	1:45	2:00	2:15	2:30	2:45	3:00	3:15	3:30	3:45	4:00	4:15	4:30	4:45	5:00	5:15	5:30
Direct Patient Care																																					
Indirect Patient Care																																					
Department Overhead																																					
B.H.H.C. Overhead																																					
Training of Others																																					
Self Education																																					
Preventive																																					
Research																																					
Receipt of Supervision																																					
Lunch, Breaks, Vacation, Sick, Comp. Time																																					
Other (Please specify)																																					

Nursing, Nutrition, Community Mental Health and Social Services. Omitted from the study were Medical Specialties because they function part-time; the Dental Department because substantial personnel changes took place during the period of study; and Physical and Speech Therapy because they were not yet fully established during the study year.

The data system generated a variety of management and evaluative information. This study primarily considers professional manpower resources, which absorb 48 per cent of the Health Center's annual expenditures; the use of nonprofessional manpower and of complementary nonlabor resources receive less attention. The real manpower input measure used (as distinguished from a monetary measure) is provider time expressed as hours and days worked per month and per year. Utilization of capital items and space was itemized, measured and related directly to individual departments for costing purposes. Departmental and general overhead expenses were allocated to individual departments by several traditional methods. Visits were used as the output measure though other measures might be equally appropriate in different settings.[7,8] Input and output data are tabulated separately for each department, disciplines within departments and even individual providers.

Encounter form and time study data were combined with personnel records and financial information for each department to show who provides what types of services to whom, to tabulate workloads of individual providers per unit of time (month, quarter or year), to look for under- or overstaffing relative to visit volumes and non-patient care activities. The data can be combined for a number of additional uses such as examining cost-effectiveness of manpower mix and resource allocations.

These information outputs were used to accomplish the following objectives:

1. To develop a profile of each department for the purpose of interdepartmental comparisons.

2. To assess manpower utilization with respect to actual and optimal workloads. For example, findings will indicate whether providers in each department can increase visit volumes, under what conditions and whether with or without reduction in non-patient care effort. Workload measures can also be translated into staffing requirements.

3. To examine manpower resource allocations relative to objectives and their respective priorities. For example, is a ten per cent resource allocation to non-patient care effort by medical departments commensurate with the importance assigned (by health center administration and/or by providers) to raising health by preventive and community efforts?

4. To analyze the costs of non-patient care activities and to separate them from the "pure" cost of patient visits. This part of the methodology facilitates computation of the average cost of visits inclusive and exclusive of the cost of community outreach, training, research and self-education.

5. To assess manpower utilization in terms of cost-effectiveness of resource allocations. For example, to the extent that both doctors and nurse practitioners are equally competent in providing certain types of visits, which type of provider produces visits at lowest cost? Furthermore, given differences in cost and practice patterns of different types of providers, what is a rational division of labor within and between departments?

The results section presents illustrative applications of the methodology in each of these areas.

RESULTS

Profiles of Departments

The utilization of manpower resources to produce patient care and non-patient care services differs between departments at the Health Center. The departments vary in size and composition of staff, in total yearly visits, in visits per man day and in visit duration (Table 1). The essence of interdepartmental differences in input-output relationships is shown in the difference (column 5, Table 1) between percentage of total staff (input) and percentage of total visits (output) for each department. In three departments—Pediatrics, Internal Medicine and Nutrition—the share of visits exceeds the share of staff. This positive differential suggests a more efficient type of production than Nursing, Community Mental Health and Social Services, where the differential is negative. However, column 5 is an oversimplification in that it is based exclusively on a single measure of output, i.e., visits. Moreover, it fails to take into account nursing inputs into Pediatrics and Internal Medicine, the heterogeneity among visits of different departments as well as interdepartmental differences in distribution of effort between patient care and non-patient care activities. Other components of the data, presented in later sections, must be examined to fully understand and use the differentials presented in column 5.

Assessment of Staffing and Workloads

The manpower evaluation methodology can be used to develop quantitative and objective criteria for staffing of the Health Center, based on delineation of input-output relations. Specific criteria for relating manpower resources of each department to its expected output had not been applied to staffing of the Health Center. We approached the issue of staffing in the following manner: first we conceptualized and defined optimal workloads; second we calculated the output capacity of present staff in each department based on optimal workloads; next we compared actual with optimal workloads; finally we developed staffing requirements based on optimal workloads and actual visit volumes during the study year. By comparing existing staff to staff requirements, each department could determine if there

302

TABLE I. PROFILES OF DEPARTMENTS

Department	No. Fulltime Equivalent Practitioners (1)	Total Visits Per Year (2)	% Distribution of Staff (3)	% Distribution of Visits (4)	Differential Between 3 & 4 (5)	Man Days Worked Per Year (6)	Average Visits Per Man Day (7)	Average Visit Duration (8)
Pediatrics	2.5	9,032	9.5	28	+ 19	560.5	16.1	18.7
Internal Medicine	2.5	7,680	9.5	23	+ 14	608.5	12.6	25.2
Nursing	9	5,795	34	18	– 16	2,043	2.8	30.7
Nutrition	1	2,331	4	7	+ 3	244	9.5	32.1
Community Mental Health	4	3,154	15	10	– 5	936	3.3	45.4
Psychiatry	1	1,163	4	4	0	231	5.0	37.3
Psychology	3	1,991	11	6	– 5	705	2.8	49.8
Social Services	7.25	4,706	28	14	– 14	1,760	2.6	57.3
Social Work	4	3,158	15	10	– 5	959	3.2	57.4
Trainees	3.25	1,548	13	4	– 9	801	1.9	57.1
Total	26.25	32,698	100	100		6,152	5.3	32.9

Sources: Reports of Evaluation Unit at Bunker Hill Health Center based on encounter forms and personnel data.

were potential for growth in visit volume, its magnitude and the conditions under which such growth could be realized.

Considerable effort was spent helping department chiefs to develop workload standards and capacity estimates geared to their own capabilities and objectives. Several times during the study year individual discussions were held with department chiefs to define optimal workloads and optimal time allocations. These discussions explored how chiefs perceived department and Health Center objectives and how they attempted to allocate resources to attain objectives. In the course of the study year actual workloads and time distributions were presented to the chiefs and revision of standards was considered.

The task of realistically specifying optimal workloads and resource allocations varied in complexity and was completed with varying degrees of success by individual department chiefs. At the beginning of the study most chiefs were not accustomed to thinking systematically and quantitatively about their resources and objectives, and required time to become oriented to a quantitative approach. Lack of consensus on a set of Health Center objectives and their priorities was an additional handicap in specifying optimal workloads.

Because the data system focused on visits as the output measure, chiefs were asked to estimate optimal workloads based on two factors: (1) the optimal time distribution between patient care and non-patient care activities, and (2) the optimal rate of visits per unit of time. Stated differently, the optimal workload depends on the portion of the workday a provider allocates to patient care and the average amount of time required for a patient visit. The first factor depends largely on the magnitude of non-patient care demands such as administrative duties and teaching. The second factor is the sum of two components: the duration of the visit and time spent on indirect patient care. Indirect patient care refers to time spent phoning, writing letters and reports, in consultations, or case conferences and in other activities related specifically to patient visits.

304

TABLE 2. ESTIMATES OF PROVIDER CAPACITIES BY DEPARTMENT

Department	Optimal Workloads: Visits Per Man Day (1)	Actual Workloads: Visits Per Man Day (2)	Differential Optimal-Actual Per Man Day (3)	Potential Yearly Visits (Based on Optimal Workloads) (4)	Actual Yearly Visits (5)	Differential Optimal-Actual Per Year (6)	Rate of Capacity Utilization (5 ÷ 4) (7)
Pediatrics	20	16.1	– 3.9	11,210	9,032	– 2,178	81%
Internal Medicine	15	12.6	– 2.4	9,127	7,680	– 1,447	84%
Nursing*	14	5.6	– 8.4	11,294	5,795	– 5,499	51%
Nutrition	10	9.5	– .5	2,440	2,331	– 109	95%
Community Mental Health	5.7	3.3	– 2.4	5,378	3,154	– 2,224	59%
Psychiatry	6.5	5.0	– 1.5	1,501	1,163	– 338	77%
Psychology	5.5	2.8	– 2.7	3,877	1,991	– 1,886	51%
Social Services	4	2.5	– 1.4	7,040	4,706	– 2,334	67%
Social Work	4	3.2	– .8	3,836	3,158	– 678	82%
Trainees	4	1.9	– 2.1	3,204	1,548	– 1,656	48%

* Based on 4.5 nurses.

305

The optimal workload is defined as the average number of visits per day that would allow the professional to provide adequate quality patient care while leaving sufficient time for the intended volume of non-patient care activities. It is important to remember that optimal workload entails the specification both of an output, the "ideal" number of visits, and of an input, intended time in non-patient care activities. It is this two-dimensional nature of the optimal workload concept that created difficulty for the chiefs, for in several instances the estimated optimal workloads were not compatible with intended time inputs into non-patient care activities. This will be seen in subsequent comparisons between optimal and actual workloads and time distributions.

Estimates of capacity for patient care (Table 2) are presented in terms of: (a) optimal workloads, e.g., visits per man day, and (b) potential yearly visit volume based on optimal workloads. Average actual workloads, actual yearly visit volumes and the differentials between optimal and actual workloads per day and per year are presented for each department. The last column of Table 2, rate of capacity utilization, is a rough measure by department of the effectiveness with which departments meet their output goals.

These capacity estimates emphasized certain issues that merited further discussion with department chiefs and illustrated the use of this approach. First optimal workload estimates were at times inconsistent with optimal time allocations as defined by the chiefs. This is illustrated by Pediatrics. The optimal visit workload as defined by the department head, combined with the average pediatric visit length implies that practically the entire workday is devoted to patient care. For example, for pediatrics:

Optimal Workload

	Visits Per Man Day	Average Duration	Total Patient Care Minutes	Total Minutes Per Man Day	Residual Minutes
Direct patient care	20 ×	18.7	= 374 min.		
Indirect patient care	20 ×	5.0	= 100 min.		
			474 min.	480	480–474 = 6

Actual Workload

Direct patient care	16.1 ×	18.7	= 301 min.		
Indirect patient care	16.1 ×	5.0	= 81 min.		
			382 min.	480	480–382 = 98

Thus a workload of twenty visits (given present visit duration) leaves six minutes of an eight-hour workday for administration, lunch, breaks and non-patient care activities. Pediatricians reported that most meetings were held before and after hours, and that lunch was consumed at the desk between patient visits. Nevertheless, the time sheets showed that 13 per cent of total pediatricians' time during the study year was spent on education, including eight per cent for self-education and five per cent for training others. The eight per cent for self-education time may well be an unintended by-product of broken appointments and a portion of the five per cent training time may overlap with patient care time, if training and patient care are jointly produced outputs. However, if pediatricians desire to allocate some time to the training of nurse practitioners and other health professionals as they indicated in interviews, and if this training either does not coincide with patient care or decreases the productivity of patient care (e.g., while the doctor acts as preceptor his patient load is reduced) 20 visits is probably an unrealistic estimate for optimal workload. The optimal workload probably lies between 16 and 20 visits, unless actual visit durations can be reduced while maintaining the same quality of patient care.

A second shortcoming of the capacity estimates is the exclusion of operational factors such as scheduling of patients and day-to-day fluctuation in visit volumes caused by walk-ins or broken visits. The capacity estimates are theoretical potentials, based on the assumption that whenever a provider is ready to see a patient a patient is waiting to be seen, and based on the assumption of constant average visit lengths, existing facilities and current modes of practice. Operational constraints such as a rigid scheduling system, a 50 per cent walk-in rate and a 30 per cent broken appointment rate in some departments can make visit volumes based on optimal workloads unrealistic targets.

The two issues just described underline the fact that accurate specification of optimal workloads and provider capacities requires an iterative process involving development of standards, comparison of performance with standards and subsequent revision of standards and performance. To specify accurately what increases in visit volumes are possible with existing staff and present allocations to non-patient care activities requires recycling of the information contained in Table 2 and an ongoing process of determination and revision of workload standards and capacity estimates.

Optimal workloads can also be translated into staffing requirements. Columns 1 and 2 of Table 3 present optimal and actual workloads per year for a full-time equivalent (FTE) provider in selected departments. Column 3 shows size of staff required to generate the study year's actual visit volumes, assuming that providers can carry optimal workloads, and column 4 shows the actual staff employed during the study year.

A reasonably good fit between existing staff and staff requirements was shown for Pediatrics, Internal Medicine and Nutrition but not for Social Services. Considering how estimated staff requirements were derived, it appears that chiefs of the first three departments were more realistic in their appraisal of current departmental capabilities than was the chief of Social Services. It was pointed out earlier that re-

308

TABLE 3. STAFFING REQUIREMENTS DEVELOPED FROM OPTIMAL WORK-
LOADS SELECTED DEPARTMENTS

	Optimal Workload Per One FTE Provider (1)	Actual Workload Per One FTE Provider During Study Year (2)	Staff Required for Study Year's Visit Volume (Optimal Workload) (3)	Actual Staff Employed During Study Year (4)
Pediatrics	4,484 visits/yr	3,612 visits/yr	2.04	2.5
Internal Medicine	3,610 visits/yr	3,072 visits/yr	2.04	2.5
Nutrition	2,444 visits/yr	2,331 visits/yr	.84	1.0
Social Services:			5.1	7.25
Social Work	959 visits/yr	788 visits/yr	3.2	4.0
Trainees	801 visits/yr	387 visits/yr	1.9	3.25

ported time spent by pediatricians in non-patient care activities exceeded the time residual associated with optimal workloads. We therefore concluded that the pediatric optimal workload is a slight overestimate. Given this bias, we infer that present staffing in Pediatrics is consistent with preliminary optimal workload estimates. A similar interpretation applies to Internal Medicine.[9]

The data for Nutrition (Table 3) also show a reasonable correspondence between the chief's estimate of optimal workload and the department's performance. Taking into account the same factors that operate in Pediatrics, such as the broken appointment rate and the joint production of training and patient care, we conclude that the Nutrition chief provided a realistic appraisal of the department's capabilities in supplying patient care and non-patient care effort. Assuming that present workload standards, non-patient care objectives, visit volumes and visit lengths are held constant, this department is adequately staffed. If, on the other hand, there is reason to expect a growing demand for visits in this department, or more effort directed into non-patient care activities, further analysis of this type can provide guidelines for future adjustments, either in staff or in visit lengths.

By contrast, in Social Services actual visits fell short of optimal workloads and the department also failed to supply the intended inputs into non-patient care activities spelled out by the chief during interviews. Further examination of Table 3

309

shows a reasonably good match between actual and optimal workloads for social workers, but a large discrepancy for trainees. Thus the poor fit between staff and staff requirements in Social Service is largely attributable to poor workload estimates for trainees, who have time distributions and work patterns notably different from those of social workers. Trainees are at the Health Center for only nine months of the year and are heavily involved in seminars and other types of educational activities. It is essential, therefore, that the iterative process of workload specification and performance measurement, particularly in regard to the trainees, be continued in this department.

Manpower Input Allocations Relative to Objectives

Despite growing interest in the rationalization of health manpower, documentation of providers' use of time has received comparatively little attention.[10-13] However, there has been increased recognition of the usefulness of such performance studies, especially since providers commonly fail to realize "how much time they actually spend in activities other than direct patient care."[14] Time study information can be particularly revealing in settings that have multiple outputs and objectives, and in settings that depart from the traditional mode of practice. Moreover, information on resource allocations can actually help department chiefs and Health Center administration define objectives and assign or reassign priorities. Finally, time study data can be used to detect dissonance among providers or between providers and administration concerning priorities of multiple objectives.

If time study data are to serve as a management tool, department chiefs and Health Center administration must understand the data and be committed to their collection. Potential users should be involved in the design and implementation of time studies, should fill in time study forms themselves and should monitor time studies for the rest of the staff. Regular feedback of the data to all providers and discussion of its im-

310

TABLE 4. AVERAGE TIME DISTRIBUTION OF PRACTITIONERS

| Department | Patient Care | | | Non-Patient Care | | | | | | % Productive Worktime Available (1+2) (3) | % Total Administration (4) | % Lunch Vacation, etc. (5) |
	% Direct Patient Care	% Indirect Patient Care	% Total Patient Care (1)	% Community Outreach (Prevention)	% Self Education	% Training Others	% Receipt Supervision	% Research	% Total Non-Patient Care (2)			
Pediatrics	51	7	58	0.3	8	5			13	72	6	22
Internal Medicine	60	12	72		2	3			5	77	4	19
Nursing	36	16	52	4	2	1	2		9	60	14	26
Nutrition	45	13	58	4	2	8	1.5	.5	16	73	13	14
Community Mental Health	32	12	44	6	7	4	1	3	21	65	14	21
Psychiatry	40	10	50	1.5	10	4			16	66	8	26
Psychology	30	12	42	7	6	5	2	4	24	66	15	19
Social Services	35	22	57	2	1.5	2.5	9		15	72	8	20
Social Work	41	25	66	2	1	1	2		6	72	8	20
Trainees	26	20	46	1	2	4	18		25	71	9	20

Sources: Time Study Reports of Evaluation Unit of the Bunker Hill Health Center.

plications are important. Only then can the data become an information base for communication about manpower resource allocations and the pursuit of objectives.

Average time distributions for the study year (Table 4) reflect interdepartmental differences in percentages of productive work time available and in time allocations to patient care and non-patient care activities. The percentage of productive time available was computed by subtracting the percentage of administration time (column 4) and of "off" time (column 5) from total time on the job. It varies between departments from 60 per cent to 77 per cent of total time. The percentage of time in patient care ranges from 44 per cent to 72 per cent and the percentage of time in non-patient care ranges from 5 per cent to 21 per cent of total time on the job.

Time study data can be useful when a department or Health Center has not defined and ranked objectives. Using time study data, an implicit set of priorities can be translated into an explicit set of objectives. For example, before implementation of time studies the chief of Community Mental Health was asked to specify the desired professional time allocation. He specified that all time, other than administration and "off" time, should be directed to patient care. Subsequent feedback of time study data indicated that Community Mental Health, in fact, allocated 21 per cent of time to non-patient care activities and only 44 per cent to patient care. Documentation of actual time allocations and visit volumes stimulated this department to think about goals and reexamine the earlier specification of optimal time distribution. Even if total productive work-time were allocated to patient care this department would handle small numbers of patients. Logically this department began to devote a growing share of manpower inputs to non-patient care activities, emphasizing preventive activities in the community.

If departments of a Health Center have explicitly formulated objectives, time study data can perform three functions; (1) they can indicate discrepancies between actual and intended

312

resource allocations, (2) they may suggest reasons for misallocations and (3) if steps are taken to shift resource allocations, these steps can be evaluated with subsequent time studies. In Nutrition, for example, objectives had been determined, and we observed the following sequence of events. Prospectively, the chief defined the intended resource allocation as follows: fifty per cent in patient care, twenty per cent prevention and training, five per cent in research and the remainder in administration and "off" time. After feedback of time study data permitted comparison of actual with intended resource allocations (Table 4) discrepancies became apparent. The comparison of actual with intended performance stimulated refinement of desired time allocations in favor of enhanced non-patient care effort.

A third use of time study data can be to suggest reallocations in patient care and non-patient care activities between different departments. For example, is it desirable that all departments engage in preventive activities in the community or are some departments more suited for this than others? However, before the tool can be applied to this type of decision-making, additional information is required on alternative divisions of labor, their relative costs and relative effectiveness. Clearly, time study data relate only to inputs. They tell nothing about outputs or about attainment of objectives. Therefore, time study data should first be combined with cost-effectiveness measures and ultimately with outcome and impact evaluations.

Allocation of Departmental Costs between Patient and Non-Patient Care Effort

The methodology presented in this paper enables management to separate the cost of non-patient care activities from the cost of patient visits. Time study data were used to separate patient care from non-patient care activities. Each department's total costs were subdivided based on departmental time distributions. For example, Community Mental Health spent six per cent of total provider time on community outreach, and thus six per cent of the yearly departmental budget was allocated as costs of community outreach. Overhead costs were similarly apportioned between each department's patient visit costs and non-patient care costs.

This allocation method facilitated computation of two sets of average visit costs for each department based on two different departmental cost totals (Table 5): the average unadjusted visit cost (column 1) based on total departmental costs divided by yearly visit volumes; and the adjusted or "pure" visit cost (column 2), computed by subtracting the costs of non-patient care activities from departmental totals before dividing by yearly visit volumes.

A further variable affecting visit costs is the cost of ancillary services such as radiology, laboratory and nursing support services, which had been prorated between nursing and medical departments according to the share each had of total visits produced by these departments. Another variable, the cost of patient care services delivered in schools and in the community, had likewise been allocated to nursing and medical departments.[15] By identifying and separating these activities, the distributions of visit cost components could be made comparable between departments (Figure 3). A second adjustment of visit costs was presented (column 5, Table 5), this one exclusive of ancillary service costs.

It can thus be seen that visit costs vary between departments for a variety of reasons. These may include heterogeneity among visits produced by different departments, interdepartmental differences in patient care/non-patient care mix, in visit volumes of providers, in visit lengths, in resource mix utilized and in input prices. For purposes of cost control, it is important to isolate the different reasons for cost variation. By separating the extent to which different departments engage in non-patient care activities and the utilization of ancillary services, departmental costs can be made more comparable.

All departments at the Health Center have multiple objectives and visits represent only one of several outputs. To make

314

TABLE 5. AVERAGE YEARLY VISIT COSTS INCLUSIVE AND EXCLUSIVE OF NON-PATIENT CARE COSTS AND AD-
JUSTED ANCILLARY COSTS

Department	Average Unadjusted Visit Costs (1)	Average Adjusted or "Pure" Visit Costs (2)	Differential between 1 and 2 (3)	Non-Patient Care Cost as a Per Cent of Average Unadjusted Visit Cost (Column 1/Column 3) (4)	Average Adjusted Visit Costs Exclusive of Ancillary Costs (5)
Pediatrics	$19.21	$17.16	$ 2.05	10%	$ 9.54
Internal Medicine	22.55	21.62	.93	4%	13.99
Nursing	20.32	19.42	.90	4%	11.76
Nutrition	11.45	9.16	2.29	20%	9.16
Community Mental Health	32.81	23.06	9.75	30%	23.06
Psychiatry	27.51	21.71	5.80	21%	21.71
Psychology	35.91	24.45	11.46	32%	24.45
Social Services	28.84	23.39	5.45	19%	23.39
Social Work	26.74	24.52	2.22	8%	24.52
Trainees	33.14	21.47	11.67	35%	21.47

Sources: Calculations provided by Evaluation Unit for this study.

315

interdepartmental visit cost comparisons that are meaningful it is essential to determine and segregate the cost of each output or activity produced by departments. Average unadjusted visit costs (column 1) are derived by allocating all departmental costs as visit costs. By adjusting the figures (column 1) for the cost of non-patient care activities in each department one can compare "pure" visit costs rather than costs of heterogeneous output bundles. Average adjusted or "pure" visit costs (column 2) show notably smaller variation between visit costs of medical and nonmedical departments. However, when the "pure" visit costs of medical and nursing departments are further deflated to eliminate the costs of ancillary services (column 5), cost differences between medical and nonmedical departments widen once more. Other factors that enter into cost variation between departments can be separated out with the above methodology, but are omitted from this discussion.

The distinction between unadjusted and "pure" visit costs has particular relevance to methods of financing the Health Center. Most departments are not separately funded for non-patient care activities; inasmuch as patient visits now constitute the primary fee-generating output of the Health Center it may be argued that all costs should be loaded on to visit costs. However, one could equally argue that the training of social workers or sex education in the schools should be financed with education rather than with health care dollars and that patient populations should not be burdened with the cost of non-patient care activities. When these issues are raised and the need to seek alternative sources of financing becomes critical, the cost of non-patient care activities will become an important piece of information.[16]

Department chiefs and Health Center administration can use these cost data to assess whether, given their costs, non-patient care activities should receive greater or lesser emphasis. The figures also enable management to develop patient fees based on "pure" visit costs.[17] Finally, when more is known about end results of patient care, training of health professionals and com-

316

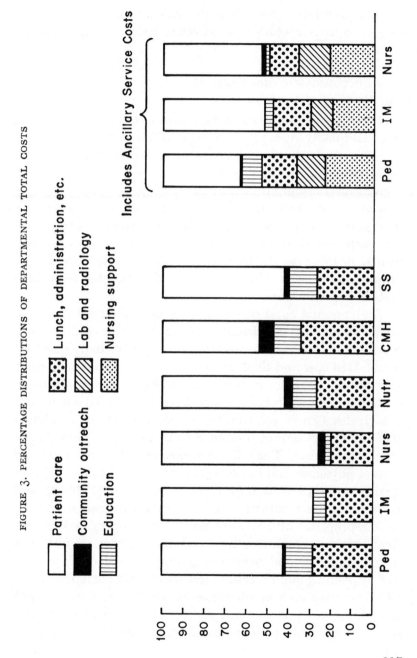

FIGURE 3. PERCENTAGE DISTRIBUTIONS OF DEPARTMENTAL TOTAL COSTS

317

munity preventive effort, cost-effectiveness studies can be conducted to suggest which types of effort yield the largest pay off per dollar.

Cost Effectiveness of Manpower Mix and Resource Allocations

A cost-effectiveness framework allows one to analyze the cost of equal quality visits produced with different manpower mixes or alternative output mixes produced with present staff size and composition. In the first approach emphasis is on maintaining a given level of output of constant quality, but producing that output at the lowest possible cost. Here one modifies the mix of inputs, moving toward least-cost combinations. The second approach represents the other side of the coin, output maximization. In this case, the focus is on achieving either the largest output or the most preferred output mix possible with fixed costs and given inputs.

The potential effect of variation in manpower mix can best be illustrated by the departments of medicine and nursing. Nurse practitioners were already working in Pediatrics and Internal Medicine and their utilization, cost and contribution to visit volume were documented during the study year. In terms of manpower resources and costs, nursing is the largest unit at the Health Center constituting 33 per cent of the combined staff and 30 per cent of combined costs, while providing 18 per cent of total visits. Time distributions, capacity utilization and costs of physicians and nurses were compared (Table 6). Nurses spent relatively less time in direct patient care (Table 4) and more in indirect patient care and administration, suggesting an inappropriate utilization of nurse practitioners. Indirect patient care and administrative functions include: clerical tasks such as ordering and maintaining supplies and equipment as well as phoning and processing test results and medical records; technical tasks such as administering diagnostic tests, medical procedures and preparations; and community health aid tasks such as prevention, patient education, case finding and patient

318

TABLE 6. COMPARISON BETWEEN NURSING AND MEDICAL DEPARTMENTS

	Nursing	Pediatrics	Internal Medicine
Per cent of productive time available	60	72	77
Per cent of time in direct patient care	36	51	60
Per cent of time in non-patient care	9	13	5
Visits per man day	5.6*	16.1	12.6
Visit duration (minutes)	30.7	18.7	25.2
Capacity utilization	51%*	81%	84%
Unadjusted average cost per visit	$20.32	$19.21	$22.55

* Based on 4.5 nurses.

follow-up. Some of these tasks can and should be performed by personnel with lower skill levels.

Nurse practitioners' capacity for patient care was estimated jointly by doctors, nurses and the evaluation staff. The judgment of doctors was weighted heavily in determining optimal workloads for nurse practitioners because doctors function as their teachers and preceptors and had given thought to performance goals. Because nurses at the Health Center have multiple functions including support functions for doctors, community health services and autonomous clinic patient care, only half of total yearly nursing days were assumed to be available for nurse practitioning. On the average, each of the 4.5 nurse practitioners generated 5.6 visits per day (compared to an optimal workload of 14 visits per day) and the rate of capacity utilization was 51 per cent. Workload indices and capacity utilization rates for nurses are based on the single output measure of visits, and it is important to suggest that were other output measures available, such as community patient care or physicians' support functions, utilization of nurses might be viewed in a different light. Given the measures we have, one cannot clearly distinguish whether nurses are underutilized (e.g., per cent of productive time available is too low), whether nursing output is undermeasured or whether nurses are inap-

319

propriately utilized by being channeled too frequently into non-output-producing tasks.

Although an hour of nursing time is less costly than an hour of physician time, the unadjusted average cost per nursing visit it slightly higher than that of the pediatric visit and slightly lower than the internal medicine visit (Table 6). The "pure" visit cost figures (Table 5) similarly show that nursing costs lie between those of Pediatrics and Internal Medicine. The relatively long duration of nurse visits and small number of visits per nurse day explain why the cost of nurse visits is not below that of physician visits.

All nurses presently employed at the Health Center are graduates of a Nurse Practitioner Training Program designed specifically to expand the role of nurses in the delivery of direct patient care. This presents an added dimension to the picture. A special investment was made in these nurses and if, subsequent to their training, they function as nurse practitioners 35 per cent of each workday (5.6 visits × 30.7 minutes = 172 minutes per day) the goals of the training program are realized only to a limited extent.

Of the total visits provided by 2.5 pediatricians, 2.5 internists and 4.5 nurse practitioners, only 25 per cent are nursing visits. It is reasonable to argue that, given the size of the present nursing staff, nurses should provide a larger share of total medical visits, and that visits should be transferred from doctors to nurses on a larger scale than is presently occurring. If there are insufficient visits of the types that nurses are qualified to handle, nurses will continue to be underutilized until visit volumes expand or until the nursing staff is reduced.

What are the prospects that increased utilization of nurse practitioners in direct patient care will reduce average visit costs or curtail rising average costs? The share of nursing visits can increase if doctors transfer cases from current patient loads, visit loads show substantial growth or the number of doctors is reduced. Any of these three changes would create opportunities for substitution of a lower for a higher priced manpower input.

320

However, only the latter two options, growth in visit volumes or reduction of physician staff, can have a cost-curtailing effect, inasmuch as a simple trade off between higher capacity utilization of nurses for lower capacity utilization of doctors will not accomplish the desired objective. If no increase in visit volumes were to occur a smaller nursing staff could reduce total nursing costs and average visit costs, but the resulting manpower mix would be more doctor intensive and therefore not represent a least-cost input combination.

The second type of cost-effectiveness question concerns maximization of output or output mix with staff held fixed in size and composition. Although output at the Health Center consists of multiple products, these may or may not constitute the best output mix relative to needs and priorities in the community. Given the present output mix, what information is available regarding output effectiveness and how can future resource allocation decisions be guided toward an optimal output mix? Outcome studies lie beyond the scope of this evaluation project but the data and analyses underscore the need for outcome evaluations.

Appropriateness of output mix has two facets: patient care versus non-patient care and the mix of non-patient care services. In reference to patient care versus non-patient care, a departmental division of labor has been established at the Health Center. Pediatrics, Internal Medicine and Nutrition make contributions to the total visit volume proportionately larger than the size of their staff; the reverse is true of Community Mental Health, Social Services and Nursing (column 5, Table 1). There is no reason to question the logic underlying this division of labor, but might or should it be extended? Medical providers spend most of their time on patient care services and produce visits in reasonably large volumes and at relatively low costs, but Mental Health and Social Service providers, who allocate somewhat more time to non-patient care services, are producing visits at low volumes and high costs. Given the style of practice presently used in these departments, the potential for growth

321

in visit volumes and reduction in visit costs is very limited, even if total productive staff time were allocated to patient care. Our data pose the question whether Mental Health and Social Service providers should allocate larger portions of time to non-patient care activities, thus increasing the volume of preventive services provided in the community. Information on outcomes, when available, can help determine the extent to which these departments should adopt the community health approach as a trade off for the individual patient care approach. It is crucial, therefore, that assessment of program effectiveness and exploration of alternative styles of practice be pursued as tasks of high priority.

The question of mix of non-patient care services is equally important, particularly when different kinds of services within this category carry benefits to different groups of people. This point is illustrated by the training program in the department of Social Services. The department is staffed with four social workers and three and one quarter trainees, and funded with traineeships from the federal government. Separate performance measures for social workers and trainees (Tables 1–5) indicate that trainees lower the departmental average for per cent of productive worktime available, per cent of time in direct patient care, visits per man day and rate of capacity utilization. The presence of trainees also raises the unadjusted average visit cost for the department. Furthermore, about 12 per cent of the 15 per cent staff time allocated to non-patient care effort is devoted to the traineeship program.

The distribution of costs and benefits of non-patient care activity is pertinent to the question of preferred mix of non-patient care effort in this department. Five overlapping groups of people are involved: society at large, the Health Center, the social workers, the patients who come to the Health Center and the Charlestown community. Society shares in the costs and benefits through subsidizing the trainees and through future services of trained social workers. The Health Center benefits by collecting fees for trainees' visits without sharing the direct cost of the trainees. (Indirectly, some costs will be incurred such as the cost of staff time, facilities and overhead.) The social workers do not incur costs, but may receive psychic benefits such as satisfaction derived from training others and enhanced prestige of the department. Last, the patients and the Charlestown community do not pay for the training program but may incur opportunity costs. The community's opportunity costs are relevant only if, in the absence of trainees, the mix of services would be different and more specifically related to needs in the community. There is no question about the desirability of training opportunities and investments to assure a future supply of social workers. The issue in question pertains to respective trade-offs and to explicit consideration of trade-offs relative to a set of priorities.

SUMMARY AND DISCUSSION

This paper has described the design of an information system and the gathering of data for evaluating manpower utilization. The purpose of the study was twofold: to produce information describing how manpower is utilized and to explore *potential* uses of the data as tools for decision-making and as instruments for achieving change. The study concentrated on procedures for initiating the goal setting process, developing performance measures, comparing actual performance to performance criteria and examining alternative courses of action. Efforts were made to involve health center administration, department chiefs and, at times, the total staff in the various stages of this process.

This methodology lends itself to further refinement and extension in a number of directions. Its most obvious shortcoming is the use of visits as the only output measure. Visits were used because they are discretely measurable output units and more easily defined and recorded than the individual services provided during visits. Nevertheless, the omission of outputs that are difficult to quantify is a serious limitation and it would have been desirable to measure the service content of visits as well as the number and kinds of health problems alleviated. Moreover, other activities such as prevention and patient education not only fail to produce visits but aim to reduce visit volumes of the Health Center. The approach taken her focused on inputs into these activities, but it is even more important to assess their contribution to health in the community. The task of developing output measures for non-patient care activities and improved output measures for patient care, though far from simple, is one that should be pursued with high priority.

The methodology concentrated on manpower utilization in a more or less static situation and focused on individual providers in separate departments. It also has potential for testing innovative uses of manpower by concentrating on interaction and collaboration of different types of providers and by assessing joint outputs and effectiveness of multiprovider care taking units or teams. Further studies should be based on before and after comparisons or on comparison between innovative and traditional models of health manpower utilization in experimental settings. It would also be desirable if this study's emphasis on process could be combined with outcome evaluation in future studies.

Furthermore, the methodology could be broadened and strengthened through application to a number of health care settings, preferably with varying manpower mixes and different patterns of manpower resource utilization. This is likely to provide further insight on the kinds of organizational structures and incentive patterns that either facilitate or impede effective manpower utilization.

An information system designed to expose problems is necessary, but not sufficient for bringing about improvements. It provides the technology but not the climate for implementation of change. Further prerequisites may include incentives for performance improvement, pressures for financial self-sufficiency and community participation in the planning process. Given that the Health Center is confronted with future demands and challenges, it is equipped to examine its options and to plan for a useful response.

REFERENCES

[1] Stimson, D. H. and Stimson, R. H., Operations Research and Systems Analysis in Hospital Administration, working paper No. 147, Berkeley, California, Institute of Urban and Regional Development, April 1971.

[2] Griffith, J. R., QUANTITATIVE TECHNIQUES FOR HOSPITAL MANAGEMENT AND CONTROL, in press.

[3] Flagle, C. D. and Young, J. P. The Applications of Operations Research and Industrial Engineering to Problems of Health Services, Hospitals and Public Health, *Journal of Industrial Engineering*, 17, 609–614, November, 1966.

[4] Smalley, H. E. and Freeman, J. R., HOSPITAL INDUSTRIAL ENGINEERING, New York, 1966.

[5] Number of registrants exceeds the number of active users of the Health Center inasmuch as registrants are entitled, but not financially or otherwise committed, to use Bunker Hill Health Center as the sole source of primary health services. Conversion of the registrant file into "active" registrants or Health Center users will be discussed by Robert L. Robertson, Gordon T. Moore and Irene Butter in their forthcoming paper on "Costs and Financing Policies at a Neighborhood Health Center."

[6] These are not outputs in a final sense, but rather intermediate output measures.

[7] Reder, M. W., Some problems in the Measurement of Productivity in the Medical Care Industry, in Fuchs, V. R. (Editor), PRODUCTION AND PRODUCTIVITY IN THE SERVICE INDUSTRIES, New York, National Bureau of Economic Research, 1969.

[8] Kovner, J. W., Measurement of Outpatient Office Visit Services, *Health Services Research*, 4, 112–127, Summer, 1969.

[9] However, these preliminary estimates imply that visits cannot be shortened when, in fact, the visit length is a function of workload.

[10] Bergman, A. B., Dassel, S. W. and Wedgwood, R. J., Time-Motion Study of Practicing Pediatricians, *Pediatrics*, 38, 254–263, August, 1960.

[11] Patterson, P. K. and Bergman, A. B., Time-Motion Study of Six Pediatric Office Assistants, *New England Journal of Medicine*, 280, 771–774, October 2, 1969.

[12] Yankauer, A., Connelly, J. P. and Feldman, F., Pediatric Practice in the United States, *Pediatrics*, March, 1970, Supplement.

[13] Donaldson, M. C. and London, C. D., Time Study of Doctors and Nurses at Two Swedish Health Centers: Swedish Health Center Doctors and Nurses, *Medical Care*, 9, 457–467, December, 1971.

325

[14] Chase, J. S. and Craig, W. R., Time and Motion Study of General Practice, unpublished, Harvard Medical School, January, 1969.

[15] More specifically, 32 per cent of total nursing time spent both at the Health Center and in the community represents patient care time, but could not be attributed to visit-specific activities. The cost of this share of nursing time was divided equally between nursing and medical visits because the activities in question are more closely related to patient care than to non-patient care functions.

[16] This issue will be discussed in more detail in a forthcoming paper by Robert L. Robertson, Gordon T. Moore and Irene Butter.

[17] See the forthcoming paper by Robertson, Moore and Butter.

ACKNOWLEDGMENTS

This investigation was supported in part by Public Health Service research grant number HF00472 from the National Center for Health Services Research and Development, Health Services and Mental Health Administration, awarded to the Harvard Center for Community Health and Medical Care, with which the authors were associated during several phases of the study. The authors acknowledge with appreciation the encouragement and constructive advice from Paul M. Densen during all phases of the study. They are also grateful to Dr. John P. Connelly, Executive Director of the Bunker Hill Health Center, for his continuous cooperation, to the staff of the Health Center for providing needed information, and to Regina Herzlinger for successfully implementing the data system at the Health Center. The authors also wish to thank Rashi Fein for many helpful comments and suggestions. Errors, omissions and interpretations are the sole responsibility of the authors.

THE SOCIAL CONTROL OF MEDICAL PRACTICE
Licensure Versus Output Monitoring

LAURENCE R. TANCREDI

AND

JOHN WOODS

The Report of the Carnegie Commission on Higher Education[1] is the most recent of a series of evaluations to highlight the acute shortage of medical manpower (doctors, dentists, nurses and so forth).[2] To meet the future needs of this country, the report strongly recommends that the number of medical school entrants should be increased from the present 9,000 to 15,300 by 1976, and to 16,400 by 1978. Such an increase should be accompanied by an average expansion of approximately 39–44 per cent in existing and developing schools by 1978. Also, the number of dental school entrants should be increased to at least 5,000 by 1976, and to 5,400 by 1980.[3]

More critical for the present, the Commission recommends that university health science centers consider the development of programs to train physician's and dentist's assistants.[4] For although the physician shortage is certainly one of the factors responsible for the crisis in the provision of medical care, it is important to recognize that at least part of the shortage may be functional, that is, attributable to the extraordinarily inefficient manner in which health manpower resources are currently being employed. One commentator has gone so far as to suggest that the major problem today is not the paucity of physicians but rather the improper use of health manpower.[5] It is becoming more apparent that there must be a dramatic change in the

327

organization of health care systems to free the doctor from many tasks that can be just as effectively performed by other types of health personnel.[6]

One of the major impediments both to the optimal utilization of existing categories of health personnel and to the development of new categories of auxiliary workers, is the body of state professional licensure laws.[7] Once the Supreme Court, in the late nineteenth century, had removed the laissez-faire doctrine of freedom of contract from the area of health care, medical practice acts were passed in all the states.[8] When written, these laws served as a means of regulating the human input into the health care delivery system by protecting the public from incompetent and unethical practitioners. The statutory mechanism of the practice acts granted a duly licensed physician an unlimited scope in the practice of medicine, and created a general prohibition on the practice of medicine by any other individual. Gradually, as other categories of medical professionals emerged, organized and exerted leverage upon the legislative process, a series of limited, narrowly defined scopes of practice were eked out of the general prohibition. As each new category took on the status and prestige of licensure, it in turn resisted the effort to be licensed of new groups that threatened to encroach upon its own perimeter of practice.[9]

It is not surprising that this mechanism has proved to be rigidly unresponsive to the sweeping technologic advances in medical care and to the huge increase in demand for health services resulting from the population explosion and societal recognition that adequate health care (subsidized by the state if necessary) is a right of every citizen.[10] What is more, the practice acts have not accomplished what they were originally intended to do—that is, maintain a minimum standard of practitioner competence. Nowhere in the statutes governing physicians, nurses and other professionals are there provisions requiring the licensee to submit the periodic re-examination or to a program of continuing education in his specialty as a condition for maintaining licensure.[11]

328

The draftsmen of the statutes did not foresee the tremendous explosion in medical knowledge beginning in the 1930's and continuing into the present, which has since subjected many a medical technique to the possibility of rapid obsolescence. Today, the renewing of licensure is a rubber-stamp procedure.[12]

No one would question that the doctor shortage could at least be mitigated by delegating those routine tasks traditionally reserved for the physician to qualified persons lower in the health care hierarchy. However, were the patient to sustain an injury at the hands of a physician's substitute and elect to bring a lawsuit for damages, two legal doctrines may come into play that hardly favor either the physician or his assistant. The first is the respondeat superior ("let the master respond") doctrine, which allows the patient to recover from the physician for the injurious actions of his negligent employee. The second is the "negligence per se" rule, which provides that mere violation of the terms of the statute is an inference of negligence or is conclusive on the issue of negligence.[13]

The consequences of delegation are even more severe if the delegatee is unlicensed. Under the practice acts, the delegatee would be criminally liable for the unlicensed practice of medicine and the professional could be prosecuted for aiding and abetting the unlicensed practice of medicine.[14] In a civil suit, of course, the unlicensed delegatee could not rely upon whatever presumption of competence a licensed worker might enjoy by virtue of his occupation's having been recognized by the legislature.

The problem of delegation is further complicated by the fact that the statutory language delineating a particular profession or occupation's scope of practice does not provide the physician with a "bright-line" distinction between what is within a subordinate's scope of practice and what is without. It is immensely difficult to apply the vaguely worded statutory terms of the various scopes of practice to complex modern-day treatment procedures that have been shaped by rapid technologic advances unforeseen at the time the statutes were enacted.

329

Thus, the uncertainty of the statutory language and the ever-present threat of civil, if not criminal, liability combine to produce a detrimental chilling effect upon any physician inclined to reallocate tasks among old and new categories of medical personnel in furtherance of the social policy of expanded medical care.[15]

Another feature of the practice acts that impedes the flexible utilization of manpower is commonly referred to as vertical (career) immobility.[16] Each licensed category of health personnel has its own set of formal educational requirements. The unlicensed aspirant, or the already-licensed worker wishing to move up to a more responsible position, may well find that his own education or experience is deemed inadequate or irrelevant to the new position, and that therefore he must undertake a costly and time-consuming formal educational program to qualify. The mechanism of the present state licensure laws also results in what is commonly referred to as horizontal (career) immobility,[17] or the power of one state medical board to refuse recognition of another state's license. A physician who has received a license in one state may not be permitted to practice medicine in an adjoining state.[18] Of course, to some extent 48 states provide some mechanism for recognition, be it through endorsement of another state's licenses (based on equivalent standards) or reciprocity (equivalence plus reciprocal recognition by both states). Yet, as shown by the Health Manpower Report, in 16 of the states all endorsements of licenses are under the control of the licensing board at its discretion, and only eight states endorse all the licenses of all other jurisdictions.

The impact of restrictions upon recognition of other states' licenses affects not only the extent of territorial coverage of the physician, but also the extent of authority for delegation of responsibilities. Consequently, a physician's assistant would likewise be prevented from providing complete medical coverage to a rural area spanning state boundaries. And, despite intense pressures for change because of the shortage of physicians, little evidence is found of significant modifications of recognition

330

policies, although there appears to be some liberalization of the reciprocity requirement as shown by the increasing number of states that have granted discretionary authority to licensing agencies for endorsing licenses of nonreciprocating states.[19]

Of the proposed alternatives to the practice acts in their present form, one planning model has been advanced that addresses itself specifically to the shortcomings of the state mandatory licensure system recounted above. That model, first put forth by Nathan Hershey[20] and later modified by Dan McAdams[21] would give state institutional licensing bodies the authority to establish job descriptions for various positions in the health care institution. The job descriptions would be broadly defined so as to provide the institutions with some flexibility for employing individuals in accordance with their self-perceived manpower needs.

To the extent that the Hershey model shifts the regulatory focus from the individual practitioner in the abstract to the individual in the context of his institutional function, it complements two other recent trends in the reorganization of the health care delivery system: (1) the growing tendency of medical care institutions to have attributed to them characteristics of responsibility and liability that have traditionally been ascribed to the individual practitioner; and (2) the move toward national standards of care, as indicated by recent malpractice case decisions and by bills currently before Congress proposing national programs of health care. Both warrant separate examination to understand the impetus they provide for a radical alteration of present licensure laws.

Despite its compatibility with these important trends in the organization of health care, the Hershey model should not be viewed as more than an interim measure. To appreciate why this is so, it is helpful to think in terms of "evolutionary stages" of health manpower regulation, defined and differentiated in terms of the regulatory mode peculiar to each stage. Though it has been 70-odd years since the demise of the freedom of contract doctrine, manpower regulation cannot be said to have

331

passed beyond its first evolutionary stage. That stage is characterized by its reliance on the screening of human *inputs* into the health care delivery system as the sole means of maintaining quality control in the practice of the healing arts. The Hershey model perpetuates this traditional reliance on input regulation; it does not, therefore, capitalize upon the results of recent research involving the entirely different idea of quality control that, when perfected, will enable manpower regulation to move into its second evolutionary stage. With the help of applied computer techniques, medical scientists will be able to quantify what were formerly crude and unsystematized articulations of treatment outcomes (outputs). Such a method of quality control portends radical reorderings not only in the manpower regime but also throughout the health care system of which it is a component. Because of its emphasis on the institutional context, the Hershey model provides an excellent bridge between the first and second evolutionary stages of manpower regulation. The point that needs to be stressed about the Hershey model—particularly in light of the fact that aspects of it have been included in the comprehensive health care bills now before Congress—is that it is transitional, no more and no less. Truly comprehensive and long-range planning for this nation's health needs must recognize the benefits to be derived in terms of flexibility from the output-measurement method of quality control.

ALTERNATIVE MODELS

Because of the inadequacies of the present licensure system, the following proposals have been suggested for reforming it:

1. Modifying existing personnel licensure laws to provide for increased task delegation and periodic re-examination of health personnel.
2. Establishing a national qualifying board to set national standards, administer national examinations and thereby eliminate the present "chaos of state's rights."[22]

3. Abolishing personnel licensure for a scheme of institutional licensing.

The first recommendation, that of strengthening existing state laws, can be achieved through exemption clauses that "loosen up" requirements for delegation of responsibility by the physician, and provisions that require re-examination and continuing education. This will result at best in mitigating the onerous aspects of respondeat superior on the full utilization of medical manpower, and in an improvement of consumer protection, but will fail to resolve other critical restrictive features of mandatory licensure—i.e., rigid categorization of personnel, and vertical and horizontal immobility.

The second proposal seems much more in keeping with contemporary trends toward national standards of care.[23] Besides improving the protection of the patient against incompetent care, a national scheme would eliminate the problems of horizontal immobility that are inherent in individual state licensure. However, it is unlikely that a national licensure of personnel per se will resolve the restrictive effects of rigid categorization of personnel, vertical immobility and physician liability under the respondeat superior doctrine. Therefore, its overall effect would probably be to hinder the optimal utilization of health manpower.

The last recommendation, that of merging the two kinds of licensing—personnel and institutional—into one system, developed out of an awareness of the incompatibility of personnel patterns established by licensing legislation and those most advantageous to the institutions for providing patient care. Nathan Hershey worked out the first principal model for this new type of licensing. In his proposal, Hershey recommends that health services institutions be invested with the responsibility for regulating health care within limits determined by a state institutional licensing agency. This agency would be empowered to establish in broad terms with the advice of health care experts, "job descriptions, including required education and work experience for specific hospital positions."[24]

The Hershey proposal is an improvement over the existing system of licensure for two reasons. First, more flexibility is provided for manpower innovation. Laws are difficult, if not impossible, to change at a rate consistent with necessary alterations in the use of health personnel. Here an agency can define the job descriptions of the institutional personnel and more easily modify the descriptions to meet new institutional needs. It has been suggested that the Hershey proposal would invest the institution with the role of "doer" in determining the distribution and quality of health care.[25] Although the institution enjoys a decidedly more active role in this system, nevertheless, it can hardly be equated with that of a "doer" for the state institutional licensing agency actually establishes the job descriptions and required qualifications with which the institution must comply.

Second, the possibility exists for circumventing the liability to physicians resulting from respondeat superior. Inasmuch as the health care institution is given major responsibility for deciding which personnel will perform which functions, it would appear reasonable to hold the institution responsible for the negligent acts of its employees. In fact, a natural consequence of this proposal might be the development of an institution-based compensation mechanism for patients injured while being treated by the institution. Such a scheme would operate in much the same manner as a workmen's compensation system, in which the negligence of the institution need not be established because specific injuries are compensated for in accordance with fixed payment schedules.[26]

By the same token, the following important problems remain unresolved:

1. Horizontal immobility: according to Hershey institutional licensure would remain a state function. In fact, because each state institutional licensing agency will establish its own pattern of job descriptions, the proposal actually compounds the legal difficulties of moving across state boundaries.

2. Consumer protection: no provision is suggested that would counteract the educational obsolescence that is not prevented by the existing state laws, unless one can assume that the institution as employer will be in a position to act against individual incompetency. Even so, the standards of care would most likely be defined on a state-by-state rather than on a nationwide basis.

3. Despite the ease of altering job descriptions, the proposal may actually continue the problem of vertical immobility engendered by the licensure laws, unless the interrelation between the "institution" and the educational system were such as to facilitate personnel in obtaining necessary training for increasing levels of responsibility within the institution.

Recognizing some of the unresolved issues in the Hershey proposal, Dan McAdams made a major modification while retaining the basic structure of institutional licensure.[27] He suggested employing a private agency, such as the Joint Commission on Accreditation of Hospitals (JCAH), to assume the role (establishing job descriptions including required education and work experience) Hershey gave to the "state institutional licensing bodies." This private agency, representing all health occupations, would function in effect as a national qualifying mechanism, and thereby provide for the horizontal mobility that is the primary advantage of a national licensure code.[28] In addition, such an agency would assure the competency of practitioners by continually reviewing the credentials of participating health care personnel.[29] Perhaps the main concern McAdams has with his recommendation is that such an institutionally based (private) agency as JCAH would not guarantee the competence of practitioners who do not operate within an institutional setting.[30] This could be remedied if some mechanism were constructed that would essentially tie all health personnel into an institutional structure.[31]

The Hershey-McAdams institutional framework for licensure

seems to be the most promising for meeting present health needs. As will be explored in the next section, it will be possible in the near future to improve upon the institutional paradigm with a system that reflects the rapidly developing technology in the monitoring of the output of health care as a method of quality control.

However, before assessing the impact of this development, considering the close association of the Hershey-McAdams proposals with the emerging trends toward the institutionalization of liability, and the establishment of national standards of care, it would be appropriate to examine these trends.

TWO CONVERGENT TRENDS IN THE ORGANIZATION OF THE HEALTH CARE SYSTEM

Institutionalization of Liability[32]

The trend toward the institutionalization of liability is most evident in several recent court cases. In the past most state courts drew a distinction between medical and administrative acts as a means for determining hospital liability. The rationale for this differentiation is twofold: that a hospital functioning as a corporation could not practice medicine in the traditional sense, and that the trained professional was an independent contractor and not "controlled" by anyone.[33] Therefore, a hospital could not be held derivatively responsible for the negligent acts of its professional employees, though it could be so held for "administrative negligence."[34]

But, the medical-administrative dichotomy is being increasingly ignored.[35] The hospital is becoming more and more liable[36] either under the theory of corporate negligence (a result of selecting or retaining incompetent employees; negligently maintaining its equipment and buildings; or for furnishing defective equipment or supplies),[37] or that of vicarious liability for the acts of its individual employees (physicians, nurses). With regard to the former, the Darling case[38] in 1965 extended considerably the scope of corporate negligence by holding the hospital liable for violation of duties it owes to the

336

patient.[39] In this now-famous case an 18-year old male was treated for a fractured leg at the emergency ward of a community hospital. A general practitioner working in the emergency ward treated the patient by applying traction and placing his leg in a cast. After a few days passed the patient complained frequently of severe pain (caused by circulatory impairment from compression) and the odor of decayed tissue was observed. But necessary attention was delayed until amputation of the leg was required.

Legal action was brought against the hospital;[40] and, although the general practitioner was not employed by the hospital, the institution nevertheless was found liable for allowing an unqualified doctor to perform orthopedic surgery, and for not requiring consultation or review of treatment. Interestingly, the court permitted the application of standards on consultation requirements in the regulations of the state hospital licensing agency, in the hospital's own bylaws, and in the private standards of expected care promulgated by the Joint Commission on Accreditation of Hospitals.[41] But, the most important feature of this case is the redefinition of the role of the institution in the practice of medicine. The court was not suggesting that the hospital must actually control the medical practice of the physician.[42] Instead, the decision emphasizes the joint responsibilities of physician and institution for the standards of patient care, and thus refutes the antiquated notion that a corporation cannot practice medicine.[43] Subsequent decisions on corporate negligence have generally followed the holdings in the Darling case, and have often added innuendoes of interpretation. For example, in Fiorentino v. Wenger, the New York Appellate Court stated that an institution may be liable if the administration knows, or should know that a physician is departing from acceptable modes of care.[44]

The second type of liability that is increasingly attributed to the hospital is vicarious liability under the doctrine of respondeat superior. This trend particularly demonstrates the shift away from the notion of the physician as "Captain-of-the-

337

Ship" toward that of the institutionalization of liability; and, concomitantly, an expanded interpretation of medical practice wherein the institution is viewed as the primary provider of care.[45] The case of French versus Fisher illustrates this new development.[46] In this case, a scrub nurse incorrectly counted the number of sponges following an abdominal operation on an infant. After a few days the child became critically ill, and it was necessary to operate and remove two-thirds of the child's small intestine because of the presence of a sponge. Under the traditional "Captain-of-the-Ship" doctrine, the surgeon would have been held liable for the nurse's negligence. However, the court abandoned this doctrine and found the hospital liable.

The shift of liability from the physician to the hospital involves another aspect of liability in addition to respondeat superior; i.e., the determination of accepted standards of care. Kapuschinsky versus U.S.[47] demonstrates the use of this determinant of liability, which has often been employed against physicians. In this case the government was found negligent for allowing an inexperienced Wave who had not been subjected to proper physical examination to come in "critical contact" with a premature baby. As a result the baby contracted staphylococcus infection of the hips, which caused residual injuries. The court ruled that it was no defense for the hospital to argue that the accepted standard of care is that prevailing within the community (the locality rule), and allowed a medical expert from outside the area to testify.

As the next section will explain, a similar move from the "locality" principle to national standards for physician practice has been operating the past several years.[48] The parallels between evaluations of standards of care expected of physicians and those of institutions, and the obvious transfer of respondeat superior from physician to institution are striking evidences of the institutionalization of medical liability.

National Standards of Care

Augmenting the impact of the move toward the institutionalization of liability on the development of an institutional framework of licensure, is an equally forceful trend toward the delineation of national standards of care. Perhaps the most significant manifestations of this trend are:

1. The development by the National Board of Medical Examiners of national examinations for determining the qualification of physicians to practice.

2. Recent court decisions involving medical malpractice that refute the traditional locality rule for acceptable standards of care.

3. Emerging proposals (bills) for a national program of health care.

Regarding the first of these manifestations, it is sufficent to say that these examinations are being accepted by virtually all the states in lieu of individual state qualifying examinations, and probably will eventually replace the state exams altogether.[49]

Recently several court cases involving medical malpractice have refuted the "locality rule" and advocated the application of national standards of physician care. One of the most important landmark cases is Brune versus Belinkoff,[50] which was decided in 1968. In this case a specialist in anesthesiology administered a high dosage of pontocaine as a spinal anesthetic to a pregnant woman. Many hours after the birth of her child the patient attempted to get out of bed, but because of numbness and weakness in her left leg she fell and injured herself. At the trial a specialist from Boston testified that the dosage of pontocaine administered was excessive, but the court charged the jury to apply the locality rule. The Supreme Court of Massachusetts, on the other hand, upheld the introduction of this testimony[51] stating that the proper standard is not whether the physician has exercised the level of care acceptable in the locality in which he practices, but rather that care and skill of the average qualified practitioner taking into account medical advances and available resources.[52]

339

The Brune versus Belinkoff case, and the line of cases that followed supporting this holding, are final breaks with the outmoded past.[53] But, from a more progressive viewpoint, they are also forerunners of a new trend that is attempting to define in a very broad sense a national concept of acceptable medical care.[54]

The last significant manifestation to be discussed is that of the current proposals for a national program of health care. These proposals are efforts to use specific payment methods to alter and expand the organization and delivery of health services. Two of these "bills"[55] in particular—"Health Securities Program" (S. 3: Kennedy Bill), and "National Health Insurance and Health Services Improvement Act of 1971" (S. 836: Javits Bill)—provide specifically for the implementation of "national standards" for health personnel. The "Health Securities Program" explicitly renders restrictive state licensure laws inoperative in determining the eligibility of otherwise qualified physicians and other health personnel for the program.[56] In addition, this bill provides for the establishment of national standards for participation of both individual and institutional providers of health services,[57] and authorizes the Health Security Board to set requirements for the continuing education of health personnel.[58]

The "Javits Bill" is similar to the "Kennedy Bill" in setting national standards, though it has no explicit provision to negate the state licensure laws. However, the "Javits Bill" does authorize the Secretary to prescribe requirements for participating physicians in the sections entitled as follows:

"A. Standards of continuing professional education

B. National minimum standards of licensure . . . [59]

C. Adherence to the standards for continuance in the program."[60]

In effect this authority circumvents the restrictions of the state licensure laws, and is not unlike that granted the Secretary in the Social Security Amendment of 1971 (Sec. 239, "Payments to Health Maintenance Organizations").[61] This provision invests the Secretary with the capability of defining national standards, but, unlike the "Javits Bill," it does not specify the requirements the Secretary can impose.[62]

It is quite likely that some national program of health will be enacted in the near future. Significant premonitory evidence of this is the recent passage of the Emergency Health Personnel Act of 1970.[63] This new law will expand the scope of activity of the Public Health Service by allowing health professionals (doctors, dentists, nurses) to enlist in the Service for the purpose of dispensing medical care in areas where demand is high, such as the rural areas and urban ghettos. Those participating in the Service will be paid on a salary basis by the federal government and be assigned at the discretion of the Secretary of Health, Education, and Welfare. In effect, this act is a major step toward the nationalization of the medical care system because it provides government involvement in direct health services to population groups long felt within the exclusive province of the private practice of medicine.[64]

All three of these signs of a shift toward national standards of care, along with those regarding changes in the role of the institution in medical care, strongly support a dynamic alteration of state licensure policies. Logically, for a new licensure policy to be compatible with these trends, it would have to emphasize the primacy of the health care institution within a nationwide context. Of those being considered at the present time, the Hershey-McAdams proposal, seems to be the one that most likely fulfills these objectives. But, as discussed earlier, it merely perpetuates the traditional reliance on input regulation and, therefore, does not recognize the important developments in outcome-measurements of health care.

THE CASE FOR NONLICENSURE

The solutions presented thus far for affording societal control over the quality of health services have continued to stress the regulation of the inputs into medical care by some form of licensure. Of these proposals, the Hershey-McAdams recommendation seems basically compatible with both the discernible trends toward the institutionalization of liability and national standards of care, and the growing need for a system that allows for a more flexible allocation of duties among health personnel. As a result, the institutional framework of licensure is presently the most acceptable plan for resolving many of the issues affecting the regulation of health care.

However, one of the most critical events of the contemporary medical scene has not been considered, and that is the introduction of computer technology. The computer has already been successfully applied to various medical tasks. It is used in diagnostic tests such as automated readings of electrocardiograms, image processing, chromosome analysis, retinograms, mammograms and electroencephalograms; and, in therapeutic activities such as monitoring cardiac patients, and delivering anesthesia during surgery. Now, because of the computer, it will be possible to monitor accurately the output of medical care, an accomplishment that will undoubtedly revolutionize the entire health care system.[65]

In an unrefined way output determinations have been operational in hospitals for several years, conducted by such groups as tissue and infection committees, utilization review committees and medical record and audit committees. The function of these groups has been to evaluate the changes in the patient's condition during his hospitalization to assure high standards of performance in the delivery of care. Assessments of care have unfortunately been predicated on imprecise criteria and are accordingly expressed in broad terms—either descriptively, or as the degree to which actual outcome approaches expected outcome, or as an accounting of the patient's maintenance, gain or loss of status.[66] However, much research is being conducted on arriving at an operational definition of health status that will provide some criteria for establishing meaningful output determinants. For example, it has been proposed that a definition for health status might be worked around the notion of

342

"function/dysfunction" based on one's ability or inability for carrying out the usual daily activities appropriate to individual social roles.[67] Alternatively, it might be based on a scale of classification of "impairment," that is along a continuum from "no impairment" to "bedridden" and "death."[68] It is expected that within the next four to five years an operational definition of "health status" will have been sufficiently researched to serve as the basis for developing output determinants.[69]

The computer is actually forcing a realignment of medical information into more sophisticated organized patterns that will be far more objective and quantifiable. The clinician is being compelled to improve the standardization of medical procedures by developing methods "for becoming more consistent in designating, more uniform in recording and more reliable in verifying symptoms and signs that are main units of clinical measurement."[70] Lawrence Weed at the Cleveland Metropolitan General Hospital has developed one of the most thoughtful approaches to organizing medical information in a manner that would be readily adaptable to computer requirements, and provide a more rational method for patient management. Weed recommends orienting the data of patients around *each medical problem,* so that as the data develop the findings can be "crystallized" into specific diagnoses that require particular therapy. Over time the "problem-oriented" medical records would result in an amount of data from various patients around specific problems sufficient enough to ensure that new "standards for reasonable numbers of tests and good care will emerge."[71] Once standards are so delineated, it would be relatively easy with the computer to set up methods for appraising the performance not only of the individual practitioner, but also that of the health care institution. A computer could be programmed to screen large amounts of data for evidence of inadequate care (diagnosis, treatment and so forth) and thereby provide information for monitoring the quality of care. This is already being done on a limited scale in several institutions throughout the country, and it is felt that the capability exists now for expand-

343

ing computer usage to the point where it will assume the primary role in the regulation of health care.[72]

The implementation of a computerized nationwide yet regionally based network for monitoring the quality of care of medical institutions would dynamically alter the utilization of health manpower. No longer would professional licensure, or "input" regulation be needed; for now it would be possible to regulate the end-product of elements, professional and institutional, that interact in the care of patients. Input regulation is at best an indirect attempt to control the output of the medical care process. From the societal standpoint it serves no other function and consequently would be rendered obsolete by the development of a reliable mechanism for regulating output.

Although having some features in common with the Hershey-McAdams institutional framework for licensure, the theoretical model of a system of output monitoring would depart in significant ways from that framework. Emphasis in the proposed model would be on the institution as the responsible agent for providing care, on the use of national rather than state standards of care and on the freedom for employing various mixes of health personnel to meet individual institutional and community needs. But, in addition, this shift of attention from "input" to "output" would have a radical impact on three crucial components of medical care: (1) consumer protection, (2) medical "professionalism" and (3) medical education.

With regard to "consumer protection" the results of a system of output regulation would be most favorable. Standards for acceptable care would have to be established on a national basis and applied through regional organizations against the "output" of individual institutions. The monitoring itself could be conducted by a private agency, which would work closely with both professional medical societies (representing all health personnel), and the federal agency responsible for financing the care. One could reasonably conjecture that the primary sanction against the institution providing inadequate care would possibly be ultimate loss of "certification" by the regulatory agency, and concomitant withdrawal of federal support.

Consumer participation would also likely be an important feature of this new system. Each institution would be forced to establish its own "regulatory" body that would periodically evaluate the activities of its health personnel in the light of current needs. Such a committee should consist of representatives from the various medical professions as well as members of the community. This regulatory committee, to respond to the requirements of the nationwide agency, would be empowered to impose sanctions on individual practitioners who are performing inadequately. Such sanctions might take the form of requiring additional education or, in the extreme, revising an individual's job description. And, the last aspect of consumer protection would be some means for compensating injuries incurred from the institution's care. Because the institution rather than the individual would be the provider of care, it would be liable for the negligence of its personnel. A natural resolution of this problem might be the implementation of some national insurance compensation scheme analogous to workman's compensation that would recompense the injured party for the institution's negligence.

The second essential component of health care that will be affected by the shift to "output" regulation is the professional identity of medicine. The salient characteristic of a profession that distinguishes it from other occupations is that society has invested it with a "legitimate" autonomy, the right to determine both who can perform its functions, and how.[73] Licensure has served a pivotal role in shaping the contours of the medical profession. Though conceived as a method for protecting the health consumer, licensure as an operating system has been forced to rely heavily on the expertise of licensed members of the profession, so that it rapidly became a powerful instrument for creating an elite that has been able to effectively exclude others from its scope of activities.

The important issue now is whether licensure of medical

345

personnel is still essential for the preservation of a professional identity. It is probably not that important, for the "core" characteristics that define the profession—specialized training in an "abstract" discipline, and a collective orientation to service—will survive without licensure.[74] The effects of "nonlicensure" might be the converse, that is that more emphasis will be appropriately placed on the educational features of the profession as reflected in the quality of performance, which will enhance the sense of identity and "collectiveness." The physician would continue as the director of the health care team. However, opportunities would be provided for vertical mobility whereby particular health workers (e.g., technologists, nurses) could conceivably, through continuing education or apprenticeship, climb a "ladder" of progressive responsibility. Throughout the medical care professions, the proper allocation of responsibilities as determined by medical training and competence should introduce significantly more incentive than has licensure for achieving optimum performance.[75]

Finally, the medical curriculum will undergo profound revisions as a result of the use of computer technology in medical care. This will occur primarily for two reasons. First, the computer's capabilities for rapid and accurate retrieval of medical information will make the current need for enormous accumulations of facts essentially superfluous. The student will be free for the first time to pursue other disciplines of increasing importance to the institutional practice of medicine, i.e., the social, economic and behavioral sciences, as well as the humanities (particularly ethics).[76] And, second, the multitudes of social, economic and medical factors that will converge at every major medical decision will require specialized personnel capable of understanding the intricate processes of "medical" decision-making. The overall impact, therefore, will be a changing of emphasis from basic medical research to the perplexing issues of health services.

For the other members of the health care team, formal education will probably be geared closer to that of the physician,

346

especially for the first few years. Even now universities are experimenting with such innovations as the development of a "core" curriculum for pharmacists, physician assistants, nurses and others.[77] The advantage of upgrading the education of other health professionals is that they will be competent to be employed with greater flexibility.

CONCLUSION

It is generally agreed that the present state mandatory licensure system, with its rigid delineation of functions for each of the respective health professions, does not allow the flexibility in manpower utilization that is required in expanding current health resources to provide comprehensive health care for every citizen. One suggested alternative to the present licensure laws, the Hershey-McAdams model, offers greater flexibility in manpower use by allowing the manpower classifications to be defined by, and in terms of the needs of, the health care institution. The Hershey model has the added advantage of complementing the general trend toward the institutionalization of health care (and the legal liability therefor) and the nationalization of the standards of that care.

Because of its sole reliance on input regulation to control the quality of practice—the trademark of the first evolutionary stage of manpower regulation—the Hershey model cannot jettison all the constrictive features of licensure. Notwithstanding its shortcomings in this respect, its institutional emphasis enables it to serve as a bridge between the first evolutionary stage of regulation and the second, the latter of which is characterized by primary reliance on the measurement of treatment outcomes to achieve quality control. Recent advances in the quantification of these outcomes, or "outputs" of the health care system, enable medical scientists to predict that such a quality control mechanism will be widely operational in five years.

Viewed in this perspective, the legislative proposals currently before Congress, which contain structural components similar

347

to the Hershey model, are the blueprints of short-range planning only. Long-range planning to meet vastly increased consumer needs requires the drafting of legislation that will incorporate the free-form innovations of quality control through outcome measurement in a system of "nonlicensure."

REFERENCES

[1] The Carnegie Commission on Higher Education, HIGHER EDUCATION AND THE NATION'S HEALTH, New York, McGraw Hill Book Company, 1970.

[2] National Advisory Commission on Health Manpower, REPORT OF THE NATIONAL ADVISORY COMMISSION ON HEALTH MANPOWER, Washington, United States Government Printing Office, 1967, Volume I, pp. 13–21; and Garfield, S., The Delivery of Medical Care, *Scientific American*, April, 1970, p. 15.

[3] The Carnegie Commission on Higher Education, *op. cit.*, pp. 44–45.

[4] *Ibid.*, p. 49.

[5] McNerney, W., Why Does Medical Care Cost so Much?, *New England Journal of Medicine*, 282, 1458, 1970.

[6] Forgotson, E. and Cook, J., Innovations and Experiments in Uses of Health Manpower: The Effect of Licensure Laws, *Law and Contemporary Problems*, 32, 731, 1967.

[7] *Ibid.*, p. 748; see also Forgotson, E., Roemer, R. and Newman, R., Licensure of Physicians, *Washington University Law Quarterly*, 249–331, Summer, 1967; National Advisory Commission on Health Manpower, *op. cit.*, Volume II, pp. 280 *et seq.*

[8] Friedman, L., Freedom of Contract and Occupational Licensing, 1890–1910: A Legal and Social Study, *California Law Review*, 53, 487, 493.

[9] *Ibid.;* and Roemer, R., Legal Systems Regulating Health Personnel: A Comparative Analysis, *Milbank Memorial Fund Quarterly*, 46, 431–471, October, 1968.

[10] Hershey, N., The Inhibiting Effect Upon Innovation of the Prevailing Licensure System, *Annals of the New York Academy of Sciences*, 166, 952, December 31, 1969.

[11] Roemer, *op. cit.*, p. 435; Forgotson and Cook, *op. cit.*, pp. 736–737.

[12] Licensing, *Yale Law Journal*, 74, 159, 1964.

[13] Forgotson, Roemer and Newman, *op. cit.*, pp. 248–331; National Advisory Commission on Health Manpower, *op. cit.*, Volume II, p. 426; Leff, A., Medical Devices and Paramedical Personnel: A Preliminary Context for Emerging Problems, *Washington University Law Quarterly*, 378, Summer, 1967.

[14] Forgotson, Roemer and Newman, *op. cit.*

15 National Advisory Commission on Health Manpower, *op. cit.*, Volume II, p. 292; Burg, C., Acts of Nurses and the Colorado Professional Nursing Practice Act, *Denver Law Journal*, 45, 467–482, 1968.

16 Hershey, N., An Alternative to Mandatory Licensure of Health Professionals, *Hospital Progress*, 50, 72, 1969.

17 National Advisory Commission on Health Manpower, *op. cit.*, Volume II, pp. 300–308.

18 Leff, *op. cit.*, p. 382.

19 National Advisory Commission on Health Manpower, *op. cit.*, Volume II, p. 312.

20 Hershey, N., An Alternative to Mandatory Licensure of Health Professionals, *Hospital Progress*, 50, 72, 1969.

21 McAdams, D., The Licensure Dilemma, *Hospital Progress*, 50, 50, 1969.

22 Derbyshire, R., MEDICAL LICENSURE AND DISCIPLINE, Baltimore, The Johns Hopkins Press, 1969.

23 See the discussion of the trend toward delineation of national standards of care in the next section of this paper.

24 Hershey, N., An Alternative to Mandatory Licensure of Health Professionals, *Hospital Progress*, 50, 72, 1969.

25 McAdams, *op. cit.*, p. 52.

26 Research on such a system for compensation is being conducted by the American Rehabilitation Foundation, Minneapolis, Minnesota.

27 McAdams, *op. cit.*, pp. 51–53; Somers, A., HOSPITAL REGULATION: THE DILEMMA OF PUBLIC POLICY, Princeton, Princeton University Press, 1969, pp. 122, 125.

28 McAdams, *op. cit.*, p. 52.

29 *Ibid.*, p. 53. The agency would be composed of representatives from each health occupation as well as from the general public and would, in effect, set standards for each discipline.

30 *Ibid.*, p. 53.

31 The Physician's Right to Hospital Staff Membership: The Public-Private Dichotomy, *Washington University Law Quarterly*, 485, December, 1966. Presently the physician's right to become a staff member of a hospital depends on whether that hospital is characterized as public or private. If it is a public institution the physician has the right to use the hospital facilities so long as he adheres to the hospital's regulations. In contrast, if it is a private hospital, the board of directors has nearly unlimited discretion in accepting or rejecting a physician for membership on the staff, and expelling him from the staff. If an institutional structure is to be effective it will be necessary to reexamine the rights of the physician in the private institution. See also, Somers, *op. cit.*, p. 18.

32 Of course recent bills being considered by Congress, which employ payment mechanisms as a means of achieving a new structure of provider services, reflect and give impetus to the institutionalization of all aspects of medical care:
a. Section 239 of the Amendment to Title XVII of the Social Security Act—
H. R. 1 (introduced by Mr. Mills, January 22, 1971, passed the House of

Representatives late June 1971): "Payments to Health Maintenance Organizations"—wherein the institution is paid on a "per capita rate for services provided for enrollees in such an organization." This emphasizes the institution over the individual physican by suggesting a mechanism other than fee-for-service. As a result, the institution becomes financially and otherwise the provider of care.

b. S. 1623, "National Health Insurance Partnership Act of 1971," introduced by Senator Wallace Bennett on April 22, 1971, on behalf of the Administration: This would require employers to make available to employees and their families a health care plan under private insurance providing specified benefits. Employees would have the option of enrolling with an approved health maintenance organization (to be paid on a per capita basis under Family Health Insurance Plan for low-income families with children not covered under a required employer plan, HMO's would be paid a prospective per capita rate equal to 95 per cent of the estimated amount needed if the service were furnished by other providers in the area) and the employers would contract with these organizations for those employees who chose to enroll.

c. "The Health Security Program" (S. 3) would stress a capitation payment mechanism allowing for fee-for-service to primary physicians. In addition, money would be distributed on a subregional fund basis determined by the size of the population. The overall effect would be toward paying larger institutions rather than individual physicians for health care, thereby resulting also in the institution as the provider of care. One senses the same potentiality for the Javits Bill (S. 836), though the details of payment have not been carefully defined.

[33] Southwick, R., Hospitals Responsibility, *Clev.—Mar. Law Review*, 17, 156, 1968.

[34] Leff, *op. cit.*, p. 369.

[35] Southwick, *op. cit.*, p. 156.

[36] Somers, *op. cit.*, pp. 37–38. Twenty-eight jurisdictions impose total liability for negligency on the hospital.

[37] Southwick, *op. cit.*, p. 151; Somers, *op. cit.*, p. 32.

[38] *Darling v. Charleston Community Hospital*, 33, Ill. 2d 326, 211 N.E. 2d 253, 1965.

[39] Southwick, *op. cit.*, p. 161; Somers, *op. cit.*, p. 32.

[40] Action also was taken against the physician, who settled the claim against him and was dismissed as a defendant. Southwick, *op. cit.*, p. 161. This is not a respondeat superior case for the negligence of the doctor was never determined in court and consequently the hospital could not be held vicariously liable.

[41] As with the "locality principle" in standard of physician care, the hospital argued that its duty is to be determined by the care customarily offered by hospitals generally in its community. However, the court applied national standards as well. See Somers, *op. cit.*, p. 33.

[42] Southwick, *op. cit.*, p. 161.

[43] *Ibid.*, pp. 160, 161.

[44] *Fiorentino v. Wenger*, 26 App. Div. 2d 693, 272 N.Y.S. 2d 557, 1966. In this case the surgeon had applied a surgical procedure that was not generally accepted treatment in the community for the patient's condition, and the child

died. The hospital was not held liable on appeal because there was no duty for it to obtain a second consent, or verify the one received. However, it could have been held liable if it knew, or should have known that an informed consent for surgical treatment was not obtained.

[45] Southwick, *op. cit.*, p. 159.

[46] *French v. Fisher,* 50 Tenn. App. 587, 362 S.W. 2d 926, 1962.

[47] *Kapuschinsky v. United States,* 248 F. Supp. 732 D.S.C., 1966.

[48] Southwick, *op. cit.*, p. 147. The courts are saying that hospitals and medical staff must adopt the "best" methods of professional standards, and not average methods or local community methods. Professional standards become a joint problem of hospital and medical staff; and the "community" has become "nationwide."

[49] Somers, *op. cit.*, p. 94.

[50] *Brune v. Belinkoff,* 354 Mass. 102, 235 N.E. 2d 793, 1968. Case overruled the 1880 case of *Small v. Howard,* 128 Mass. 131, which established in Massachusetts the "locality rule."

[51] Landau, D., Medical Malpractice: Overturning Locality Rule Used in Determining a Physician's Standard of Skill and Care, *Boston University Law Review,* 48, 710.

[52] *Brune v. Belinkoff, op, cit.,* The court also included a statement about the expected care from the general practitioner. The court said that the specialist should be held to the standard of skill of the average member of the profession practicing the specialty.

[53] Landau, *op. cit.*, p. 711.

[54] *Ibid.,* pp. 712, 713. One of the very real practical consequences of the *Brune v. Belinkoff* case (and similar ones) is that the decision represents a determined effort by the court to mitigate the burden on plaintiffs in malpractice cases. It attempts to do this by: (1) raising the professional standards of care to that of a major medical center, subject to some qualifications; (2) permitting expert medical witnesses to be obtained from other than "similar community;" (3) removing geographic limitations on the admissibility of medical treatises and books.

[55] The proposal endorsed by the American Medical Association is H.R. 4960, the "Health Care Insurance Act of 1971," introduced by Representative Richard Fulton on February 25, 1971. This bill is referred to as the Medicredit proposal. In the Medicredit proposal of 1970 (and the Fisher Bill—H.R. 1283— of 1971) utilization of the existing peer-review procedures was stressed. The "Health Care Insurance Act of 1971" deleted the provision that established Professional Review Organizations (PRO) to review charges and utilization. Of course, with the implementation of the AMA tax credit scheme it would be natural to include ultimately basic quality standards. The "National Healthcare Act of 1971," H.R. 4349, introduced by Representative Omar Burleson on February 17, 1971, is endorsed by the Health Insurance Association of America. This Bill provides for setting standards for providers of services, be they Institutions (hospitals, extended care facilities and home health agencies); health maintenance organizations, or physicians and dentists.

Therefore, though not explicitly supporting national standards of care, all of the major types of proposals for a national program of health care seem implicitly to support the imposition of national standards. See: Report of A Special Committee on The Provision of Health Services, AMERIPLAN: A PROPOSAL FOR THE DELIVERY AND FINANCING OF HEALTH SERVICES IN THE UNITED STATES, Chicago, American Hospital Association, 1970. From the standpoint of licensure of personnel, AMERIPLAN embodies the Hershey-McAdams model by investing the Health Care Corporation (the organizational entity that is capable of providing comprehensive health care to a defined population) with the authority for control over the use and development of personnel. In addition, AMERIPLAN provides for the establishment of national standards of care through a National Health Commission whose function would be to promulgate federal regulations for the Health Care Corporation. The state health commissions would be concerned with assuring that the Health Care Corporation complies with the national regulations.

[56] S. 3 ("The Health Security Program").

[57] *Ibid.,* Sx. 56 (a): (1), (3), (4).

[58] S. 3, Sx. 54, "Consideration of Professional Association Standards:" ". . . the Board shall take into consideration standards or criteria established or recommended by any appropriate professional or other association or organization."

[59] See "Javits Bill," S. 836, Sx. 141 A and B.

[60] *Ibid.,* Sx. 141 C.

[61] H.R. 1, Sx. 239 (To add to Title XVIII of the Social Security Act Sx. 1976, "Payments to Health Maintenance Organizations").

[62] H.R. 1, Sx. 239 (Sx. 1876 [4]), "demonstrates to the satisfaction of the Secretary proof of financial responsibility and proof of capability to provide comprehensive health care services, including institutional services, efficiently and economically;" and 6: ". . . that services measure up to quality standards which it establishes in accordance with regulations."

[63] Emergency Health Personnel Act of 1970, P.L. 91–623 (42 *USC* Sx 254b).

[64] Professionals will serve in such areas at the request of state health authorities and county medical societies, and participate in programs of Model Cities and Office of Economic Opportunity (in addition to traditional programs such as the Indian Health Service, Coast Guard Health Service, Public Health Service Hospitals that treat merchant seamen and so forth). This enlistment will be in lieu of military service.

[65] Schwartz, W., Medicine and the Computer: The Promise and Problems of Change, *New England Journal of Medicine,* 283, 1257, 1970.

[66] Kelman, H., Camerman, E. and Conrad, H. C., Monitoring Patient Care, *Medical Care,* 7, 2, 1969; see also, Sanazaro, P., and Williamson, J., End Results of Patient Care: A Provisional Classification Based on Reports by Internists, *Medical Care,* 6, 128–130, 1968; Morehead, M., Evaluating Quality of Medical Care in the Neighborhood Health Center Program of the Office of Economic Opportunity, *Medical Care,* 8, 113–131, 1970.

[67] Fanshel, S. and Bush, J., A Health-Status Index and Its Application to Health Services Outcomes, *Operations Research,* 18, 1021–1022, 1970.

352

[68] Williamson, J., Outcomes of Health Care: Key to Health Improvement, in Hopkins, C. E. and Breslow, L. (Editors), OUTCOMES CONFERENCE I–II, Washington, United States Department of Health, Education, and Welfare, December, 1969, pp. 75–101.

[69] Williamson, J. W., personal correspondence.

[70] Feinstein, A., CLINICAL JUDGMENT, Baltimore, The Williams & Wilkins Co., 1967, p. 329.

[71] Weed, L., Medical Records that Guide and Teach, *New England Journal of Medicine*, 278, 593–600, 1968.

[72] Schwartz, *op. cit.*, p. 1260. Drug control section (25) of the Kennedy Bill attempts to use drug treatment as a means of establishing standard treatments for various diseases. The Javits Bill also provides for a similar control. X Sx.25 (S. 3): "The Board . . . shall establish and disseminate (and review and if necessary revise, at least annually) (1) a list of drugs for use in participating institutions and comprehensive health service organizations, and (2) a list (for use outside such institutions and organizations) of diseases and conditions for the treatment of which drugs may be furnished as a covered service, and specification of the drugs that may be so furnished for each disease or condition listed."

[73] Freidson, E., PROFESSION OF MEDICINE: A STUDY OF THE SOCIOLOGY OF APPLIED KNOWLEDGE, New York, Dodd, Mead & Co., 1970, pp. 354–357.

[74] *Ibid.*, pp. 71–73.

[75] Drucker, P., THE PRACTICE OF MANAGEMENT, New York, Harper & Row, Publishers, 1954, Chapter 23.

[76] Schwartz, *op. cit.*, p. 1260.

[77] An example of such a curriculum is the pharmacist clinician program at the University of California, San Francisco.